The Complete HIV/AIDS Teaching Kit

with **CD-ROM**

About the Authors

Josefina J. Card, PhD, is Founder, President, and CEO of Sociometrics Corporation, an applied social science research and development (R&D) company based in Los Altos, CA. Dr. Card is a nationally recognized social scientist and an expert in the establishment and operation of research-based social science resources, products, and services. She has served as Principal Investigator of over 70 research-to-practice R&D projects, most of them funded by the U.S. National Institutes of Health. These R&D projects have resulted in the development of several hundred social science-based commercial products, including the exemplary data sets, effective intervention programs, and evaluation and training materials comprising the Social Science Electronic Data Library; the Program Archive on Sexuality, Health and Adolescence; the HIV/AIDS Prevention Program Archive; and the Institute for Program Development and Evaluation. These resources have been used by thousands of academic as well as health practitioner customers in schools, clinics, and communities across the country. Alongside her track record as a project manager, Dr. Card has established a solid track record as a health and population scientist. She has authored over 80 books, monographs, and journal articles. Her work is noted for its integration of behavioral, social, psychological, and demographic perspectives. Throughout her career, Dr. Card has recognized the importance of communicating scientific findings to scientists as well as to other professionals (service providers, policy makers, health practitioners) and lay citizens who could benefit from the body of knowledge. Dr. Card also has devoted a significant portion of her career to facilitating the development and scientific evaluation of social intervention programs. She has served as a member of many federal advisory committees, including the NIH (National Institutes of Health) Study Section for Social Sciences and Population, the NICHD (National Institute on Child Health and Human Development) Population Research Committee, and the NICHD Advisory Council. Dr. Card is also active in the community. While her children were in school, she served as PTA officer, founded the Gunn High School Parent Community Service Boosters, and chaired the Gunn Parent-Teacher Wish List Fund. She also served as Chair of the Palo Alto Unified School District Housing Options for Teachers project, aimed at bringing and keeping outstanding teachers in the award-winning PAUSD school district. From 1999 to 2003, she worked with the Packard Foundation, the Santa Clara County Public Health Department, and the Adolescent Pregnancy Prevention Network in an effort that lowered the County's teen pregnancy and birth rates by over 40%, surpassing the also impressive performances by the state and nation in this regard. Currently Dr. Card, a native of the Philippines, is working with Pathways Philippines and with the Ayala Foundation USA to raise funds to allow outstanding graduates of Philippine public high schools to go to college.

Angela Amarillas, MA, is a program manager at the California Healthy Kids Resource Center where she reviews instructional materials and research to determine and disseminate the highest quality, research-based school health and health education resources to be implemented in California schools, K–12. In addition, Ms. Amarillas co-teaches a course at Stanford University (Human Biology 95Q: Gender,

Culture, and HIV/AIDS) that explores how gender and culture affect the transmission of HIV and the impact of AIDS. Many of her students have gone on from this class to perform sponsored research in HIV and women's health issues. Previously, as a health educator at Stanford, Ms. Amarillas founded and directed student health education programs and projects including the Residential Peer Health Education program, disordered eating and body image awareness initiatives, HIV/AIDS prevention programs, and the Peer Nutrition Education program. After graduating with a Master's degree in Education from Stanford, Ms. Amarillas was a Research Associate with Sociometrics Corporation, a Bay Area social science research and development firm, where she developed research-based health-related curricula and other resources that bridge social science research and public health practice for students and practitioners. Ms. Amarillas is also known internationally as a teacher and performer of historical and vernacular social couple dance.

Alana Conner, PhD, is the senior editor of the *Stanford Social Innovation Review*, a quarterly publication of the Stanford Graduate School of Business that presents new ideas for social change to nonprofit, business, and government leaders. Dr. Conner earned her PhD in social psychology at Stanford University, where she studied how ethnic and class cultures shape people's notions of who they are and why they do the things they do. As a postdoctoral scholar at the University of California, San Francisco, medical center, she expanded her research to explore the cultural grounding of health and disease. She published her research in *Journal of Personality and Social Psychology, Psychological Science, Journal of Cross-Cultural Psychology, Current Directions in Psychological Science*, and other peer-reviewed journals. She then applied her knowledge as a senior research associate at Sociometrics Corporation, where she helped create Web-based products about HIV/AIDS and its prevention. In addition to working her day jobs, Conner has written about social science and health for National Geographic Television, the *New York Times Magazine, Static,* and other venues. She is currently authoring a book about cultural psychology.

Diana Dull Akers, PhD, is a Senior Research Associate at Sociometrics Corporation where she has served as Principal Investigator for a number of federally funded projects concerning adolescent reproductive health and adult HIV/AIDS prevention. This work has included the development and testing of several computer-based HIV/AIDS personal risk assessment and education tools, designed in both English and Spanish for use in diverse clinic settings. She has also served as Project Director for Sociometrics' Institute for Program Development and Evaluation, sponsored by the National Institute of Child Health and Human Development, and for the Program Archive on Sexuality, Health and Adolescence (PASHA), cosponsored by the National Institute of Child Health and Human Development and the United States Office of Population Affairs. Dr. Dull Akers earned her PhD in Sociology at the University of California, Santa Cruz. Before joining Sociometrics in 1999, Dr. Dull Akers held a joint teaching appointment for the departments of Sociology and Gender Studies at Sonoma State University. Her research, publications, and teaching focus on social-behavioral approaches to health and illness, gender, sexuality, domestic violence, and aging.

Julie Solomon, PhD, serves as a Senior Research Associate and the Director of Training Support at Sociometrics Corporation. As a Senior Research Associate, she has directed R&D, evaluation, and consulting projects in diverse behavioral health areas, including HIV, STI, and teen pregnancy prevention; substance abuse prevention; violence prevention; and clinician–patient communication in the context of (patient) communication disorders. These projects have been funded by a variety of public and private entities, including the National Institutes of Health (NIH), the David & Lucile Packard Foundation, Johnson & Johnson Corporate Contributions, the California Healthy Kids Resource Center, and the Santa Clara County

(California) Public Health Department. As Director of Training Support at Sociometrics, Dr. Solomon develops and delivers workshops on program planning and evaluation for diverse audiences, principally practitioners in the sexual and reproductive health fields. Dr. Solomon joined Sociometrics in 1999 after completing a PhD in linguistics at Stanford University. While in graduate school, she taught in several departments and also worked for ETR Associates, the American Institutes for Research (AIR), and the Palo Alto Medical Foundation Research Institute on projects addressing sexual behavior and HIV risk among Latino youth and adults in California. A common thread that runs through much of Dr. Solomon's work is a desire to empower health and social service providers to carry out appropriate cultural adaptation and successful replication of empirically validated prevention programs. She has recently published on these topics through the National Campaign to Prevent Teen Pregnancy and in the journal *Evaluation and the Health Professions*. In addition to coauthoring *The Complete HIV/AIDS Teaching Kit*, she is also a coauthor of *Tools for Building Culturally Competent HIV Prevention Programs* (Springer Publishing Company, 2007).

Ralph J. DiClemente, PhD, is Charles Howard Candler Professor of Public Health and Associate Director, Emory/Atlanta Center for AIDS Research. He holds concurrent appointments as Professor in the School of Medicine, in the Division of Infectious Diseases and the Department of Pediatrics, in the Division of Epidemiology, Infectious Diseases and Immunology, and the Department of Psychiatry. He was, most recently, Chair, Department of Behavioral Sciences and Health Education at the Rollins School of Public Health, Emory University. Dr. DiClemente was trained as a Health Psychologist at the University of California San Francisco, where he received his PhD in 1984 after completing an MS in Behavioral Sciences at the Harvard School of Public Health and his undergraduate degree at the City University of New York. Dr. DiClemente is an internationally recognized expert on the development and evaluation of prevention programs tailored to African American adolescents and young adults. He is particularly well versed in designing programs that use peer-based models of implementation and that are culturally and developmentally appropriate. He has published extensively in the area of HIV/STD prevention, particularly among African American adolescents and young adults. He also has published extensively in the area of partner violence. He is the author of more than 200 publications, including the following recent books: *Handbook of Health Promotion and Disease Prevention*; *Handbook of Adolescent Health Risk Behaviors*; *Handbook of HIV Prevention*; *Adolescents and AIDS: A Generation in Jeopardy*; *Preventing HIV Infection in Developing Countries: Biomedical and Behavioral Interventions; Women's Sexual and Reproductive Health: Social, Psychological and Public Health Perspectives*; and *Emerging Theories in Health Promotion Research and Practice.*

The Complete HIV/AIDS Teaching Kit

with **CD-ROM**

AUTHORS

Josefina J. Card, PhD
Angela Amarillas, MA
Alana Conner, PhD
Diana Dull Akers, PhD
Julie Solomon, PhD
Ralph J. DiClemente, PhD

SPRINGER PUBLISHING COMPANY
New York

Springer Publishing Company, LLC
11 West 42nd Street
New York, NY 10036-8002
www.springerpub.com

Acquisitions Editor: Jennifer Perillo
Managing Editor: Mary Ann McLaughlin
Production Editor: Shana Meyer
Cover Design: Joanne E. Honigman
Composition: Aptara, Inc.

07 08 09 10/ 5 4 3 2 1

Library of Congress Cataloging-in-Publication Data

The complete HIV/AIDS teaching kit : with CD-ROM / Josefina J. Card . . . [et al.].
p. ; cm.
Includes bibliographical references and index.
ISBN 978-0-8261-0316-1 (softcover)
1. AIDS (Disease)—Study and teaching. HIV infections—Study and teaching. I. Card, Josefina J.
[DNLM: 1. HIV Infections. 2. Teaching—methods. 3. Acquired Immunodeficiency Syndrome. 4. Health Education—methods. WC 18 C737 2007]

RA643.8.C654 2007
616.97′920071–dc22

2007021151

Printed in the United States of America by Bang Printing.

Dedication

This book is dedicated to all the brave and generous men and women fighting the spread of HIV/AIDS around the world. It is also dedicated to our Project Officer at the National Institutes of Health, Dr. Louis Steinberg, a steadfast champion of the HIV/AIDS cause, who died before the book he strongly supported was completed.

Acknowledgments

The authors thank our editor, Jennifer Perillo, who designed many of the elements that will increase the usefulness of this book and whose generous assistance and encouragement inspired us all; Sheri Sussman, our acquisitions editor, who had faith in this effort when it was just an idea; Nancy Brown and Robert Siegel, who provided expert input on the book's content; Jessica Sales and Robin Milhausen, for their invaluable assistance in preparing the PowerPoint slides on the CD-ROM; Allison Hoff and Tabitha Benner, who provided extremely useful production assistance; and Tamara Kuhn, who designed and produced the CD-ROM. Your contributions are acknowledged with gratitude and appreciation.

Contents

PART I

HIV/AIDS: THE EPIDEMIC

PART II

PREVENTING HIV

PART III

LIVING WITH HIV/AIDS

Introduction

HIV/AIDS has rapidly emerged as one of the greatest threats to human health in the 21st century. There were an estimated 4.3 million new HIV infections (*incident* infections) in 2006; about half of those newly infected were young people ages 15–25. As of the end of 2006, the number of people living with HIV/AIDS (HIV/AIDS *prevalence*) was estimated at 39.5 million, close to two-thirds of whom were living in sub-Saharan Africa (Henry J. Kaiser Family Foundation, 2006). Women accounted for 48% of those living with HIV. Over 25 million people have died since the beginning of the AIDS epidemic. Currently, over 7,500 people die from AIDS each day—about five people every minute (UNAIDS, 2006).

In the last 2 decades, there have been significant advances in the control and treatment of HIV/AIDS, but still no cure. Prevention thus remains a critically important strategy for reducing the impact of this global pandemic. Science has shown that HIV is transmitted from person to person by a known set of risk behaviors and transmission routes, including unprotected sex with an infected partner, the sharing of equipment used to inject both illegal and legal drugs, and mother-to-child transmission.[1]

In the charged debates about HIV/AIDS, HIV risk behaviors are often described in simplistic terms as a matter of "human choice," with little attention paid to the complex social, environmental, cultural, and economic factors impacting these choices. It is critically important to understand not only the science of this disease but also the behavioral and sociocultural influences that both *facilitate* and *prevent* the spread of HIV. *The Complete HIV/AIDS Teaching Kit*—a research-based resource for diverse audiences, including academic and health professionals—was written to facilitate such understanding.

The book offers an overview of what science knows about the incidence, prevalence, antecedents, consequences, prevention, and treatment of HIV/AIDS, in a manner that is uniquely focused through a sociocultural lens. The text is organized into four parts.

Part 1—HIV/AIDS: THE EPIDEMIC provides an overview of both the virology of HIV and the biomedical aspects of AIDS, and reviews the natural and social history of the epidemic. Part 1 also details how HIV is transmitted and explores the biological, psychological, demographic, sociological, and cultural risk factors that influence the likelihood of acquiring and transmitting HIV.

HIV is deadly, but preventable. Although HIV transmission largely results from individual behaviors, individual behaviors themselves are the result of a variety of influences. Part 2—PREVENTING HIV outlines prevention strategies that address these influences on the individual level, the community level, and the societal level.

[1] Standardized protective measures for screening blood and guarding against HIV transmission are employed by health and occupational workers throughout much of the world. However, *in the absence of such protective measures*, HIV transmission can still occur through several additional routes, including: occupational exposure to contaminated blood, blood transfusions, and the sharing of equipment used for body piercings, tattooing, and other body modification practices involving potential blood-to-blood exposure.

In addition, Part 2 surveys the scientific theories of behavior change that have been applied to HIV prevention and summarizes how prevention interventions are best developed, implemented, evaluated, adapted, and replicated.

Although HIV-positive (HIV+) people are living longer, healthier lives in large part because of advances in anti-HIV drug therapies, living with (and dying from) HIV/AIDS can be an emotional and physical roller coaster of hope and disappointment. Part 3—LIVING WITH HIV/AIDS offers a synopsis of the medical issues as well as the psychological and social challenges of living with HIV and AIDS. Because the transmission of HIV invariably involves an individual who is HIV+, Part 3 also includes a discussion of prevention strategies for people living with HIV and AIDS to avoid passing their infection on to others, while protecting their sexual health, avoiding new sexually transmitted infections, and delaying disease progression.

When it was first reported, the unknown disease that later came to be called AIDS seemed to infect only gay men. This has changed. The HIV infection rates and death toll from AIDS are evident among people of all ages, gender, sexual orientation, socioeconomic status, race, and ethnicity. Part 4—GENDER, CULTURE, AND HIV/AIDS examines how gender-based and cultural factors come together to increase an individual's risk of becoming infected with HIV, and how gender and culture influence how individuals and societies are affected by AIDS.

Each of the four parts of the book can be used as a separate, standalone entity. Occasionally, material is repeated for this effect.

Given the devastating human toll of the HIV/AIDS epidemic, it is imperative that prevention education efforts continue and that accessible prevention and treatment information be widely and routinely disseminated. *The Complete HIV/AIDS Teaching Kit* was designed for academic and health professionals in classroom and community settings who want to integrate social and behavioral research on HIV/AIDS into their work. Both academic and service provider audiences will appreciate *The Complete HIV/AIDS Teaching Kit*'s highly accessible format, content, and supplemental resources. These value-added features of the book include:

- learning objectives and key terms at the beginning of each chapter
- an instructor resources section at the end of each chapter, with learning activities, discussion questions, quizzes, Web resources, recommended readings, and PowerPoint slides for classroom use
- a helpful glossary at the end of the book clarifying key science/medical terms

Additionally, the enclosed CD-ROM contains electronic versions of the supplemental resources, including:

- PowerPoint slides for use in your milieu; the slides can be mixed, matched, and edited to suit a variety of topics (the slides on the CD-ROM include similar content as those printed in the book; however, they contain additional visuals and graphics and are in color)
- Discussion topics and "learn-by-doing" activities that can be used as in-class exercises, supplementary homework, or as the basis for outside-the-classroom, real-world learning
- Recommended reading lists
- Links to important Web resources for learning more about HIV/AIDS

The remainder of this introduction will show academic instructors and practitioners how they can use *The Complete HIV/AIDS Teaching Kit* to instruct their students and clients.

TIPS FOR HEALTH AND SOCIAL SCIENCE EDUCATORS AND STUDENTS

Professors and students at advanced high school, undergraduate, and Master's levels can use *The Complete HIV/AIDS Teaching Kit* and its companion CD-ROM as a primary or secondary textbook in general health education courses, as well as any course including an HIV-focus.

The Complete HIV/AIDS Teaching Kit can be used as a resource across a variety of courses and academic disciplines. For example:

> An instructor of a college-level training course for undergraduate peer health educators could draw on *The Complete HIV/AIDS Teaching Kit* to help students practice integrating HIV content into their sexual health education efforts (Part 1, chapters 3 and 4).
>
> A health education instructor might drawn on *The Complete HIV/AIDS Teaching Kit* to help students better understand HIV transmission routes, HIV risks, and HIV risk reduction strategies (Part 2, chapter 7).
>
> A social psychology professor could draw on *The Complete HIV/AIDS Teaching Kit* to augment a lecture on stigma, focusing on why HIV/AIDS has emerged as one of the most stigmatizing medical conditions in modern history (Part 3, chapter 13).
>
> Educators in the fields of sociology or gender studies might draw on *The Complete HIV/AIDS Teaching Kit* to help students explore the dynamic relationship between gender, risk behaviors and health, using HIV/AIDS as a case study (Part 4, chapter 17).

SAMPLE SYLLABI

In short, *The Complete HIV/AIDS Teaching Kit* offers academics and students a vast array of research-based HIV/AIDS resources in multiple, user-friendly formats. These resources can be readily accessed to bolster course content, enhance classroom learning strategies, and support oral and written presentations by instructors and students alike. The following sample syllabi show how the book's material can be adapted to various courses at different academic levels.

Sample Syllabus 1:

Integrating HIV/AIDS Content Into a Public Health Course

Kathleen Roth teaches an introductory public health course in a graduate school of public health. Although she is particularly interested in adding an HIV/AIDS unit to her course, she knows her students come from varied backgrounds and scholarly disciplines offering different exposure to the topic of HIV/AIDS. Dr. Roth's challenge is to develop a presentation that is readily understandable by all of her students. To accomplish this task, she decides to use content and PowerPoint slides from *The Complete HIV/AIDS Teaching Kit* to construct a new three-session unit on HIV/AIDS.

In her first session, Dr. Roth uses content from Part 1 to describe the natural and social history of the discovery and spread of HIV since it was first identified in the early 1980s. To encourage interactive learning, she asks students to break into small work groups to complete the "HIV/AIDS Timeline" assignment found in the Learning Activities section of chapter 2.

For her second session, Dr. Roth draws on information from chapter 3 of *The Complete HIV/AIDS Teaching Kit* to help students explore some of the ways that biology, behavior, psychological factors, sociocultural factors, and demographic characteristics influence people's HIV risk levels as well as their preventive behavior. Dr. Roth then guides students in a discussion of common myths and misconceptions about how this virus is passed from person to person.

In the third and final session, Dr. Roth uses Part 2, chapters 6 and 7 to outline HIV prevention strategies from a public health perspective. She and her students discuss both the screening of blood to avoid transmission of HIV during blood transfusions and the development and dissemination of effective behavior change prevention interventions designed to reduce HIV-associated drug and sexual risk behaviors. For the final class assignment, Dr. Roth's students complete the "Theories in Action" writing assignment described in the Learning Activities section (Part 2, chapter 6) in which they propose their own theory-based prevention program.

***The Complete HIV/AIDS Teaching Kit* resources used in this public health course:**

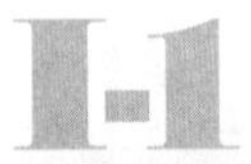

Intro Table I-1

TOPIC	RESOURCES FOR LECTURE PREPARATION	ACTIVITIES AND ASSIGNMENTS
Natural and Social History of HIV/AIDS	Part 1, chapters 1 and 2	*Assignment:* HIV/AIDS Timeline (Part 1, chapter 2)
HIV Risk and Transmission	Part 1, chapters 3 and 4	*Group Activity:* Transmission Case Studies—Scenarios of Risk (Part 1, chapter 4)
HIV/AIDS Prevention From a Public Health Perspective	Part 2, chapters 6 and 7	*Assignment:* Theories in Action (Part 2, chapter 6)

Sample Syllabus 2:

Integrating HIV/AIDS-Related Content Into a Human Biology Course

Professor Diana Tally teaches a university level human biology course. She is interested in integrating new content and learning activities that focus on the ways in which gender and cultural factors affect health. Dr. Tally likes the idea of using HIV/AIDS as a case study focus for this new course because the topic is timely and relevant.

Drawing on content and materials from Part 4, Dr. Tally and her students consider how an individual's risk of becoming infected with HIV is affected by gender and cultural factors. To begin this unit, Dr. Tally uses an activity called "Is it Sex or Gender?" (Part 4, chapter 15) to help students better conceptualize gender as a socially constructed category. She then uses content and slides from Part 4, chapter 15 to explore domestic and international trends concerning HIV/AIDS rates for women.

To further develop her course's gender, health, and HIV focus, Dr. Tally reworks an existing lecture on disease transmission. Adding content from Part 4, chapters 15 and 16, Dr. Tally and her students consider how biological differences between women and men affect the acquisition and transmission of HIV. Professor Tally has her students complete the "Gender in the Real World" assignment, then share their reactions to this unconventional exercise. The assignment helps students to analyze how gender- and culture-based inequalities are causally linked to the spread and impact of disease.

In her next lecture, Professor Tally wants to focus on the ways inequality affects health, looking in particular at the intersections of gender-, culture-, and economic-based inequality. She uses content and slides from Part 4, chapter 17 to teach about the impact of women's economic dependency on men and how this might lead to engaging in high-risk sexual behaviors that increase the likelihood of acquiring HIV. She and her students also explore the reasons why HIV/AIDS is concentrated in economically disadvantaged and marginalized communities. To assess her students' learning, Dr. Tally concludes this unit with a writing assignment called "Gender Inequality and HIV/AIDS" that she finds in the Learning Activities for Part 4, chapter 17.

***The Complete HIV/AIDS Teaching Kit* resources used in this human biology course:**

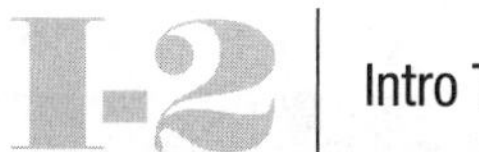

Intro Table I-2

TOPIC	RESOURCES FOR LECTURE PREPARATION	ACTIVITIES AND ASSIGNMENTS
Introduction: Gender, Culture, and Health	Part 4, chapter 15	*Group Activity:* Is It Sex or Gender? (Part 4, chapter 15)
Biological Vulnerability, Gender Roles, and Disease	Part 4, chapters 15 and 16	*Assignment:* Gender in the Real World (Part 4, chapter 16)
Gender- and Culture-Based Inequality and Health	Part 4, chapter 17	*Assignment:* Gender Inequality and HIV/AIDS (Part 4, chapter 17)

TIPS FOR HEALTH AND SOCIAL SERVICE PROVIDERS

The far reach and dynamic nature of the HIV/AIDS epidemic in the United States present complex challenges to health professionals and social service providers who work in HIV prevention programs in community-based organizations, clinics, and schools. These professionals are at the frontline of the fight against the disease. They educate citizens of various racial/ethnic, socioeconomic, sexual orientation, regional, and cultural backgrounds on what HIV is and what science now knows about how to prevent the spread of the disease.

These health and social service providers—often overworked and underfunded—can benefit from accessible, user-friendly resources that help them perform their work. *The Complete HIV/AIDS Teaching Kit's* comprehensive, science-based content, teaching aids, and CD-ROM offer health and service providers one such resource.

For those who specialize in HIV/AIDS prevention and treatment, there is increasing urgency to identify, implement, and sustain cost-effective programs and services that make a difference. For practitioners in other fields, such as sexual and reproductive health, substance abuse prevention and treatment, mental health, and domestic violence prevention, there is a growing need to integrate an HIV/AIDS focus into their own programs and services.

What follows are suggestions for how health and HIV/AIDS practitioners can use this book and CD-ROM as a "one-stop shopping" resource to meet their HIV/AIDS-related program needs. The suggested uses are followed by an illustrative practitioner application of how *The Complete HIV/AIDS Teaching Kit* might be used to achieve service provision-related goals.

HOW TO USE *THE COMPLETE HIV/AIDS TEACHING KIT* AS A SELF-PACED RESOURCE FOR INCREASING STAFF'S KNOWLEDGE OF "HIV/AIDS BASICS"

For practitioners who *do not* specialize in HIV/AIDS-related services, *The Complete HIV/AIDS Teaching Kit* is an excellent, self-paced resource for learning basic information about the nature, extent, causes, and consequences of HIV/AIDS, as well as the social and behavioral aspects of prevention and treatment. This information can help practitioners consider how best to address the HIV/AIDS-related needs of their clients and communities, whether through new in-house services or referrals to other agencies.

For providers who *do* specialize in HIV/AIDS prevention or treatment, *The Complete HIV/AIDS Teaching Kit* can provide a helpful review or refresher on "HIV/AIDS basics." Those working in the prevention arena can use the book to increase their basic knowledge of treatment, whereas those who specialize in treatment can increase their understanding of prevention issues among HIV+ populations.

Practitioners using *The Complete HIV/AIDS Teaching Kit* to learn or brush up on HIV/AIDS basics will find Part 1 particularly useful. Other parts of the book provide helpful overviews of topics such as prevention and treatment approaches, social and psychological aspects of living with HIV, and the relationship between gender and HIV.

HOW TO USE *THE COMPLETE HIV/AIDS TEACHING KIT* AS A SOURCE OF INFORMATION ON SCIENCE-BASED BEST PRACTICES IN HIV/AIDS PREVENTION AND TREATMENT PROGRAMMING, WRITTEN FOR NONSCIENTISTS

For providers who are planning or delivering HIV/AIDS prevention and treatment programs or services, the ability to apply science-based best practices effectively in the context of practical resource constraints is crucial to program success and sustainability. However, the findings of scientific research are often not presented in ways that are accessible to nonscientist professionals. *The Complete HIV/AIDS Teaching Kit* can help to bridge the gap between science and practice. For example, providers may choose to utilize Part 2 and Part 3 to explore theories, approaches, and characteristics of effective prevention and treatment efforts.

HOW TO USE *THE COMPLETE HIV/AIDS TEACHING KIT* AS A SOURCE OF READY-TO-USE MATERIALS FOR DELIVERING STAFF TRAINING WORKSHOPS ON HIV/AIDS AND HIV/AIDS-RELATED PROGRAMMING, BASED ON THE LATEST BEHAVIORAL AND SOCIAL RESEARCH

Agency staff—both paid and volunteer—can benefit from training workshops in HIV/AIDS-related topics for several reasons. First, this type of training can build staff's knowledge, skills, and self-confidence to plan, implement, and sustain successful intervention efforts. Second, it can help staff interact in a more informed and effective manner with clients, community members, and other key stakeholders. *The Complete HIV/AIDS Teaching Kit* includes resources that can be adapted or used as is to meet training goals. Trainers can use the PowerPoint slides to present the latest research findings on the social and behavioral causes and consequences of HIV/AIDS, and science-based best practices in prevention and treatment programming.

The book's mix-and-match options help practitioners tailor these materials as needed for different workshop formats, topics, and audiences.

Trainers also will appreciate the individual and group learning activities offered in each part of the book. These activities can be used in workshops or seminars to reinforce service providers' knowledge, afford skills practice, and increase motivation to apply their understanding and proficiency to programming and service delivery work. For example, the group activity "Controversies in Positive Prevention" (Part 3), can help participants identify and consider ethical principles that guide effective prevention among HIV+ people.

HOW TO USE *THE COMPLETE HIV/AIDS TEACHING KIT* AS A SOURCE OF INFORMATIONAL AND SKILLS-BUILDING ACTIVITIES THAT CAN BE INCORPORATED INTO HIV/AIDS-RELATED CLIENT INTERVENTIONS

Practitioners who are developing HIV/AIDS-related interventions can save time and effort by incorporating relevant program activities developed by others. Every chapter in each of the four parts of *The Complete HIV/AIDS Teaching Kit* offers learning activities of diverse lengths, formats, and topical foci. Practitioners can pick and choose activities that are most relevant for their goals, strategies, and target populations.

For example, "Myths About HIV and AIDS" is a 30-minute interactive group activity (offered in chapter 1, Activity 1 of *The Complete HIV/AIDS Teaching Kit*) that helps participants to dispel myths and understand facts about HIV.

For practitioners seeking a longer activity, "Eliminating Barriers: Identify, Prioritize, Create Solutions" is a 30-minute group exercise found in Part 2 (chapter 7, Activity 4). This activity increases participants' skill in identifying and addressing barriers to STI/HIV risk reduction.

The Complete HIV/AIDS Teaching Kit has something to offer to a range of health and social service providers working in diverse agency and community contexts. One illustrative example of how this book might be used to address specific needs is presented here.

PRACTITIONER CASE STUDY:

Discussing HIV/AIDS Issues With HIV+ clients

Maria Santiago is a community health nurse who provides medication, support, and other care-related services for HIV+ individuals in her community. To provide her patients with badly needed science-based information about the disease, Ms. Santiago decides to create an all-day educational workshop for her patients. Following the workshop, she will ask her patients if they believe the same workshop might be helpful to their family members, friends, and caregivers. She will take her patients' postworkshop suggestions and use them to give the same workshop to her patients' family and friends.

Ms. Santiago begins the workshop by ensuring that participants understand "HIV/AIDS basics." She uses the following PowerPoint slides from Part 1:

- Transmission of HIV
- The path from HIV to AIDS
- HIV/AIDS prevalence rates in the United States for men and women, different racial/ethnic groups, and different regions of the country

Ms. Santiago also wants her patients to better understand some of the medical, social, and psychological challenges they face. She wants them to be aware of scientific advances in treatment of HIV. She reads Part 3 and then organizes her presentation using PowerPoint slides on the following topics:

- Psychological and social challenges of living with HIV/AIDS
  - HIV-related stigma and discrimination
  - HIV-related grief, stress, and uncertainty
  - Social support services for those living with HIV/AIDS

- The medical side of living with HIV/AIDS
  - HIV/AIDS treatment approaches
  - Treatment challenges for HIV-positive people
  - Opportunistic infections associated with HIV/AIDS

In strategizing group exercises for her workshop, Ms. Santiago takes note of an exercise concerning HIV/AIDS grief and loss described in the "Additional Resources" section of Part 3. She adapts this exercise by inviting one of her patients to speak to the other workshop participants about his experience making an AIDS memorial quilt panel for his partner.

To close the workshop, Ms. Santiago plans to ask the guest speaker to comment on a key theme in Part 3 of *The Complete HIV/AIDS Teaching Kit*—the importance of social support services like hers for those living with HIV/AIDS.

Following the workshop, Ms. Santiago will ask her patients if they believe the same workshop might be helpful to their family members, friends, and caregivers, so they might better understand some of the issues faced by people living with HIV. With her patients' encouragement and support, she will take their suggestions and use them to tailor future workshops for this larger audience.

***The Complete HIV/AIDS Teaching Kit* resources used for this workshop:**

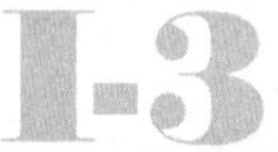

Intro Table I-3

TRAINING EXERCISE	POWERPOINT SLIDES
Group Activity: The NAMES Project: AIDS-Related Grief (Part 3, chapter 13)	■ How HIV is transmitted (Part 1, chapter 4) ■ The path from HIV to AIDS (Part 1, chapter 2) ■ HIV/AIDS prevalence rates, United States, by gender, race/ethnicity, and region (Part 1, chapter 1) ■ HIV/AIDS treatment approaches/adherence (Part 3, chapter 12) ■ Opportunistic infections (Part 3, chapter 12) ■ HIV-related stigma and discrimination (Part 3, chapter 13) ■ HIV-related grief, stress, and uncertainty (Part 3, chapter 13) ■ Social support services for HIV+ people (Part 3, chapter 13)

REFERENCES

Henry J. Kaiser Family Foundation (2006). *HIV/AIDS policy fact sheet: The global HIV/AIDS epidemic*. Washington, DC: Henry J. Kaiser Family Foundation.

United Nations Programme on HIV/AIDS (UNAIDS). (2006). *2006 report on the global AIDS epidemic*. Geneva, Switzerland: UNAIDS.

PART I

HIV/AIDS: The Epidemic

Acquired immune deficiency syndrome, AIDS, is one of the greatest threats to human health in the 21st century. Part 1 provides an overview of this deadly disease and of the human immunodeficiency virus (HIV) that causes AIDS. Part 1 begins by recounting the worldwide destruction wrought by AIDS since it was first identified in the early 1980s. It then describes in detail how infection with HIV leads to AIDS, and how biological features, behaviors, psychological tendencies, demographic characteristics, and social and cultural factors affect people's chances of infection. Finally, Part 1 describes how HIV is transmitted.

Acquired immune deficiency syndrome, AIDS, is one of the greatest threats to human health in the 21st century. According to the Joint United Nations Programme on HIV/AIDS (UNAIDS) 2006 Report on the Global AIDS epidemic:

Every day, over **7,500 people die** from AIDS.

Every hour, more than **300 people die** from AIDS.

Every minute, another **5 people die** from AIDS.

Learning Objectives

- Define HIV and AIDS
- Explain how HIV and AIDS are diagnosed
- Identify key historical moments in the discovery of, and response to, HIV/AIDS
- Understand the medications most commonly used to treat HIV
- Discuss which populations are currently most affected by HIV/AIDS and why
- Distinguish between AIDS incidence, prevalence, and mortality

Key Terms

AIDS
antiretroviral therapy
CDC
HAART
HIV
incidence
mortality
MSM
NIH
opportunistic infections
prevalence
seroconversion
surveillance
virus

An Overview of the HIV/AIDS Epidemic

HIV/AIDS has been identified in virtually every region of the world, reaching epidemic levels and affecting the lives of millions of men, women, and children of all ages, races, ethnicities, religions, and sexual orientations. Despite its widespread devastation, HIV/AIDS is a relatively new illness. Chapter 1 first describes HIV and AIDS, then outlines how HIV and AIDS were discovered and increasingly understood. Chapter 1 goes on to describe the epidemiology of the HIV/AIDS epidemic, presenting data on the number of people living with and dying from AIDS. Chapter 1 closes with a brief overview of useful epidemiological terms.

WHAT ARE HIV AND AIDS?

HIV stands for *human immunodeficiency virus*. HIV infects only *humans*, creates *deficiencies* in the body's *immune* system, which normally protects the body against illness, and is a *virus*. Viruses are tiny substances that enter the body's cells and cause illness.

AIDS stands for *acquired immune deficiency syndrome*. People do not inherit AIDS through their genes. Instead, they *acquire* AIDS through contact with HIV. AIDS is primarily a sickness of the body's *immune* system—the very system that is designed to defend the body against sickness. People with AIDS have a *deficiency* in their immune systems, meaning that the immune system no longer works properly. Without a healthy immune system, people infected with HIV get sick with other diseases much more easily, and get well much more slowly, if at all. AIDS causes many different diseases and opportunistic infections, so it is not just one illness but a *syndrome* made up of many symptoms and illnesses.

Acquired immune deficiency syndrome, AIDS, is one of the greatest threats to human health in the 21st century. According to the Joint United Nations Programme on HIV/AIDS (UNAIDS) 2006 Report on the Global AIDS epidemic:

Every day, more than **7,500 people die** from AIDS.

Every hour, more than **300 people die** from AIDS.

Every minute, another **5 people die** from AIDS.

Defining and Diagnosing HIV

To diagnose an HIV infection, health care providers examine a person's blood or body tissues for the virus using tests designed and licensed for this purpose. A person who has HIV in his or her body is said to be *HIV positive* (HIV+ or *seropositive for HIV*). Because HIV causes subtle changes in the immune system long before the infected person feels sick, the term *HIV disease* is used to cover the time spanning from initial infection with the HIV virus to the diagnosis of AIDS. AIDS is the late stage of infection with HIV. In the absence of HIV treatment, most, if not all, HIV+ people will develop AIDS.

Diagnosing AIDS

To diagnose AIDS in the United States, health care workers use criteria established by the Centers for Disease Control and Prevention (CDC). People are diagnosed with AIDS if they are HIV+ and have at least one of certain diseases, called *opportunistic infections*, which take advantage of HIV+ people's weakened immune system. There are 26 opportunistic diseases associated with AIDS, including pneumonia, *Kaposi's sarcoma* (a cancer), invasive cervical cancer, and pulmonary tuberculosis (i.e., tuberculosis of the lungs). People are also diagnosed with AIDS if they are HIV+ and have very low levels of certain kinds of white blood cells called *T-cells*. T-cells are some of the most important cells of the immune system. They protect from viral infections, help other cells produce antibodies, fight bacterial infections, and fight cancers.

People with AIDS often are called just that, or by the acronym *PWAs*. In recent years, the more optimistic term *people living with AIDS* (*PLWAs*) has become preferred by some AIDS activist groups.

HIV/AIDS AND SCIENCE: A SELECT TIMELINE

In the early 1980s, the first cases of two rare illnesses, Kaposi's sarcoma and pneumocystic pneumonia, were reported in California and New York. Around this same time, health care providers began to report an unusual immune system failure among gay men in the United States. Epidemiologists generally were baffled by the variety of symptoms that they were seeing among male homosexuals. Some used phrases such as *gay cancer* and *gay plague* to describe this new disease (Kanabus & Fredricksson, n.d.a).

Although not fully understood at the time, it is now believed that the HIV/AIDS epidemic actually gained momentum in the mid- to late 1970s. Researchers have since identified HIV-infected people and blood samples that existed before 1970 (Mann, 1989). The past 2 decades of scientific responses to the HIV/AIDS epidemic have been marked by rapid progress leading to important discoveries. Yet, many of the answers to critical questions about this disease either remain unknown or are jeopardized by diverse political agendas.

Key Moments in Our Understanding of—and Responses to—HIV/AIDS

1980–1983

- **1982.** After it is known as *gay cancer, new pneumonia,* and *Gay-Related Immune Deficiency (GRID)*, the syndrome is renamed acquired immune deficiency syndrome (AIDS) by the CDC when it becomes clear that the epidemic is affecting broader populations than originally thought (Stine, 1993).
- **1982.** The CDC releases its first AIDS case definition, which "defines a case of AIDS as a disease, at least moderately predictive of a defect in cell-mediated immunity, occurring in a person with no known cause for diminished resistance to that disease" (AIDS ACTION, n.d.).
- **1982.** The National Institutes of Health (NIH) rejects a proposal for a research study to determine whether women get AIDS (AIDS ACTION, n.d.).

- **1983.** Dr. Luc Montagnier and his team at the Institute Pasteur in Paris, France, isolate a new virus linked to AIDS (Barre-Sinoussi et al., 1983; Kanabus & Fredricksson, n.d.a). The first governmental AIDS hotline is established by the federal Department of Health and Human Services. The first woman is diagnosed with AIDS (in San Francisco) (AIDS ACTION, n.d.).

1984–1985

- **1984.** Dr. Robert Gallo and colleagues at the U.S. National Cancer Institute also isolate an AIDS-causing virus. Scientists later conclude that Drs. Montagnier and Gallo discovered the same virus, which is named HIV (human immunodeficiency virus) (Stine, 1993). Later epidemiological evidence continues to strongly support the argument that AIDS is caused by a virus (Cohen, 1998).
- **1985.** The first International AIDS Conference is held in Atlanta, Georgia. At the conference, the CDC lists the signs and symptoms of AIDS so that health care providers and researchers can identify and report cases, determine the extent of the epidemic, and figure out the cause of AIDS (Cohen, 1998).
- **1985.** Researchers discover a second retrovirus in West Africa that is closely related to HIV. The virus is spread from person to person in ways similar to HIV, and it is related to many of the same symptoms and sicknesses as HIV (Stine, 1993). To distinguish the two highly similar viruses, the first discovered retrovirus is named *human immunodeficiency virus type 1* (*HIV-1*) and the second *human immunodeficiency virus type 2* (*HIV-2*). (In common usage, "HIV" usually indicates HIV-1 because HIV-2 is rare in most parts of the world [Cohen, 1998].)
- **1985.** The first test to detect HIV antibodies (called *Enzyme-Linked Immunosorbent Assay,* or *ELISA*) is approved in the United States (Stine, 1993). The test makes it possible to screen blood products, to detect HIV infection in people who have not yet developed AIDS, and to identify *seroconversion* (the time when the body's immune system begins reacting to HIV, often with flu-like symptoms) in newly infected individuals (Cohen, 1998).
- **1985.** Research leads to a description of the stages of HIV/AIDS. Although researchers initially believe that during the earliest (latent) stage of infection, HIV is more or less dominant, they later learn that, during this stage, virus particles are actively replicating in people's lymphoid organs (which produce white blood cells that protect the body against disease [Cohen, 1998]).

1986–1989

- **1986.** The Surgeon General issues a landmark federal report to the Reagan administration and to the public that calls for AIDS education and condom use to prevent the transmission of HIV.
- **1986.** Early tests show that a drug called *azidothymidine* (AZT), originally developed in 1964 as a possible anticancer drug, slows down HIV's attack on the immune system (AIDS ACTION, n.d.).
- **1987.** The U.S. Food and Drug Administration (FDA) approves AZT as the first drug for HIV infection (Kanabus & Fredricksson, n.d.b). AZT works by interrupting HIV's invasion of a person's healthy cells.

1990–1993

- **1990.** The political AIDS activism group ACT UP conducts a protest at the National Institutes of Health (NIH), demanding more HIV treatments and the expansion of clinical trials to include more women and people of color.

- **1991.** *DDL* (*didanosine*) becomes the second drug approved by the FDA for the treatment of AIDS. It is to be used in combination with AZT by adult patients with advanced HIV infection. This is the first successful use of a combination of drugs to treat HIV infection (Kanabus & Fredricksson, n.d.b).
- **1993.** Reports show that some people infected with HIV who have never taken AZT already have resistance to the drug. This occurs because people transmitting the HIV have themselves taken AZT and are transmitting a variant of HIV that is already resistant to AZT (Kanabus & Fredricksson, n.d.c).
- **1993.** The *female condom*, a polyurethane (plastic) sheath worn by a woman inside the vagina during sex, is approved by the FDA, offering women a new way to protect themselves against contracting HIV.
- **1993.** In recognition of the increasingly diverse populations affected by HIV/AIDS, the CDC revises the AIDS case definition to be more inclusive of women and injection drug users; therefore, the number of documented AIDS cases goes up in these populations. Similarly, the NIH implements new guidelines requiring that women and minorities are included in all clinical trials involving human subjects, unless there are scientific reasons not to do so.

1994–1996

- **1994.** The CDC announces that AIDS is the leading cause of death among 25- to 44-year-old Americans (AIDS ACTION, n.d.).
- **1994.** The first HIV saliva test (OraSure) is approved by the FDA for use in clinical settings (AIDS ACTION, n.d.).
- **1995.** *Saquinavir*, the first protease inhibitor (a new class of *antiretroviral treatment*), is approved (AIDS ACTION, n.d.). Antiretroviral treatment for HIV infection consists of drugs that work against HIV infection itself by slowing down the replication of HIV in the body.
- **1996.** The use of three antiretroviral medications used in combination becomes the new standard of HIV care. This approach to HIV treatment is sometimes called *Highly Active Antiretroviral Therapy (HAART)*, or simply *antiretroviral therapy*. The drugs used in HAART target different stages of the HIV reproductive cycle, making the HIV less likely to reproduce and to mutate.

1997–1999

- **1997.** The effect of new treatments is clearly seen as the number of Americans newly diagnosed with AIDS drops for the first time since the epidemic began. HIV+ people in some countries are able to return to work as a result of the improvement in their health as a result of antiretroviral therapy (Kanabus & Fredricksson, n.d.c).
- **1998.** The number of American AIDS deaths drops 47% from the previous year; the drop is credited to the effectiveness of HAART. Nonetheless, problems with HAART are noted. Many patients experience difficult side effects, including nausea, kidney failure, body shape changes, and even hallucinations. Health care professionals note that adherence to the complicated HAART treatment is a major concern in their communities (AIDS ACTION, n.d.).
- **1999.** The CDC begins funding the "Prevention for HIV Infected Persons Project" (PHIPP), asking certain jurisdictions to make prevention for HIV+ people (e.g., preventing further infection to themselves and others) a priority. Grants are awarded to five health departments around the country.

2000–2003

- **2000.** *Nonoxynol-9* (N-9), a common spermicide formerly believed to be a potentially effective barrier against HIV, is shown to significantly increase the risk of HIV transmission. Before this discovery, prevention efforts actively encouraged individuals to use products containing N-9, assuming it had some microbicidal effect against HIV (AIDS ACTION, n.d.).
- **2001.** In a historic session of the United Nations General Assembly on the AIDS epidemic, participants unanimously pass a resolution declaring AIDS a global catastrophe and calling for worldwide commitment to end the epidemic.
- **2003.** The CDC announces a new initiative to target people who are living with HIV to address their prevention, transmission, and care needs. Of the 40,000 new infections that occur each year in the United States, 27,000 are estimated to be the result of transmission from people who are unaware that they are infected, whereas 13,000 are the result of contact with people who are aware of their HIV+ status.
- **2003.** The Bill and Melinda Gates Foundation awards $60 million to the International Partnership for Microbicides, the largest grant ever awarded to support work in this field.

2004–Today

- Combinations of anti-HIV medications are credited with declines in HIV-related sickness and death (Simoni, Frick, Pantalone, & Turner, 2003).
- Drug therapy is also found to reduce the spread of HIV from mother to child when given to the mother from the second trimester of pregnancy until delivery, during labor and delivery, and to the baby for 6 weeks after birth (Cohan, 2003).
- Antiretroviral therapy remains expensive. As a result, although HIV disease rates have fallen in many industrialized countries, they continue to rise in those parts of the world that cannot afford antiretroviral therapy.
- Today in the United States, the two groups most affected by AIDS are men who have sex with men and injection drug users (IDUs). Other high-risk groups include hemophiliacs, heterosexual partners of people infected with HIV, blood transfusion recipients, Central Africans, infants of HIV-infected mothers, and infants of injection drug–using mothers (Cohen, 1998; Kanki & Essex, 2000).
- Currently, ethnic and racial minorities represent the majority of new AIDS cases, the majority of Americans living with AIDS, and the majority of deaths among persons with AIDS in the United States (Henry J. Kaiser Family Foundation, 2004). Women also account for a growing proportion of cumulative reported AIDS cases (CDC, 2005).

GLOBAL INCIDENCE AND PREVALENCE OF HIV/AIDS TODAY

There were an estimated 4.3 million new HIV infections (*incident* infections) worldwide as of the end of 2006, about two-thirds of which occurred in sub-Saharan Africa (Henry J. Kaiser Family Foundation, 2006) (see Figure 1-1). About half of those infected were young people ages 15–25 (UNAIDS, 2006).

As of the end of 2006, the number of people living with HIV/AIDS (HIV/AIDS *prevalence*) was estimated at 39.5 million, close to two-thirds of whom were living in sub-Saharan Africa (Henry J. Kaiser Family Foundation, 2006) (see Figure 1-1). Women accounted for 48% of those living with HIV (UNAIDS, 2006).

Region	Total No. (%) Living With HIV/AIDS, end of 2006	Newly Infected in 2006	Adult (aged 15-49) Prevalence Rate, 2006
Global Total	**39.5 million (100%)**	**4.3 million**	**1.0%**
Sub-Saharan Africa	24.7 million (62.5%)	2.8 million	5.9%
South/South-East Asia	7.8 million (19.7%)	860,000	0.6%
Eastern Europe/Central Asia	1.7 million (4.3%)	270,000	0.9%
Latin America	1.7 million (4.3%)	140,000	0.5%
North America	1.4 million (3.5%)	43,000	0.8%
East Asia	750,000 (1.9%)	100,000	0.1%
Western/Central Europe	740,000 (1.9%)	22,000	0.3%
Middle East/North Africa	460,000 (1.2%)	68,000	0.2%
Caribbean	250,000 (0.6%)	27,000	1.2%
Oceania	81,000 (0.2%)	7,100	0.4%

Figure 1-1 HIV prevalence and incidence by region (Henry J. Kaiser Foundation, 2006).

Over 25 million people have died since the beginning of the AIDS epidemic. Currently, over 7,500 people die from AIDS each day—about 5 people every minute (UNAIDS, 2006).

Statistics such as those offered earlier are based on *surveillance* data. Surveillance is the ongoing, systematic collection, analysis, interpretation, and sharing of health data. These data not only show patterns of disease incidence, prevalence, and mortality but also help predict how much a disease will affect a specific population.

Global data about HIV/AIDS are collected by many different sources and compiled by a few key international organizations. These include the Joint United Nations Programme on HIV/AIDS (UNAIDS) and the World Health Organization (WHO). UNAIDS and WHO estimate global HIV/AIDS morbidity and mortality rates using all available data, including surveys of pregnant women and population-based surveys, such as household surveys conducted in Kenya, Mali, Zambia, and Zimbabwe (UNAIDS, n.d.). UNAIDS and WHO also publish updated country estimates biannually.

HIV/AIDS IN THE UNITED STATES TODAY

One of the major collectors and distributors of data about the HIV/AIDS epidemic is the CDC. The CDC collects two sets of data to track the HIV/AIDS epidemic in the United States: results from HIV surveillance and results from AIDS surveillance.

HIV Surveillance

Twenty-nine states and the U.S. Virgin Islands have been reporting new HIV infections to the CDC since 1998. In more recent years, additional areas have joined the reporting system, facilitating the monitoring of HIV trends over time and better understanding of the behaviors that increase HIV infection risk in the United States and its territories (CDC, 2003, n.d.e). The HIV data collected by CDC (such as those shown in Figure 1-2) are statistically adjusted to take into consideration reporting delays.

AIDS Surveillance

AIDS diagnoses are reported to the CDC by all U.S. states and territories. These data are statistically adjusted for reporting delays and are used to look at AIDS trends in

Reported Cases of HIV Infection (not AIDS), by Age Group at Diagnosis, Cumulative through 2004—42 Areas

Age (years)	HIV Infection (not AIDS) No.	HIV Infection (not AIDS) %
<13	4,814	2
13–14	393	<1
15–24	35,630	16
25–34	81,231	35
35–44	70,437	31
45–54	27,591	12
55–64	7,170	3
≥65	2,145	<1
Total	229,411	

Note. Data from 42 areas with confidential name-based HIV infection reporting as of December 2004.

Figure 1-2 Cases of HIV infection (not AIDS) by age at diagnosis through 2004—42 areas (CDC, n.d.e).

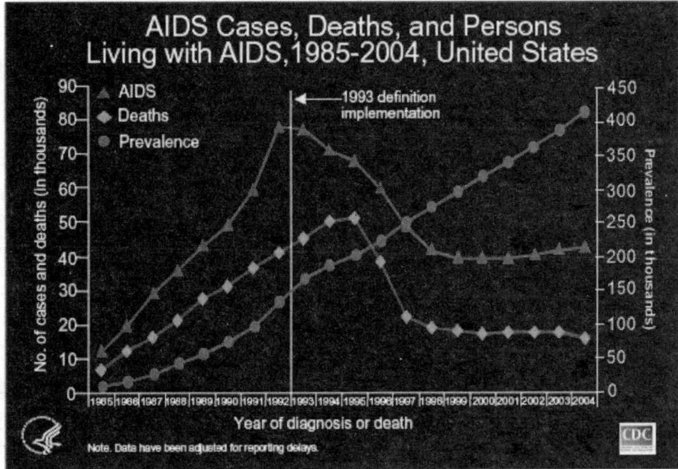

Figure 1-3 Number of AIDS cases, AIDS deaths, and people living with AIDS, 1985–2004, United States (CDC, n.d.a).

the United States (CDC, 2003). For example, as the line marked by triangles in Figure 1-3 shows, the number of new AIDS cases (i.e., AIDS *incidence*) has been decreasing since 1993. In 1993, approximately 80,000 adults and adolescents were diagnosed with AIDS. By 1998, that number had dropped by about 50%, to approximately 40,000 cases. Decreases in incidence were partly a result of better HIV prevention, such as organizations testing their blood supplies for HIV and individuals practicing safer sex. They also were in large part a result of the introduction of HAART in 1996. HAART interferes in the HIV reproductive cycle, making HIV less likely to reproduce in the body and lead to AIDS.

Because HAART slows the progression of AIDS, its use also has contributed to a decrease in AIDS-related deaths and a corresponding increase in the number of people living with AIDS (i.e., AIDS *prevalence*) (Osmond, 1998). As is seen in the graph line in Figure 1-3 marked with circles, in 1993, under 150,000 people were living with AIDS in the United States. By 2003, U.S. AIDS prevalence had increased to around 400,000 people.

The graph line marked with diamonds shows AIDS *mortality*—the number of people who died from AIDS in a given year. Mortality began to drop markedly after the introduction of HAART in 1996. New and more effective medications for *opportunistic infections* (infections that take advantage of HIV+ people's weakened immune systems) also may have contributed to this decrease.

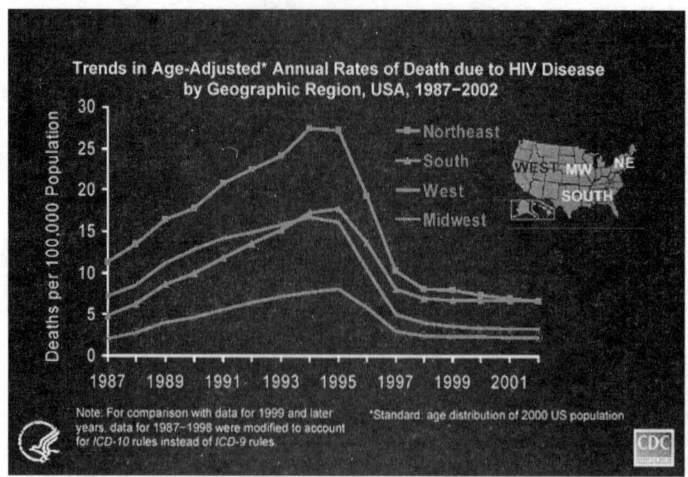

Figure 1-4 Deaths due to HIV disease by U.S. region, 1987–2002 (CDC, n.d.f).

Although new therapies for treating HIV/AIDS have been responsible for decreasing AIDS-related mortality, treating AIDS can be very complicated and difficult. People with HIV/AIDS often take many medications, and the appropriate dosage of these medications must be taken on a specific time schedule. Unfortunately, the medicines, although effective, sometimes have unpleasant side effects that may discourage people from taking them as prescribed. In addition, if not taken properly, HIV may become resistant to the medicines, meaning that the medicines no longer work as well. Thus, AIDS mortality may not continue to decrease until new and improved treatments are available.

U.S. Regional Disparities in AIDS Death Rates

As shown in Figure 1-4, before the introduction of HAART, the age-adjusted rate of death as a result of AIDS (HIV disease) increased most rapidly in the South and Northeast regions of the United States. The rate decreased rapidly in 1996 and 1997 in all regions but not as sharply in the South. By 2002, the Northeast and South had the same death rate from HIV disease.

However, of the people who died of HIV disease from 1987 to 2002, the proportion who resided in the South increased from 28 to 49%, whereas the proportions who resided in other regions decreased or remained relatively unchanged (CDC, n.d.g).

THE CHANGING FACE OF THE HIV/AIDS EPIDEMIC

> To face the HIV/AIDS epidemic is to see the many faces of the epidemic.

Despite great strides in HIV prevention, the HIV/AIDS epidemic continues to evolve and grow, challenging researchers, practitioners, and policy makers to adapt to its changing face. One key challenge is that the populations who most need prevention interventions continue to shift.

Although men who have sex with men (MSM) remain the largest exposure group in the United States, racial and ethnic minorities (especially people of color) represent the majority of new HIV infections, the majority of Americans living with HIV/AIDS, and the majority of deaths among HIV+ people in the United States (CDC, 2005; Kaiser Family Foundation, 2004). For example, although African Americans and Latinos represent 12% and 13% of the U.S. population (Grieco & Cassidy, 2001), African Americans accounted for 50% of all HIV/AIDS cases diagnosed in 2004 (CDC, 2005). The number of African Americans living with AIDS as of 2004 far exceeded that of any other ethnic group (CDC, n.d.c), as shown in Figure 1-5.

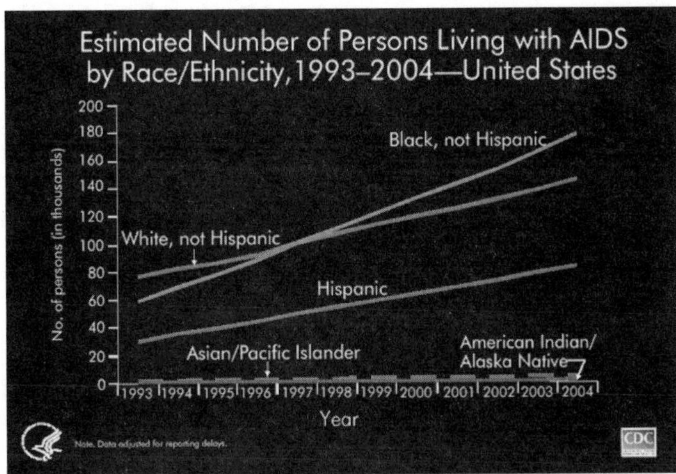

Figure 1-5 Number of people living with AIDS by race/ethnicity, 1993–2004—United States (CDC, n.d.c).

The HIV/AIDS epidemic also is increasingly affecting women and heterosexuals. Women accounted for 7% of the AIDS cases diagnosed in the United States in 1986 (CDC, n.d.b). In 2004, women accounted for approximately 27% of all newly diagnosed AIDS cases in the United States (CDC, n.d.c). Among women, 78% of HIV/AIDS cases in 2004 were from heterosexual exposure (CDC, n.d.d). Further discussion of the increasing impact of HIV/AIDS on women worldwide may be found in Part 4 of this book.

REFERENCES

AIDS ACTION. (n.d.). *Keeping time: Social and governmental developments in HIV*. Retrieved October 4, 2004, from http://www.aidsaction.org/sitemap/timeline/index.htm

Barre-Sinoussi, F., Chermann, J. C., Rey, F., Nugeyre, M. T., Chamaret, S., Gruest, J., et al. (1983). Isolation of a T-lymphotropic retrovirus from a patient at risk for acquired immune deficiency syndrome (AIDS). *Science, 220*, 868–871.

Centers for Disease Control and Prevention (CDC). (2003). *Fact sheet: HIV/AIDS among African Americans*. Atlanta, GA: CDC.

Centers for Disease Control and Prevention (CDC). (2005). *HIV/AIDS surveillance report, 2004*. Atlanta, GA: CDC.

Centers for Disease Control and Prevention (CDC). (n.d.a). Estimated number of AIDS cases, deaths, and persons living with AIDS, 1985–2004, United States. In *HIV/AIDS surveillance—Trends L207 through 2003* [Slide series], slide 1. Atlanta, GA: CDC.

Centers for Disease Control and Prevention (CDC). (n.d.b). Estimated number of adults and adolescents living with AIDS, by sex, 1993–2004, United States. In *HIV/AIDS surveillance—General epidemiology (through 2004)* [Slide series], slide 4. Atlanta, GA: CDC.

Centers for Disease Control and Prevention (CDC). (n.d.c). Estimated number of persons living with AIDS by race/ethnicity, 1993–2004, United States. In *HIV/AIDS surveillance—General epidemiology (through 2004)* [Slide series], slide 5. Atlanta, GA: CDC.

Centers for Disease Control and Prevention (CDC). (n.d.d). Proportion of HIV/AIDS cases among adults and adolescents, by sex and transmission category, 2004—35 areas. In *HIV/AIDS surveillance—General epidemiology (through 2004)* [Slide series], slide 4. Atlanta, GA: CDC.

Centers for Disease Control and Prevention (CDC). (n.d.e). Reported cases of HIV infection (not AIDS), by age group at diagnosis, cumulative through 2004—42 areas. In *HIV/AIDS surveillance—General epidemiology (through 2004)* [Slide series], slide 19. Atlanta, GA: CDC.

Centers for Disease Control and Prevention (CDC). (n.d.f). Trends in age-adjusted annual rates of death due to HIV disease by geographic region, USA, 1987–2002. In *Mortality L285 through 2002* [Slide series], slide 12. Atlanta, GA: CDC.

Centers for Disease Control and Prevention (CDC). (n.d.g). Trends in the percentage distribution of deaths due to HIV disease by geographic region, USA, 1987–2002. In *Mortality L285 through 2002* [Slide series], slide 13. Atlanta, GA: CDC.

Cohan, D. (2003). Perinatal HIV: Special considerations. *Topics in HIV Medicine, 11*(6), 200–213.

Cohen, P. T. (1998). Clinical overview of HIV disease. In L. Pieperl, S. Coffey, O. Bacon, & P. Volberding (Eds.), *HIV InSite knowledge base*. San Francisco: Center for HIV Information, University of California, San Francisco.

Grieco, E. M., & Cassidy, R. C. (2001). *Overview of race and Hispanic origin: Census 2000 brief.* Washington, DC: U.S. Department of Commerce, Economic and Statistics Administration, U.S. Census Bureau.

Henry J. Kaiser Family Foundation (2004). *HIV/AIDS policy fact sheet: The HIV/AIDS epidemic in the United States*. Washington, DC: Henry J. Kaiser Family Foundation.

Henry J. Kaiser Family Foundation (2006). *HIV/AIDS policy fact sheet: The global HIV/AIDS epidemic*. Washington, DC: Henry J. Kaiser Family Foundation.

Kanabus, A., & Fredricksson, J. (n.d.a). *The history of AIDS 1981–1986*. Horsham, UK: AVERT.org. Retrieved September 26, 2003, from http://www.avert.org/his81_86.htm

Kanabus, A., & Fredricksson, J. (n.d.b). *The history of AIDS 1987–1992*. Horsham, UK: AVERT.org. Retrieved February 4, 2004, from http://www.avert.org/his87_92.htm

Kanabus, A., & Fredricksson, J. (n.d.c). *The history of AIDS 1993–1997*. Horsham, UK: AVERT.org. Retrieved February 4, 2004, from http://www.avert.org/his93_97.htm

Kanki, P. J., & Essex, M. E. (2000). The past and future of HIV/AIDS. In K. H. Mayer & H. F. Pizer (Eds.), *The emergence of AIDS: The impact on immunology, microbiology, and public health* (pp. 3–32). Washington, DC: American Public Health Association.

Mann, J. M. (1989). AIDS: A worldwide pandemic. In M. S. Gottlieb, D. J. Jeffries, D. Mildvan, A. J. Pinching, T. C. Quinn, & R. A. Weiss (Eds.), *Current topics in AIDS, Vol. 2* (pp. 1–10). New York: John Wiley & Sons.

National Institute of Allergy and Infectious Diseases (NIAID). (2001). *How HIV causes AIDS.* Bethesda, MD: NIAID.

Osmond, D. H. (1998). Epidemiology of HIV/AIDS in the United States. In L. Pieperl, S. Coffey, O. Bacon, & P. Volberding (Eds.), *HIV InSite knowledge base*. San Francisco: Center for HIV Information, University of California, San Francisco.

Simoni, J. M., Frick, P. A., Pantalone, D. W., & Turner, B. J. (2003). Antiretroviral adherence interventions: A review of current literature and ongoing studies. *Topics in HIV Medicine, 11*(6), 185–198.

Stine, G. J. (1993). *Acquired immune deficiency syndrome: Biological, medical, social, and legal issues*. Englewood Cliffs, NJ: Prentice Hall.

United Nations Programme on HIV/AIDS (UNAIDS). (2006). *2006 report on the global AIDS epidemic.* Geneva, Switzerland: UNAIDS.

United Nations Programme on HIV/AIDS (UNAIDS). (n.d.). *How do UNAIDS/WHO arrive at estimates?* Geneva, Switzerland: UNAIDS.

Instructor Resources

LEARNING ACTIVITIES

ACTIVITY 1:

Group Activity: Myths About HIV and AIDS

Objective: To dispel common myths about HIV/AIDS transmission and risk.

Minimum Time: 30 minutes

View a detailed guide for this activity on the CD-ROM.

ACTIVITY 2:

Assignment: HIV/AIDS Timeline

Objective: To understand the history of HIV/AIDS in the United States.

Since first recognized as a distinct infectious disease in 1981, HIV/AIDS has created a tremendous burden of illness and death in the United States. Create a visual timeline presenting the major events and advances in the HIV/AIDS epidemic in the United States.

ACTIVITY 3:

Assignment: The Origins of HIV

Objective: To understand how the HIV virus originated.

There have been many theories about the origins of HIV, including conspiracy theories (e.g., HIV was manufactured by the CIA) and theories about transmission from wild chimpanzees to humans. Write a research-based paper defending or refuting the following statement:

> The HIV virus originated in Africa.

DISCUSSION QUESTIONS

1. AIDS originally was considered a "gay cancer" that affected gay men only. How did that misconception impact early HIV/AIDS incidence, research, and treatment?
2. What are some drawbacks of antiretroviral therapies, and why are they important to address?

3. Why might ethnic and racial minorities represent the majority of new AIDS cases?
4. Why is it important for local, national, and international authorities to track and share HIV/AIDS surveillance data?

QUIZ

1. How many people have died from AIDS since the beginning of the epidemic?
   a) Over 8 million
   b) Over 17 million
   c) Over 20 million
   d) Over 25 million
2. 1997 marked the first year since the discovery of AIDS that the number of Americans newly diagnosed with AIDS dropped. What was the reason for the decrease?
   a) The drug azidothymidine (AZT)
   b) The combination of AZT and didanosine (DDL)
   c) Highly Active Antiretroviral Therapy (HAART)
   d) The use of nonoxynol-9 as a spermicide
3. The majority of new AIDS cases appear in which population?
   a) Men who have sex with men
   b) Women
   c) Racial and ethnic minorities
   d) Young people aged 15–25
4. List two opportunistic infections that may lead to a diagnosis of AIDS.
5. Name at least two ways that HIV transmission can be prevented.
6. Why is surveillance data important?
7. Of the 40,000 new HIV infections that occur each year in the United States, roughly how many are estimated to be from people who are unaware that they are HIV+?
   a) One-quarter
   b) One-third
   c) One-half
   d) Two-thirds

ANSWERS

1. **D.** Over 25 million people have died since the beginning of the AIDS epidemic; that figure is larger than the population of Cuba, Greece, Venezuela, North Korea, Uganda, or Saudi Arabia.
2. **C.** Highly Active Antiretroviral Therapy (HAART)—a combination of three antiretroviral medications—became the new standard of HIV care in 1996 and led to the first decrease in new diagnoses the following year.
3. **C.** Although men who have sex with men remain the largest exposure group in the United States, racial and ethnic minorities (especially people of color) represent the majority of new HIV infections, the majority of Americans living with HIV/AIDS, and the majority of deaths among HIV+ people in the United States.
4. There are 26 opportunistic diseases associated with AIDS, including pneumonia, *Kaposi's sarcoma* (a cancer), invasive cervical cancer, and pulmonary tubercu-

losis (tuberculosis of the lungs). A full list of opportunistic infections appears in chapter 2.

5. HIV transmission can be prevented by proper condom use (by males or females); by drug therapy for pregnant women who are HIV+; and by testing blood supplies for HIV. (More prevention techniques will be discussed in Part 2 of this book.)
6. Surveillance (the ongoing, systematic collection, analysis, interpretation, and sharing of health data) is important because it helps predict how much a disease will affect a specific population. This is particularly important in the case of HIV/AIDS, as the populations who most need prevention interventions continue to shift.
7. **D.** Of the 40,000 new HIV infections that occur each year in the United States, 27,000 are estimated to be from people who are unaware that they are HIV+.

WEB RESOURCES

History of Scientific Discovery and HIV/AIDS

In Their Own Words: NIH Researchers Recall the Early Years of AIDS (NIH)

http://aidshistory.nih.gov/

The National Institutes of Health (NIH) launched this Web site to commemorate the 20th anniversary of the first publication about AIDS ("Pneumocystis Pneumonia—Los Angeles," by Michael Gottlieb et al., *Morbidity and Mortality Weekly Report, 30* (June 5, 1981: 250–252). This Web site features compelling stories told through interviews of physicians, scientists, nurses, and administrators involved in AIDS research at NIH. The voices of some of them can be heard in audio clips, in which they discuss their first encounters with AIDS patients, the discovery of HIV, the search for treatments, and other aspects of AIDS treatment and research. In addition to the oral history transcripts and brief biographies, the site features a 1981–1988 timeline of key events in AIDS history, focused mainly on NIH and other federal agencies, as well as document and image archives. The document archive includes selected press releases, articles authored by Dr. Harden, as well as copies of the AIDS Memorandum, which was a fast-track way to circulate unpublished observations and data among NIH AIDS researchers in the early 1980s.

HIV/AIDS Surveillance and Statistics

Global and U.S. HIV/AIDS Surveillance and Statistics (HIV Insite—University of California, San Francisco)

http://hivinsite.ucsf.edu/InSite?page=li-12-01

Comprehensive list of links to global and U.S. HIV/AIDS surveillance and statistics.

Links to global research data include:

- **HIV InSite: Countries and Regions**
  http://www.hivinsite.com/InSite.jsp?page=kb-01&doc=cr-00-00

Global, regional, and country-level information on HIV/AIDS, including statistics, key indicators, maps, reports, and links.

- **Joint United Nations Programme on HIV/AIDS (UNAIDS): Epidemiology http://www.unaids.org/en/HIV_data/Epidemiology/default.asp**

Includes global and country reports on the state of the pandemic, and archives of documents on estimates, projections, surveillance, and reporting.

- **World Health Organization (WHO): Epidemiological Fact Sheets http://www.who.int/hiv/pub/epidemiology/pubfacts/en/**

Compilations of the available serological and behavioral data in a country.

- **WHO: Global Atlas of Infectious Disease http://www.who.int/globalatlas/**

Standardized data and statistics for infectious diseases at country, regional, and global levels. Resource includes interactive database and mapping interface.

- **UNAIDS/WHO: Facts and Figures on International HIV/AIDS Prevalence and Incidence http://www.who.int/hiv/facts/en/**

A listing of UNAIDS and WHO reports and resources on prevalence and incidence of HIV/AIDS around the world.

Links to national (U.S.) research data include:

- **Centers for Disease Control and Prevention: HIV/AIDS Surveillance Report http://www.cdc.gov/hiv/topics/surveillance/resources/reports/index.htm**

Links to the most current U.S. HIV/AIDS surveillance data published annually.

- **Centers for Disease Control and Prevention: Statistics and Trends in HIV and AIDS in the United States http://www.cdc.gov/hiv/topics/surveillance/basic.htm**

Includes basic statistics and links to slide sets (pdf and PowerPoint) that display visual summaries of U.S. HIV/AIDS trends and statistics.

- **Kaiser Family Foundation: State Health Facts Online http://www.statehealthfacts.kff.org/**

Contains the latest state-level data on demographics, health, and health policy, including HIV/AIDS, health coverage, access, financing, and state legislation.

RECOMMENDED READING

The HIV/AIDS Epidemic's History of Scientific Discovery

The Emergence of AIDS: The Impact on Immunology, Microbiology, and Public Health

Searching for the cause of AIDS led to dozens of discoveries that would otherwise have been delayed for years, particularly those related to the human immune system. These chapters, in *The Emergence of AIDS: The Impact on Immunology, Microbiology, and Public Health,* review the scientific discoveries, advances in laboratory techniques, and innovations in collaborative research between epidemiologists, clinicians, and scientists that have come out of the quest for understanding HIV/AIDS.

Kanki, P. J., & Essex, M. E. (2000). The past and future of HIV. In K. H. Mayer & H. F. Pizer (Eds.), *The emergence of AIDS: The impact on immunology, microbiology, and public health.* Washington, DC: American Public Health Association.

Laurence, J. (2000). The virus versus the immune system. In K. H. Mayer & H. F. Pizer (Eds.), *The emergence of AIDS: The impact on immunology, microbiology, and public health.* Washington, DC: American Public Health Association.

Mayer, K. (2000). How infectious is infectious? In K. H. Mayer & H. F. Pizer (Eds.), *The emergence of AIDS: The impact on immunology, microbiology, and public health.* Washington, DC: American Public Health Association.

DeGruttola, V. (2000). The response of quantitative scientists to challenges posed by the AIDS epidemic. In K. H. Mayer & H. F. Pizer (Eds.), *The emergence of AIDS: The impact on immunology, microbiology, and public health.* Washington, DC: American Public Health Association.

HIV/AIDS Epidemiology

Epidemiology of HIV/AIDS in the United States (Osmond, 2003)

Summarizes the history of HIV/AIDS surveillance and reviews the methods and results of the efforts to understand the prevalence and incidence of HIV/AIDS in the United States.

Available online at http://www.hivinsite.com/InSite.jsp?page=kb-01&doc=kb-01-03

Current Worldwide HIV/AIDS Statistics: AIDS Epidemic Update (UNAIDS)

This report, published annually in December by WHO and UNAIDS, contains up-to-date information and statistics about the global pandemic.

Available online at http://www.unaids.org/en/HIV_data/Epidemiology/default.asp

Current U.S. HIV/AIDS Statistics: HIV/AIDS Surveillance Report (CDC)

This report, published annually by the Centers for Disease Control, contains up-to-date information and statistics about the epidemic in the United States.

Available online at http://www.cdc.gov/hiv/topics/surveillance/resources/reports/index.htm

Second-Generation HIV Surveillance: Better Data for Decision-Making (WHO, 2004)

Rehle, T., Lazzari, S., Dallabetta, G., & Asamoah-Odei, E. (2004). Second-generation HIV surveillance: Better data for decision-making. Bulletin of the World Health Organization, *82(2):121–127.*

This paper explains the benefits of using second-generation surveillance systems in providing comprehensive, cost-effective, and appropriate response to HIV/AIDS control programs. Second-generation systems focus on improving and expanding existing surveillance methods and combine them in ways that have the greatest explanatory power. The authors emphasize improvements in the current surveillance methodologies, and discuss in detail crucial issues such as the validity of HIV prevalence data measured in pregnant women and linking HIV surveillance and behavioral data collection.

Methods and Tools for HIV/AIDS Estimates and Projections (Ward, Walker, & Ghys, 2004)

Ward, H., Walker, N., & Ghys, P. D. (Eds.). (2004). Methods and tools for HIV/AIDS estimates and projections. Sexually Transmitted Infections, 80*(Suppl 1).*

The August 2004 supplement to the journal *Sexually Transmitted Infections* presents seven articles that describe some of the tools generated by researchers to assist with HIV surveillance systems.

Principles of Epidemiology

U.S. Department of Health and Human Services. (1998). CDC principles of epidemiology *(2nd ed.). Atlanta, GA: Centers for Disease Control and Prevention.*

Principles of Epidemiology is an excellent introductory text and is used extensively by public health agencies to train personnel in epidemiology. It is a publication of the Centers for Disease Control and Prevention, the primary federal agency involved in HIV/AIDS surveillance.

POWERPOINT SLIDES

(Note: A full-color version of these slides, with graphics, is also available on the CD-ROM.)

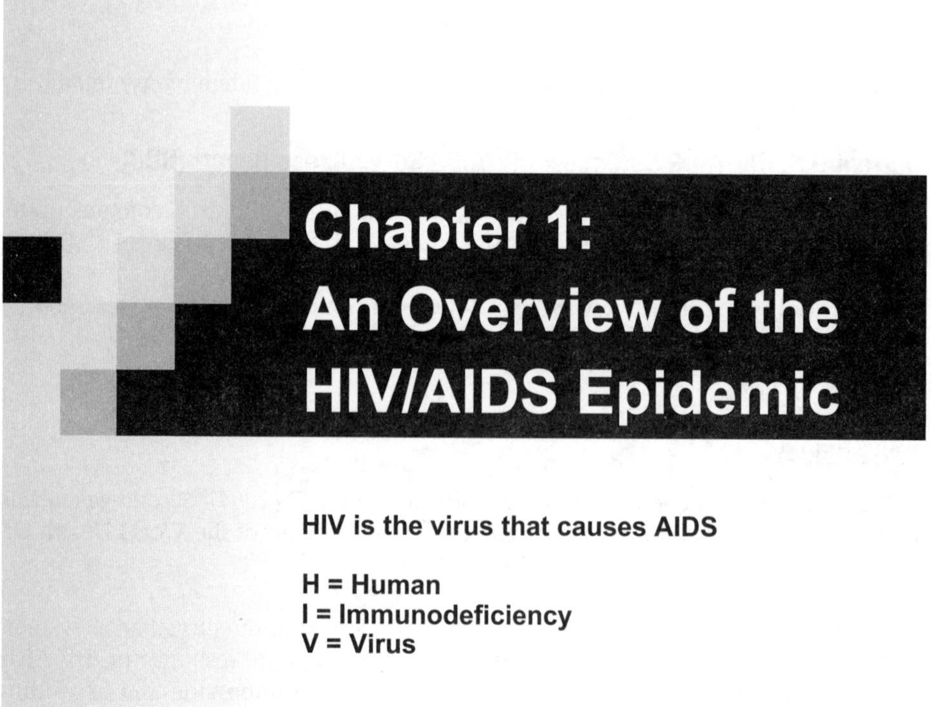

An Epidemic Emerges...

- 1980–1983: After being known as Gay-Related Immune Deficiency (GRID), the syndrome is renamed acquired immune deficiency syndrome (AIDS).
- 1984–1985: The first test (ELISA) to detect HIV antibodies is approved in the United States.
- 1986–1989: A drug called azidothymidine (AZT) slows down HIV's attack on the immune system.
- 1990–1993: CDC revises its definition of AIDS cases to be more inclusive of women and injection drug users.

An Epidemic Emerges...(continued)

- 1994–1996: Highly Active Antiretroviral Therapy (HAART) becomes the new standard of HIV care.
- 1997–1999: Number of American AIDS deaths drops 47% from the previous year.
- 2000–2003: The UN General Assembly on the AIDS epidemic passes a resolution declaring AIDS a global catastrophe.
- 2004–present: Drug therapy is found to reduce the spread of HIV from mother to child.

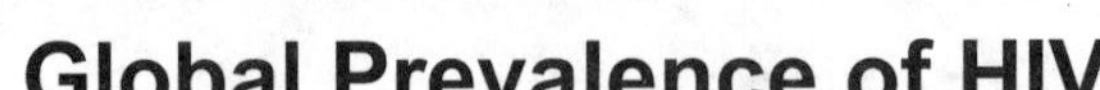

Global Prevalence of HIV

HIV Prevalence and Incidence by Region
(Henry J. Kaiser Foundation, 2006)

Region	Total No. (%) Living With HIV/AIDS, end of 2006	Newly Infected in 2006	Adult (aged 15-49) Prevalence Rate, 2006
Global Total	**39.5 million (100%)**	**4.3 million**	**1.0%**
Sub-Saharan Africa	24.7 million (62.5%)	2.8 million	5.9%
South/South-East Asia	7.8 million (19.7%)	860,000	0.6%
Eastern Europe/Central Asia	1.7 million (4.3%)	270,000	0.9%
Latin America	1.7 million (4.3%)	140,000	0.5%
North America	1.4 million (3.5%)	43,000	0.8%
East Asia	750,000 (1.9%)	100,000	0.1%
Western/Central Europe	740,000 (1.9%)	22,000	0.3%
Middle East/North Africa	460,000 (1.2%)	68,000	0.2%
Caribbean	250,000 (0.6%)	27,000	1.2%
Oceania	81,000 (0.2%)	7,100	0.4%

Reported Cases of U.S. HIV Infection

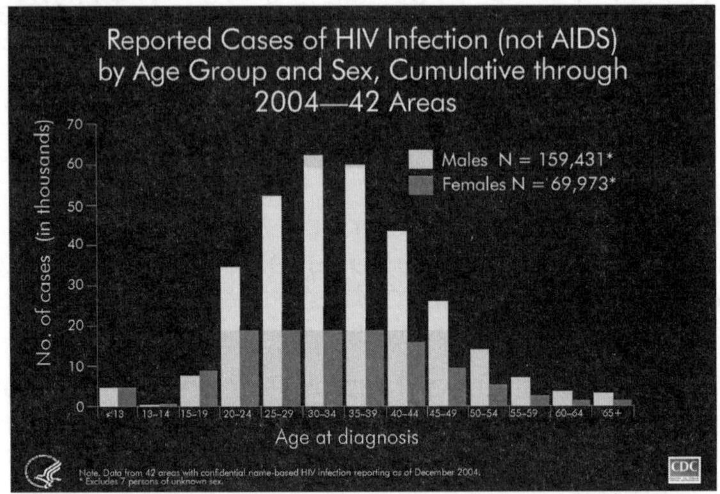

U.S. AIDS Cases, Deaths, and Overall Prevalence

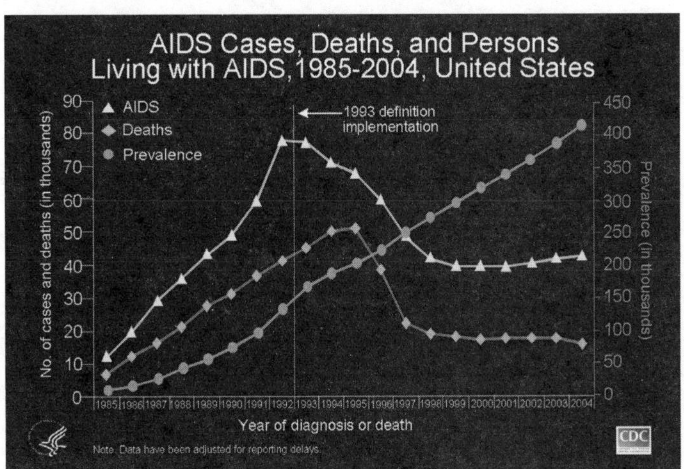

Deaths due to HIV Disease by U.S. Region

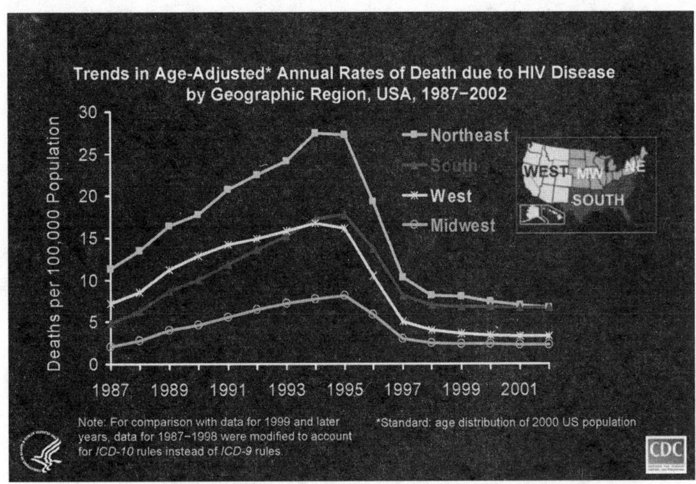

U.S. AIDS Prevalence by Race and Ethnicity

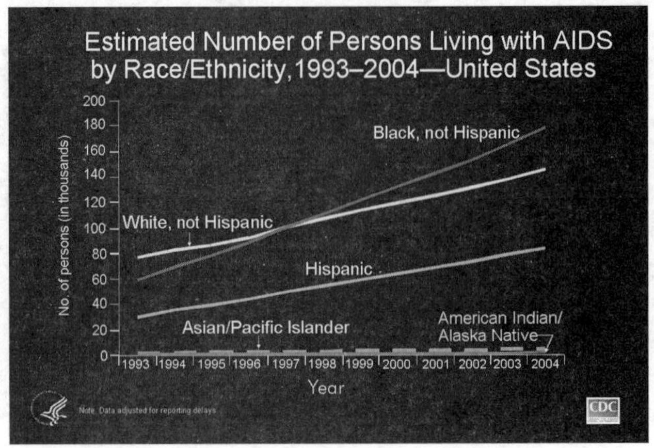

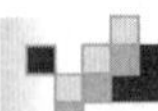

U.S. AIDS Prevalence by Gender

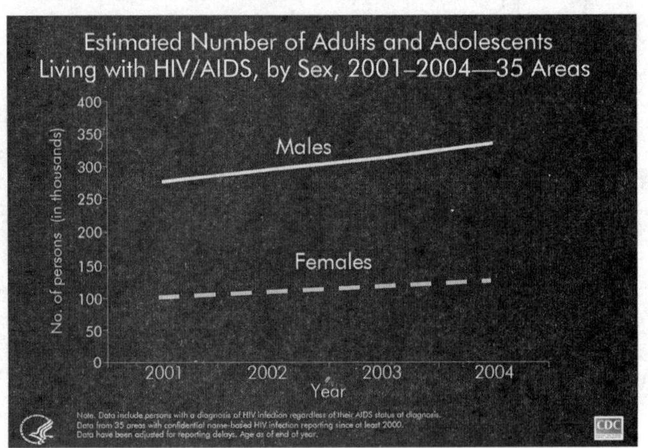

Learning Objectives

- Explain the structure and components of an HIV particle
- Describe the process by which an HIV infection occurs
- Describe what happens in the human body after HIV infects cells
- Compare and contrast the available HIV tests and describe the benefits of testing
- List and describe the stages and symptoms of HIV disease

Key Terms

acute HIV syndrome
antibodies
asymptomatic period
CD4+ cell
clinical latency
DNA
lentivirus
lymphatic system
lymphocyte
primary infection
protease
protease inhibitor
replication
retrovirus
reverse transcriptase
RNA
seroconversion
T-cell
viral envelope
virus
white blood cell

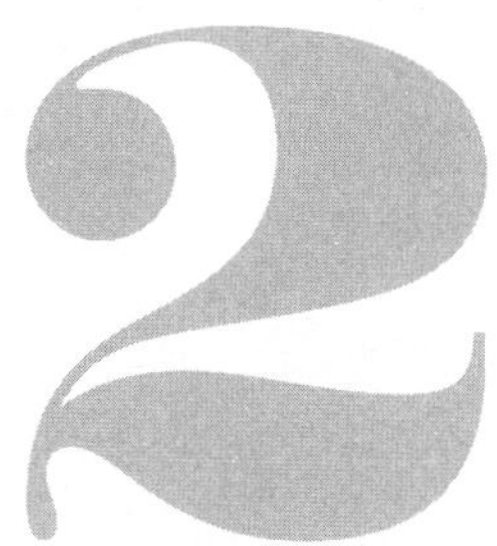

The Path From HIV to AIDS

HIV is a virus that infects the human body and causes AIDS. This chapter examines how this tiny virus wreaks so much havoc on the human body. Beginning at the molecular and cellular levels, this chapter first explores what HIV is made of and how it infects people. It then describes the stages and symptoms of HIV/AIDS.

THE BIOLOGY OF HIV

HIV Is a Virus

A *virus* is a tiny, relatively simple, nonliving organism, usually made up of little more than a few strands of genetic material and a protein shell. HIV is a virus that infects only people and creates a deficiency in their body's immune system. Viruses similar to HIV affect other animals, including cats and monkeys.

HIV belongs to a family of viruses called *retroviruses*. Unlike regular viruses, which have DNA (*deoxyribonucleic acid*) as their genetic material, retroviruses have RNA (*ribonucleic acid*). Retroviruses also contain an enzyme called *reverse transcriptase*, which allows the retrovirus's genetic material to infiltrate the host cell's genetic material.

In comparison to cells and DNA-based viruses, retroviruses *mutate* (that is, their genetic code changes) very quickly. When retroviruses mutate, a person's immune system often does not have any defenses against the new version of the retrovirus. As a result, retroviruses are more difficult to fight than normal viruses.

Retroviruses mutate more quickly than other viruses because of the way they reproduce. When cells and normal viruses reproduce, an enzyme "proofreads" the resulting genetic material. The equivalent enzyme involved in retroviruses' reproduction—reverse transcriptase—does not proofread the new genes. As a result, new batches of retroviruses are more likely to have errors, or mutations, in their genes than are new batches of normal viruses or cells.

The human immunodeficiency virus also belongs to a subfamily of retroviruses called *lentiviruses*. *Lenti* means "slow," so lentiviruses are retroviruses that have a long delay between the time they initially infect a person and the time the person starts to show serious symptoms (Anderson, 1992).

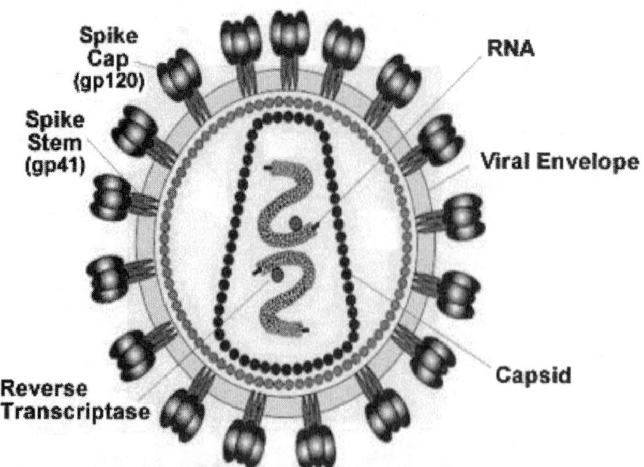

Figure 2-1 The structure of HIV-1 (National Institute of Allergy and Infectious Diseases [NIAID], 2001).

Although deadly to the cell it attacks, a single human immunodeficiency virus (or viral particle) is much smaller than a human cell. HIV particles have a diameter of only 1/10,000 of a millimeter, compared to the average human cell size of 1/10 of a millimeter. HIV particles are also much simpler in structure than human cells. HIV particles are made up of the following parts:

The Viral Envelope

The outer coat of the virus is called the *viral envelope*, or *lipid membrane* (see Figure 2.1). The viral envelope is composed of two layers of fat molecules (*lipid* means fat). HIV gets its outer envelope from its host. As newly formed HIV particles break through a host cell's surface in a process called "budding," they wrap themselves in fat molecules from the host's outer membrane (NIAID, 2001).

The Spikes

The complex proteins that protrude through the surface of the viral envelope are frequently called *spikes* (see Figure 2.1). These spikes are HIV's landing gear, attaching the virus to a host cell and fusing the two together. Each HIV has average of 72 spikes. Each spike is made up of two parts: a stem and a cap. Each stem consists of three glycoprotein 41 (gp41) molecules, and each cap consists of three glycoprotein 120 (gp120) molecules. The stem anchors the spike to the viral envelope.

The Capsid and Its Contents: RNA and Reverse Transcriptase

Within the envelope of a mature HIV particle is a bullet-shaped core, called the *capsid* (see Figure 2.1). The capsid surrounds two single strands of HIV's single-strand genetic material, ribonucleic acid (RNA). Each strand of RNA has a copy of the virus's genes. These genes contain the information that HIV uses to make new virus particles. HIV has only nine genes, in comparison to human cells, which have an average of 30,000–50,000 genes. The capsid also houses two molecules of HIV *reverse transcriptase*. Reverse transcriptase is an enzyme that allows the HIV's RNA to change into double-strand *deoxyribonucleic acid (DNA)*, so that it can pass into the host cell's nucleus, commandeer the host cell, and begin reproducing itself (NIAID, 2001).

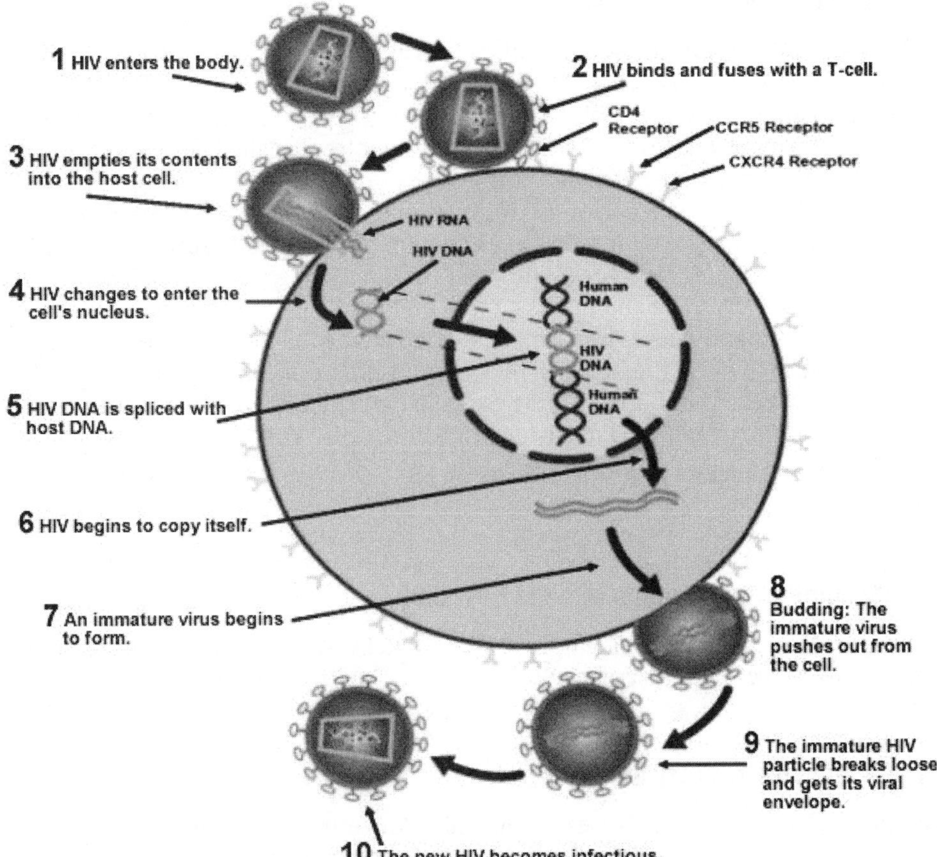

Figure 2-2 How HIV infects cells (Adapted from AIDS InfoNet, 2005).

HOW HIV MAKES PEOPLE SICK

How HIV Infects People

Figure 2.2 provides an overview of how HIV infects cells in the body. Further description of each step in the process is provided below.

1. HIV Enters the Body

HIV particles are transmitted to uninfected people through infected body fluids. These body fluids include blood and blood products, semen, vaginal fluid, other body fluids that contain blood, breast milk, brain and spinal cord fluid, fluid around bone joints, and amniotic fluid. HIV-infected body fluids may enter an uninfected person's body in the following ways:

- Having sex (anal, vaginal, or oral) with an infected person.
- Being stuck or pierced with a needle or other sharp object that contains HIV-infected blood.
- Receiving a blood transfusion or organ or tissue transplant from an infected person.
- HIV-positive women can pass HIV to their children during pregnancy, childbirth, or breast-feeding.

(For further details on HIV transmission, see chapter 4.)

2. HIV Binds and Fuses With a T-cell

Although HIV can infect a number of cells in the body, its main targets are *T-cells* called *CD4 positive* (*CD4+*) cells. T-cells are a kind of *lymphocyte*, which are cells that the body's immune system makes to fight off dangerous invaders. (Lymphocytes are also called *white blood cells*.) T-cells that have a molecule called cluster designation 4 (CD4) on their surfaces are called *CD4+*, or *T-helper* cells.

To bind to the CD4+ cell, a gp120 molecule (on the cap of an HIV spike) first forms a chemical bond with a CD4 molecule on the host cell's surface. The gp120 then binds to another receptor on the host cell's surface, such as CCR5 or CXCR4. The HIV's viral envelope and the host cell's membrane then fuse together, allowing the virus's RNA and *reverse transcriptase*—an enzyme that enables the virus's RNA genetic code—to enter the host cell and turn into DNA once inside the host cell.

The newest class of anti-HIV drugs, called *entry inhibitors*, works by keeping these spikes from binding and fusing with host cells. There is currently just one entry inhibitor available, called *enfuvirtide* (or T-20), but researchers are studying many others.

3. HIV Empties Its Contents Into the Host Cell

These contents include two identical strands of RNA—HIV's genetic code—and two molecules of reverse transcriptase.

4. HIV Changes to Enter the Cell's Nucleus

In most cells and normal viruses, DNA is first converted to RNA in a process called transcription, and then RNA is turned into proteins in a process called *translation*. HIV is different, though, and must first convert its RNA into DNA in a process called *reverse transcription*. For reverse transcription, HIV uses an enzyme called reverse transcriptase. The viral DNA that results from reverse transcription contains the instructions HIV needs to hijack a T-cell's genetic machinery and begin reproducing itself (GlaxoSmithKline, 2001; Pieribone, 2002/2003).

Most of the drugs approved in the United States for the treatment of people infected with HIV work by interfering with reverse transcriptase's ability to change RNA to DNA. These drugs, called *reverse transcriptase inhibitors*, include *zidovudine* (AZT), *nevirapine*, *abacavir*, and *efavirenz*, among others.

5. HIV DNA Is Spliced With Host DNA

The newly reverse-transcripted HIV DNA next makes its way into the host cell's nucleus. Once inside, the HIV DNA is spliced into strands of the host cell DNA, with the aid of an enzyme called integrase. This process is called *integration* (GlaxoSmithKline, 2001; Pieribone, 2002/2003). HIV DNA that enters the host cell DNA is called a provirus.

6. HIV Begins to Copy Itself

In order to survive, the HIV provirus must eventually make copies of itself, or *replicate*. The first step to replication is a process called *transcription*. Transcription creates a strand of genetic code that the host cell's protein-making machinery can read. During transcription, an enzyme called *RNA polymerase* separates the two halves of DNA like a zipper. One of these halves is then used to create a new strand of RNA, called *messenger RNA* (mRNA). HIV's genes may actually accelerate the process of transcription.

During translation, structures in the host cell's *cytoplasm* (that is, the area outside of the nucleus) use the mRNA as a blueprint for building proteins and enzymes. These new proteins and enzymes will eventually come together to make a new HIV particle.

7. An Immature Virus Begins to Form

The newly made proteins and enzymes, as well as viral RNA, come together just inside the host cell's membrane.

8. The Immature Virus Is Pushed out from the Cell

Proteins, enzymes, and RNA form a bud on the surface of the host cell membrane.

9. The Immature HIV Particle Breaks Loose and Gets Its Viral Envelope

As the viral particle pushes off from the infected host cell, it takes proteins from the host cell membrane that will become the particle's viral envelope. The core of the virus is still immature, so the HIV particle cannot yet infect other host cells.

10. The New HIV Becomes Infectious

At the last step of the viral cycle, a viral enzyme called *protease* cuts the long chains of proteins and enzymes in the HIV particle core, making the particle infectious. At this stage, the HIV particle is said to be mature. Drugs called *protease inhibitors* interfere with this last step of the viral life cycle (GlaxoSmithKline, 2001; Pieribone, 2002/2003).

What Happens After HIV Infects Cells

Once HIV enters the body and infects cells, it replicates rapidly and spreads widely. Two to four weeks after exposure, most HIV-infected people suffer flu-like symptoms, as their immune systems fight off the initial HIV infection. This first immune response may dramatically reduce HIV levels (Pieribone, 2002/2003). As a result, the number of CD4+ T-cells in a person's body may rebound after the first, acute infection, and may even approach their original levels. The HIV+ person may then remain free of HIV-related symptoms for years.

Meanwhile, however, the virus continues replicating in the organs and tissues of the body's *lymphatic system*, which is the system that produces, stores, and carries white blood cells to fight infection and disease. These organs and tissues include the spleen, thymus, lymph nodes, tonsils, and adenoids. Although HIV is confined to a person's lymphatic system, it may not be readily detectable in his or her blood. Ultimately, however, the accumulated HIV overwhelms the person's system, and large quantities of virus enter the bloodstream.

HIV infections usually progress to AIDS for two reasons. First, HIV evades the immune system, so the body stops fighting it. Although the body's immune system is usually strong enough to wipe out most viral infections, it cannot fight what it cannot detect. HIV is a fast-mutating virus, meaning that its genetic makeup changes often. HIV's many mutations make some of its particles invisible to the body's immune system, so that they continue to replicate and cause damage. HIV can also hide in the genetic material of an infected cell, where it is shielded from the immune system's radar.

A second reason that HIV infection generally leads to AIDS is that HIV damages the immune system, so the body cannot fight it. During HIV's life cycle,

CD4+ cells change, get damaged, and die. Over time, there are not enough healthy CD4+ cells to defend the body. Without enough CD4+ cells, the body's immune system is unable to defend itself against many infections. When the immune system is so weak that it can no longer defend against opportunistic infections, a person is said to have AIDS.

HOW HIV IS DIAGNOSED

As the body fights a particular virus, it creates substances called *antibodies* to that virus. Tests for HIV usually measure the presence of HIV antibodies in blood, urine, or saliva, rather than testing for the presence of HIV itself (San Francisco AIDS Foundation [SFAF], 1998a).

Main Types of HIV Tests

Several different types of tests can be used to detect HIV. An *Enzyme-Linked Immunosorbent Assay* (*ELISA*) determines HIV antibodies' presence in blood or oral fluids. When people show HIV antibodies on two or more ELISA tests, they undergo an independent, highly specific supplemental test (most commonly, the *Western Blot test*) to confirm ELISA's results (Constantine, n.d.). Western Blot is a highly specific supplemental test that detects the presence of HIV antibodies in the blood. The Western Blot test is less sensitive than the ELISA test, but it hardly ever gives a false positive result; therefore, it is used for confirming the ELISA test. *Rapid serum HIV antibody tests, saliva- and urine-based antibody tests,* and *home HIV antibody testing kits* also have been approved by the Food and Drug Administration (FDA) and are commercially available (Constantine, n.d.). The rapid HIV tests can be administered outside of a traditional laboratory setting and processed in as little as 20 minutes (CDC, 2003b, 2006). *HIV RNA tests* are being used in research and health care settings to diagnose HIV infection very early after exposure, before antibodies are even formed (Constantine, n.d.). These tests look for bits of HIV RNA in the blood.

Benefits of HIV Testing

Most HIV testing is combined with HIV risk-reduction counseling and referral for HIV/AIDS treatment (if the person does have HIV). This combination of services is known as *Counseling, Testing, and Referral* (*CTR*) or *Voluntary Counseling and Testing* (*VCT*). VCT offers a number of benefits. When HIV-infected people learn of their positive serostatus, they may be able to obtain treatment that can reduce their symptoms and increase their life spans. HIV testing and accompanying counseling also can help people who are HIV+ to initiate behavioral changes that will reduce the likelihood of their being infected with a different strain of HIV or of passing HIV to others. HIV-negative (HIV− or *seronegative for HIV*) people also can benefit from testing and accompanying counseling, as it may provide them with the knowledge and motivation that they need to take further steps to protect themselves from HIV. In addition, the data that researchers and health care workers obtain from analyzing HIV test results help them to learn more about HIV epidemiology and mechanisms of transmission (CDC, 2001, 2006; Family Health International [FHI], 2003; Roland, Fine, & Volberding, 1998).

Increasing Access to HIV Testing

In the United States, many HIV-infected individuals do not get tested until late in their infections. As a result, they are already very sick when they first learn that they are HIV+. For example, of the 104,780 people who tested positive for HIV between 1994 and 1999, 41% developed AIDS within 1 year (CDC, 2003a).

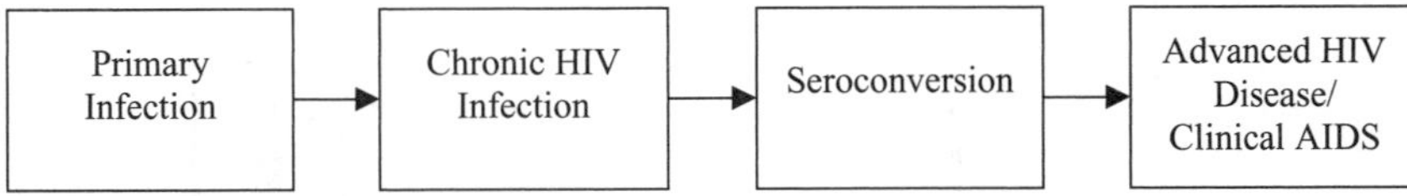

Figure 2-3 Stages of HIV disease.

Additionally, people who are tested do not necessarily return to learn their test results. For example, in 2000, of an estimated 2 million CDC-funded HIV tests, approximately 18,000 tests represented new HIV diagnoses. During 2000, of persons with positive tests for HIV, 31% did not return for their test results (CDC, 2003a).

An emphasis on expanding access to testing and on providing prevention and care services for people infected with HIV can reduce new infections and lead to reductions in HIV-associated morbidity and mortality (CDC, 2003a). Strategies to increase access to HIV testing include making HIV testing a routine part of medical care and implementing new models for diagnosing HIV infections outside medical settings (CDC, 2003b).

THE STAGES AND SYMPTOMS OF HIV DISEASE

Primary Infection

Primary infection (see Figure 2.3) is the first stage of HIV disease, when the virus first establishes itself in the body (SFAF, 1998b). Two to four weeks after exposure to the virus, up to 87% of HIV-infected persons suffer flu-like symptoms for a few days, indicating that their immune systems are fighting the newly introduced HIV. This sickness is called *acute HIV syndrome*. Its symptoms include fevers, chills, headaches, night sweats, rashes, and swollen glands (Bradley Hare, 2004).

It usually takes 6–12 weeks for the immune system to produce antibodies to fight against the virus. This means that a newly infected person's blood may not test positive for HIV antibodies in the first few weeks after becoming infected. Newly infected people are highly contagious during primary infection because large quantities of HIV are present in their genital fluids (NIAID, 2003).

Seroconversion

Seroconversion describes the time when the body begins producing antibodies to the virus. Most people develop antibodies within 3 months. Some people can take up to 6 months to develop antibodies to HIV (SFAF, 1998b).

Chronic HIV Infection

After the primary infection, HIV+ people then enter an *asymptomatic period* (that is, a time when they have no signs or symptoms of HIV disease). This period is also called *clinical latency*. The duration of people's asymptomatic period varies and is influenced by their overall health and immune system functioning.

How long does it take people to develop symptoms of HIV disease? There is no one answer to this question. Some people may develop symptoms within a few months, whereas others may not have symptoms for more than 10 years. The average person with HIV is symptom-free for 7–8 years. It is important to know that even in the absence of clinical symptoms, the virus continues to multiply, infecting and killing immune system cells.

Although HIV+ people have no symptoms during the asymptomatic period, their immune systems are already suffering from the presence of HIV. The virus is actively multiplying, and infecting and killing immune system cells (NIAID, 2003). HIV levels (often referred to as *plasma viral load*) in an HIV+ person's body correlate with the rate of CD4+ cell decline (immune system decline). This means that the

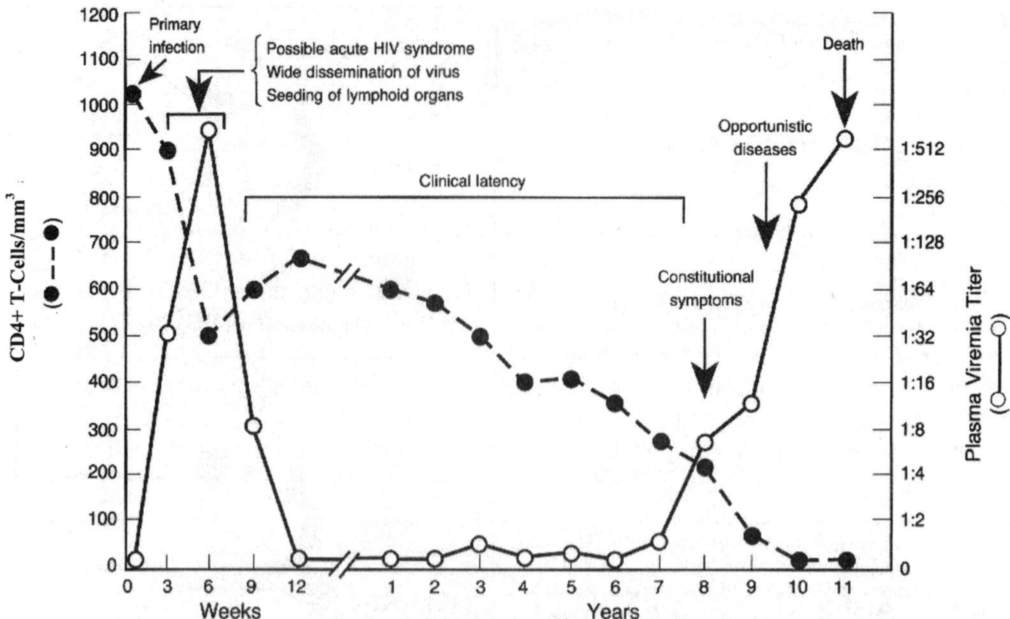

Figure 2-4 CD4+ T-cell count, viral load, and HIV disease symptoms over time (Pantaleo, Graziosi, & Fauci, 1993).

more HIV a person has in his or her body—that is, the higher the plasma viral load—the lower his or her number of health-protecting CD4+ cells. The more HIV levels increase and numbers of CD4+ cells decrease, the faster a person progresses to AIDS and death (NIAID, 2003).

Figure 2.4 shows how the average person with HIV CD4+ cell counts and plasma viral loads (*plasma viremia tier* in the figure) changes over the course of HIV disease. As the graph shows, the natural progression of HIV disease (in the absence of treatment) is fairly slow, taking a decade or more from infection to the development of severe immunodeficiency (NIAID, 2003). The line with closed circles on it charts the average number of CD4+ cells (the immune cells that HIV attacks) in HIV+ people's bodies over time. The line with open circles on it charts the average number of HIV particles in HIV+ people's bodies over time.

Once the immune system is damaged, many people will begin to experience some relatively mild symptoms that are not specific to HIV infection. These include:

- Swollen lymph nodes that persist for more than 3 months
- Fatigue
- Weight loss
- Frequent fevers and sweats
- Persistent or frequent yeast infections (oral and vaginal)
- Persistent skin rashes and flaky skin
- Pelvic inflammatory disease (PID) that does not respond to treatment
- Short-term memory loss
- Frequent or severe herpes infections with oral, genital, or anal sores
- Shingles (a nerve disease)

Advanced HIV Disease/Clinical AIDS

During advanced HIV disease, people experience more severe symptoms, including opportunistic infections and diseases. The Centers for Disease Control and Prevention (CDC) has two different sets of criteria for diagnosing AIDS. Both sets of criteria include the presence of HIV or HIV antibodies in the blood or tissues. The first set of criteria also specifies the number of CD4+ cells that signals AIDS. The second set of criteria specifies the 26 opportunistic infections that signal AIDS.

CDC AIDS Criteria: Set 1:

An HIV infection, confirmed by testing, plus a CD4+ T-cell count of less than 200 per cubic millimeter of blood (healthy adults usually have CD4+ T-cell counts of 1,000 or more) (CDC, 1992).

CDC AIDS Criteria: Set 2:

An HIV infection, confirmed by testing, plus one of 25 clinical conditions, primarily *opportunistic infections* that do not normally affect healthy people, including certain kinds of pneumonia or tuberculosis (CDC, 2003a). In people with AIDS, these infections are often severe and sometimes fatal because of the people's compromised immune systems.

Opportunistic infections are infections that are caused by bacteria, funguses, or viruses that may not cause illness in people with normal immune systems. In HIV+ people, however, these disease-causing agents take the "opportunity" to flourish in the absence of a normal immune response.

Opportunistic infections that—accompanied by a positive HIV test—indicate AIDS include:

- Pneumocystis Carinii Pneumonia (PCP) (a kind of pneumonia)
- Kaposi's sarcoma (KS) (a kind of cancer)
- HIV wasting syndrome (extreme weight loss)
- Non-Hodgkin's lymphoma (a kind of cancer)
- *Cryptococcosis*, extrapulmonary (a parasitic infection, initially of the lungs, that spreads to other parts of the body)
- *HIV encephalopathy* (AIDS Dementia)
- *Mycobacterium Avium Complex Intracellulare* (MAC/MAI) (a bacterial infection of the lungs)
- *Candidiasis* (yeast infection) of the trachea, bronchi, or lungs
- *Candidiasis* (yeast infection) of the esophagus
- *Cryptosporidiosis*, chronic intestinal (a bacterial infection of the intestines)
- *Cytomegalovirus* (CMV) disease (CMV is a virus in the herpes family)
- Tuberculosis (outside of the lungs)
- Herpes simplex virus infection
- *Progressive Multifocal Leukoencephalopathy* (PML) (a nervous system disorder)
- Primary lymphoma of the brain (a cancer)
- *Toxoplasmosis* of the brain (a parasitic infection of the brain)
- *Histoplasmosis* (a fungal infection that often scars the lungs)
- *Isoporiasis*, chronic intestinal (protozoa, or tiny parasitic organisms, that infect the intestines)
- *Coccidioidomycosis* (a fungal infection)
- *Salmonella septicemia* (a bacterial infection)
- Bacterial infections, recurrent
- *Lymphoid interstitial pneumonia/pulmonary lymphoid hyperplasia* (lung diseases)
- Pulmonary tuberculosis
- Recurrent bacterial pneumonia (two or more episodes in 1 year)
- Invasive cervical cancer

Symptoms of opportunistic infections common in people with AIDS include:

- Coughing and shortness of breath
- Seizures and lack of coordination
- Difficult or painful swallowing
- Mental symptoms such as confusion and forgetfulness
- Severe and persistent diarrhea
- Fever
- Vision loss
- Nausea, abdominal cramps, and vomiting
- Weight loss and extreme fatigue
- Severe headaches
- Coma

The Course of HIV Disease in Children

In the early stages of HIV disease, children who are HIV+ may be frequently ill or have slowed growth. At later stages, children get opportunistic infections just as adults do, although the incidence of various infections differs between children and adults. In particular, serious bacterial infections occur more frequently in HIV+ children than in HIV+ adults. These children also suffer from the usual childhood infections, such as pink eye (*conjunctivitis*), more severely than uninfected children do. These infections can lead to seizures, pneumonia, diarrhea, dehydration, and other critical health problems (NIAID, 2004).

REFERENCES

AIDS InfoNet. (2005, April 20). *Fact sheet 106, HIV life cycle.* Retrieved December 7, 2006, from http://www.aidsinfonet.org/factsheet˙detail.php?fsnumber=106

Anderson, K. (Ed.). (1992). *Mosby's medical, nursing, and allied health dictionary* (4th ed.). St. Louis, MO: Mosby-Year Book.

Bradley Hare, C. (2004). Clinical overview of HIV disease. In L. Pieperl, S. Coffey, O. Bacon, & P. Volberding (Eds.), *HIV InSite knowledge base.* San Francisco: Center for HIV Information, University of California, San Francisco.

Centers for Disease Control and Prevention (CDC). (1992). 1993 revised classification system for HIV infection and expanded surveillance case definition for AIDS among adolescents and adults. *Morbidity and Mortality Weekly Report, 41*(RR-17), 1–19.

Centers for Disease Control and Prevention (CDC). (2001). Revised guidelines for HIV counseling, testing, and referral. *Morbidity and Mortality Weekly Report, 50*(RR19), 1–58.

Centers for Disease Control and Prevention (CDC). (2003a). Advancing HIV prevention: New strategies for a changing epidemic—United States, 2003. *Morbidity and Mortality Weekly Report, 52*(15), 329–332.

Centers for Disease Control and Prevention (CDC). (2003b). *Advancing HIV prevention: The science behind the new initiative.* Atlanta, GA: CDC.

Centers for Disease Control and Prevention (CDC). (2006). Evolution of HIV/AIDS prevention programs—United States, 1981–2006. *Morbidity and Mortality Weekly Report, 55*(21), 597–603.

Constantine, N. (2003). HIV antibody assays. In L. Pieperl, S. Coffey, O. Bacon, & P. Volberding (Eds.), *HIV InSite knowledge base.* San Francisco: Center for HIV Information, University of California, San Francisco.

Family Health International (FHI). (2003). *Fact sheet: Voluntary counseling and testing for HIV.* Arlington, VA: FHI.

GlaxoSmithKline. (2001). *How HIV works in your body.* Research Triangle Park, NC: GlaxoSmith-Kline.

National Institute of Allergy and Infectious Diseases (NIAID). (2001). *How HIV causes AIDS.* Bethesda, MD: NIAID.

National Institute of Allergy and Infectious Diseases (NIAID). (2003). *HIV infection and AIDS: An overview.* Bethesda, MD: NIAID.

National Institute of Allergy and Infectious Diseases (NIAID). (2004). *HIV infection in infants and children.* Bethesda, MD: NIAID.

Pantaleo, G., Graziosi, C., & Fauci, A.S. (1993). The immunopathogenesis of human immunodeficiency virus infection. *New England Journal of Medicine, 328*(5), 327–335.

Pieribone, D. (2002/2003, Winter). The HIV life cycle. *ACRIA Update, 12*(1).

Roland, M. E., Fine, R., & Volberding, P. (1998). HIV antibody testing: Indications and interpretations. In L. Pieperl, S. Coffey, O. Bacon, & P. Volberding (Eds.), *HIV InSite knowledge base*. San Francisco: Center for HIV Information, University of California, San Francisco.

San Francisco AIDS Foundation (SFAF). (1998a). HIV testing. In *AIDS 101: Guide to HIV basics*. Retrieved January 15, 2004, from http://www.sfaf.org/aids101/hiv_testing.html

San Francisco AIDS Foundation (SFAF). (1998b). The stages of HIV disease. In *AIDS 101: Guide to HIV basics*. Retrieved January 15, 2004, from http://www.sfaf.org/aids101/hiv_disease.html

Instructor Resources

LEARNING ACTIVITIES

ACTIVITY

Assignment: Trends in HIV/AIDS Incidence: The Difference Between Men and Women

Objective: To understand how HIV/AIDS incidence differs between men and women.

According to the Centers for Disease Control and Prevention, the annual rate of death among HIV infected individuals in the United States peaked in 1995, decreased through 1997, and leveled after 1998.

Write a detailed report summarizing the HIV/AIDS surveillance data on HIV/AIDS mortality rates in the United States from the 1980s through today, and respond to the following questions:

- What accounted for the decline in the number of new AIDS cases for both men and women in the United States in the late 1990s?
- Why has the number of newly reported AIDS cases in American women not declined at the same rate as that of men?

(NOTE: Good sources of U.S. HIV/AIDS-related surveillance data and reports are the Centers for Disease Control and Prevention [http://www.cdc.gov] and the Henry J. Kaiser Family Foundation [http://www.kff.org].)

DISCUSSION QUESTIONS

1. HIV is classified as a retrovirus. How are retroviruses different from regular viruses, and what implication does this have for HIV disease progression and treatment?
2. HIV is also classified as a lentivirus. How are lentiviruses different than other retroviruses, and what implication does this have for HIV disease testing, diagnosis, and progression?
3. In the United States, many HIV-infected individuals do not get tested until late in their infections. Why? What can be done to change this?

QUIZ

1. True or False: A virus can reproduce itself on its own.
2. How quickly can an HIV test detect HIV antibodies in the blood?

a) 1–3 months after exposure, although in some cases it may take up to 6 months
b) 3–6 months after exposure, although in some cases it may take up to a year
c) 1–2 months after exposure, although in some cases it may take up to a month

3. Lentiviruses differ from other retroviruses in which way?
a) They mutate quickly.
b) They have a long delay period between infection and the display of symptoms.
c) They have DNA (rather than RNA) as their genetic material.
d) They have RNA (rather than DNA) as their genetic material.

4. Match the HIV component with its function:

a) viral envelope	1) Anchors the spike to the viral envelope.
b) spikes	2) Surrounds the RNA.
c) stem	3) Coats the virus.
d) capsid	4) Attaches the virus to a host cell.
e) reverse transcriptase	5) Allows the RNA to change into DNA.

5. List any five bodily fluids through which HIV particles may be transmitted.

6. List four ways through which HIV-infected body fluids may enter an uninfected person's body.

7. Which is *not* a main target of HIV?
a) CD4+ cells
b) T-cells
c) lymphocytes
d) red blood cells

8. Match the process with its definition:

a) translation	1) The process in which DNA is converted to RNA
b) transcription	2) The process in which RNA is coverted to proteins
c) replication	3) The process in which HIV DNA is spliced into host cell DNA
d) integration	4) The process in which HIV makes copies of itself

9. After infection, HIV replicates in the organs and tissues of the________ system.
a) reproductive
b) digestive
c) lymphatic
d) circulatory

10. Match the stage of HIV disease with the correct description.

a) Primary infection	1) During this stage, the body shows no signs of HIV disease.
b) Acute HIV syndrome	2) During this stage, the body begins producing antibodies to the virus.
c) Seroconversion	3) Opportunistic infections and diseases may appear during this stage.
d) Clinical latency	4) The stage in which the virus first establishes itself in the body.
e) Advanced HIV disease	5) Flu-like symptoms may occur during this stage.

11. The average person with HIV is symptom-free for how long?
a) 1–2 years
b) 3–5 years
c) 7–8 years
d) more than 10 years

12. True or False: HIV lies dormant during the asymptomatic period.

ANSWERS

1. **False.** Unlike living things, viruses cannot reproduce on their own. Instead, viruses make copies of themselves by hijacking the cells of a living being (the virus's host), infiltrating the host cells' genetic material, and converting the host cells' activities to virus production. In this process, viruses often damage the host's cells and cause disease in the host.
2. **A.** Tests can usually detect HIV antibodies in the blood 1–3 months after exposure to the virus, although in some cases it may take up to 6 months.
3. **B.** *Lenti* means "slow," so lentiviruses are retroviruses that have a long delay between the time they initially infect a person and the time the person starts to show serious symptoms.
4. **A–3; B–4; C–1; D–2; E–5.** The outer coat of the virus is called the viral envelope, or lipid membrane. The spikes are HIV's landing gear, attaching the virus to a host cell and fusing the two together. Each spike is made up of two parts: a stem and a cap. The stem anchors the spike to the viral envelope. Within the envelope of a mature HIV particle is a bullet-shaped core, called the capsid, which surrounds two single strands of HIV's genetic material, ribonucleic acid (RNA). The capsid also houses two molecules of HIV reverse transcriptase, an enzyme that allows the HIV's RNA to change into double-strand deoxyribonucleic acid (DNA).
5. Body fluids include blood and blood products, semen, vaginal fluid, other body fluids that contain blood, breast milk, brain and spinal cord fluid, fluid around bone joints, and amniotic fluid.
6. HIV-infected body fluids may enter the body through sex (anal, vaginal, or oral) with an infected person; being stuck or pierced with a needle or other sharp object that contains HIV-infected blood; receiving a blood transfusion or organ or tissue transplant from an infected person; and during pregnancy, childbirth, or breast-feeding.
7. **D.** Although HIV can infect a number of cells in the body, its main targets are *T-cells* called *CD4 positive* (*CD4+*) cells. T-cells are a kind of *lymphocyte*, which are cells that the body's immune system makes to fight off dangerous invaders. (Lymphocytes are also called *white blood cells.*) T-cells that have a molecule called cluster designation 4 (CD4) on their surfaces are called *CD4+*, or *T-helper* cells.
8. **A–2; B–1; C–4; D–3.** In most cells and normal viruses, DNA is first converted to RNA in a process called transcription, and then RNA is turned into proteins in a process called translation. Once inside a host cell, the HIV DNA is spliced into strands of the host cell DNA, with the aid of an enzyme called integrase. This process is called integration. In order to survive, the HIV provirus must eventually make copies of itself, or replicate.
9. **C.** The virus replicates in the organs and tissues of the lymphatic system, which is the system that produces, stores, and carries white blood cells to fight infection and disease.
10. **A–4; B–5; C–2; D–1; E–3.** Primary infection is the first stage of HIV disease, when the virus first establishes itself in the body. Two to four weeks after exposure to the virus, up to 87% of HIV-infected persons suffer flu-like symptoms for a few days, indicating that their immune systems are fighting the newly introduced HIV. This sickness is called acute HIV syndrome. Seroconversion describes the time when the body begins producing antibodies to the virus.

Most people develop antibodies within 3 to 6 months. After the primary infection, HIV+ people then enter an asymptomatic period (that is, a time when they have no signs or symptoms of HIV disease). This period is also called clinical latency. During advanced HIV disease, people experience more severe symptoms, including opportunistic infections and diseases.

11. **C.** The average person with HIV is symptom-free for 7–8 years. However, some people may develop symptoms within a few months, whereas others may not have symptoms for more than 10 years.

12. **False.** Although people have no signs or symptoms of HIV disease during the asymptomatic period, the virus is multiplying and their immune systems are already suffering from the presence of HIV.

WEB RESOURCES

Virology and Natural History of HIV/AIDS

CELLS alive!

http://www.cellsalive.com

CELLS alive! allows teachers and students to use their images in class reports, projects, homework, lectures, and handouts. The site includes interactive and animated diagrams of the intracellular events of HIV infection, from initial attachment of a viral particle to a CD4+ cell, through budding of new viruses from that cell. (http://www.cellsalive.com/hiv0.htm)

How AIDS Works (How Stuff Works 2001)

http://health.howstuffworks.com/aids3.htm

An easy-to-understand description of the mechanics of HIV with animated drawings.

Surviving AIDS. See HIV in Action (Nova Online 1999)

http://www.pbs.org/wgbh/nova/aids/action.html

In a series of sophisticated color graphics and QuickTime movies, AIDS researcher José Assouline guides viewers through the life cycle of HIV. From “Surviving AIDS” (http://www.pbs.org/wgbh/nova/aids/), a PBS/Nova Online production.

AIDS: The War Within—Illustrations of the AIDS Life Cycle (1996)

http://www.msichicago.org/exhibit/AIDS/AIDSlc1.html

Images from an exhibit from the Museum of Science and Industry in Chicago on the AIDS life cycle.

RECOMMENDED READING

Virology of HIV/AIDS

How HIV Works in Your Body (GlaxoSmithKline)

A cartoon approach to understanding what HIV does once it is inside the body. Available online at http://www.thebody.com/glaxo/howhiv/howhiv.html

The Link Between HIV and AIDS

Fact Sheet: The Evidence That HIV Causes AIDS (NIAID 2003)

This document summarizes the abundant evidence that HIV causes AIDS. Questions and answers at the end of this document address the specific claims of those who assert that HIV is not the cause of AIDS.
Available online at http://www.niaid.nih.gov/factsheets/evidhiv.htm

The Origin of HIV

The Past and Future of HIV

Kanki, P. J., & Essex, M. E. (2000). The past and future of HIV. In K. H. Mayer & H. F. Pizer (Eds.), The emergence of AIDS: The impact on immunology, microbiology, and public health. *Washington, DC: American Public Health Association.*
This chapter discusses the origins of HIV, reviewing the findings from the first 20 years of epidemiological research.

POWERPOINT SLIDES

(Note: A full-color version of these slides, with graphics, is also available on the CD-ROM.)

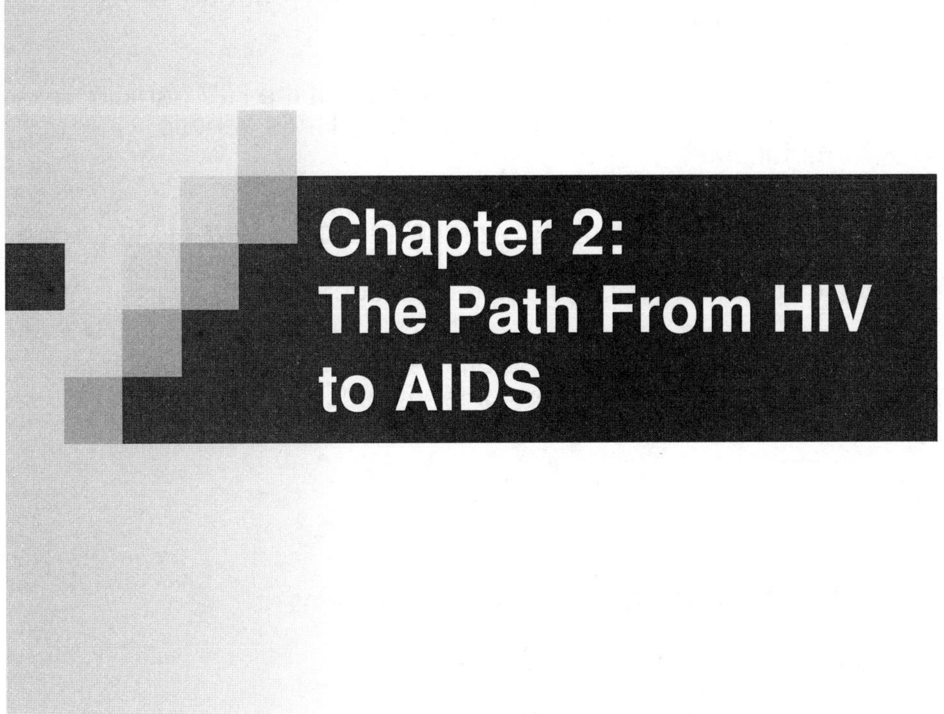

The Path From HIV to AIDS

- HIV infects only humans and creates a deficiency in the body's immune system.
- HIV belongs to a family of viruses called retroviruses.
- Because retroviruses mutate very quickly, a person's immune system does not have any defenses against the new version of the virus.
- HIV is also a lentivirus—a virus with a long delay between initial infection and the time the infected person starts to show symptoms.

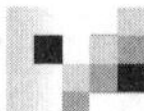

The Structure of HIV-1

- The Spikes: The complex proteins that protrude through the surface of the viral envelope
- The Capsid: The bullet-shaped core of the HIV particle that surrounds two single strands of HIV's genetic material
- Reverse Transcriptase: An enzyme that allows HIV's RNA to change into DNA so that it can pass into the host cell's nucleus to begin reproducing itself
- The Viral Envelope: The outer coat of the virus, which is composed of two layers of fat molecules

What Happens After HIV Infects Cells?

- Once in the body, HIV replicates and spreads widely.
- 2-4 weeks after exposure, most HIV-infected people suffer flu-like symptoms, as their immune systems fight off the initial HIV infection.
- This immune response may dramatically reduce HIV levels.
- The number of CD4+ T-cells in a person's body may rebound after the first, acute infection.

What Happens After HIV Infects Cells? (continued)

- The HIV+ person may remain free of HIV-related symptoms for years.
- The virus continues replicating.
- Eventually, HIV overwhelms the person's system and large quantities of the virus enter the bloodstream.

Why Do HIV Infections Almost Always Progress to AIDS?

1. HIV *eludes* the immune system so that the body stops fighting it.
   - HIV's many mutations make some of its particles invisible to the body's immune system.

2. HIV *damages* the immune system, so that the body can't fight it.
   - Not enough healthy CD4+ cells to defend the body against infections
   - When the immune system can no longer defend against opportunistic infections, the person has AIDS.

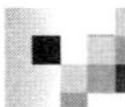

Diagnosing HIV Infection

Main Types of HIV Tests:

- **ELISA** (Enzyme-Linked Immunosorbent Assay): determines if HIV antibodies are present in blood or oral fluids
- **Western Blot:** A highly specific test that is used for confirming the ELISA test
- **Rapid HIV tests:** Saliva-based, urine-based, and home HIV antibody testing kits
- **HIV RNA tests:** Diagnose HIV infection very early, before antibodies are even formed

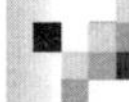

The Stages and Symptoms of HIV Disease

Primary Infection:

- The first stage of HIV disease
- 2 to 4 weeks after infection, 87% of HIV+ persons suffer flu-like symptoms (acute HIV syndrome).
- It usually takes 6 to 12 weeks for the immune system to develop antibodies to fight the virus.
- Seroconversion is the time when the body begins producing antibodies; this can take up to 6 months.

The Stages and Symptoms of HIV Disease (continued)

Chronic HIV Infection:

- Asymptomatic Period
  - Also called clinical latency—person has no signs or symptoms of HIV disease
  - Although individual shows no symptoms, the virus is actively multiplying and infecting and killing immune system cells.
- Immune System Decline
  - The more HIV a person has (the plasma viral load), the lower the number of CD4+ cells; ultimately results in the rapid decline of immune system

Immune System Decline

Mild, Non-specific Symptoms

- When the immune system is damaged, people begin to experience mild symptoms:
  - Swollen lymph nodes
  - Fatigue
  - Weight loss
  - Frequent fevers and sweats
  - Frequent or persistent yeast infections
  - Persistent skin rashes
  - Shingles

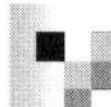

Advanced HIV Disease/ Clinical AIDS

- The CDC has two sets of criteria for diagnosing AIDS:
  - **Set 1**—An HIV infection, confirmed by testing, plus a CD4+ T-cell count of less than 200 per cubic millimeter of blood
  - **Set 2**—An HIV infection, confirmed by testing, plus one of 26 clinical conditions, primarily opportunistic infections that do not normally affect healthy people

Opportunistic Infections

Infections that do not cause disease in people with healthy immune systems, for example:

- Pneumocystis Carinii Pneumonia (PCP) (a kind of pneumonia)
- Kaposi's sarcoma (KS) (a kind of cancer)
- HIV wasting syndrome (extreme weight loss)
- Non-Hodgkin's lymphoma (a kind of cancer)
- HIV encephalopathy (AIDS dementia)
- Candidiasis (yeast infection) of the trachea, bronchi, or lungs
- Candidiasis (yeast infection) of the esophagus

Learning Objectives

- Understand the biological risk factors for HIV
- Understand the psychological risk factors for HIV
- Understand how demographic characteristics impact risk of HIV
- Understand the social and cultural risk factors for HIV
- Understand the behavioral risk factors for HIV

Key Terms

gender
sex
SES
STD
STI
transgender
viral load

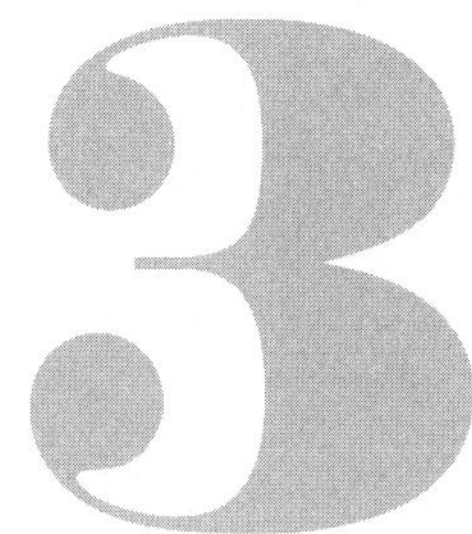

Correlates of HIV Infection Risk

Unlike many viruses, which pass easily through air, water, food, and casual contact, HIV usually requires risky behaviors such as unprotected sex and drug use for its transmission. People do not perform these risky behaviors in a vacuum. Instead, biological, psychological, demographic, and sociocultural factors affect both the likelihood and the consequences of these behaviors, as is represented in Figure 3-1 (Farmer, Walton, & Furin, 2000).

This chapter discusses these key factors and the specific behaviors that can lead to HIV transmission. (Part 4 will discuss demographic and sociocultural issues surrounding HIV/AIDS in greater detail.)

"People become infected with HIV through behaviors, not because of membership in any particular 'high risk group.' HIV infection is a possibility for almost everyone, but an inevitability for almost no one" (Smith, 1998).

BIOLOGICAL RISK FACTORS FOR HIV

There are a number of biological factors (both one's own and those of one's partners) that make it easier or more difficult for HIV to enter the body. These include the presence of other *sexually transmitted diseases/infections* (*STDs/STIs*), tissue/membrane vulnerability, and viral load (Kalichman, 1998).

Certain characteristics of people's bodies can increase their chances of getting or giving HIV when they engage in risky behaviors.

Presence of STIs/STDs

HIV is transmitted through bodily fluids. Biological features that increase an uninfected person's contact with infected body fluids will therefore increase that person's chances of contracting HIV. One such biological feature is having an STI/STD. In some studies, HIV– people with an STI/STD who had sex with an HIV+ partner were 10 times more likely to contract HIV than were HIV– people without an STI/STD (Chin, 2000; Osmond, 1998).

HIV+ people with STIs/STDs are also more likely to shed blood and pus through genital sores, exposing their sexual partners to HIV. In addition, the immune systems of people with STIs/STDs sends immune cells to these genital lesions to fight the infections there. These immune cells—CD4+ cells—are precisely the cells to which HIV attaches. As a result, HIV+ men and women with STIs/STDs have many more HIV particles concentrated near their penis and vagina, respectively,

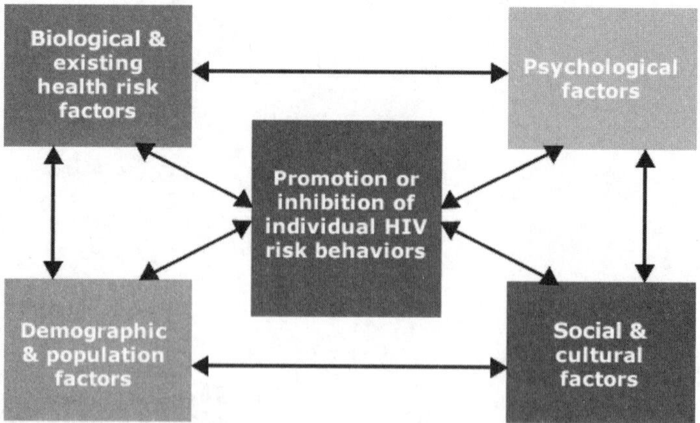

Figure 3-1 Interaction of risk factors for getting and giving HIV/AIDS.

than do HIV+ people without STIs/STDs. For example, one study found that HIV+ men with STIs/STDs had 8 times more HIV in their semen than did HIV+ men without STIs/STDs (Osmond, 1998). Thus, having an STI/STD not only makes HIV+ people more likely to expose uninfected partners to their bodily fluids, but it also makes their bodily fluids more contagious (i.e., the fluids have more HIV particles).

Tissue/Membrane Vulnerability

Uninfected people may contract HIV through the cuts and scrapes that they get during vaginal intercourse. In particular, the biological risk of contracting HIV through heterosexual sex is greater for women than for men for several reasons (Volberding, 1998; World Health Organization [WHO], 2000):

- The vagina has larger areas of exposed, sensitive skin than does the penis.
- HIV has an easier time surviving in the vagina than it does on the surface of the penis.
- There are more copies of the virus in a man's semen than there are in the fluids of a woman's vagina.

HIV also can be transmitted through the tearing that can take place during anal intercourse. In heterosexual anal intercourse, the biological risk of contracting HIV is greater for women than for men, as the anus has larger areas of exposed, sensitive skin than does the penis, and as the HIV is more likely to survive in the anus than on the penis (Volberding, 1998; WHO, 2000). Moreover, men's semen has more HIV than do women's anal fluids (WHO, 2000). For these same reasons, among men who have sex with men, receptive anal sex (i.e., being the person who is penetrated by a partner) is riskier than insertive anal sex (Osmond, 2004) (see also chapter 4).

Additionally, studies have shown that uncircumcised men are at greater risk of acquiring HIV and of transmitting HIV than circumcised men. The inner surface of the penis's foreskin contains cells called *Langerhans cells* that are particularly receptive to the HIV virus. These cells are likely to be the primary point of viral entry into the penis of an uncircumcised man. Male circumcision, which surgically removes all or part of the foreskin, has been shown in several studies to reduce the likelihood that an HIV– man will become infected with HIV or that an HIV+ man will transmit HIV. Male circumcision also can reduce the likelihood of infection with other STIs/STDs that can facilitate HIV transmission (CDC, 2006; Szabo & Short, 2000).

Viral Load

Higher concentrations of HIV are found in blood and semen during the first stage of HIV disease—that is, during acute infection—than at later stages of disease (Lawn, Butera, & Folks, 2001). The more HIV a person has (i.e., the greater a person's viral load), the more likely he or she is to transmit HIV to someone else.

PSYCHOLOGICAL RISK FACTORS FOR HIV

How people think and feel influences how they behave. Psychological factors such as risk perception, personality characteristics, and psychological states influence the extent to which people engage in high- or low-risk behaviors.

Beliefs and Risk Perception

People who think AIDS is a relatively minor or remote problem are less likely to take steps to reduce their risks. In addition, people who think that they personally are not at risk for HIV infection are more likely to engage in risky behaviors.

Personality Characteristics

Other psychological risk factors, including personality characteristics such as low self-esteem, *narcissism* (preoccupation with the self), antisocial personality, *impulsivity* (the tendency to do things suddenly, without thinking about the consequences of the action), tendency to take risks, and tendency to seek out new sensations, are related to sexual risk-taking behavior (Kalichman, 1998). Coping responses also influence risk behavior. To escape from or relieve stress, some people engage in high-risk sexual behaviors or use drugs and alcohol, just as others may smoke cigarettes or overeat (Kalichman, 1998; Zierler & Krieger, 2000).

Psychological States

Psychological disorders such as personality disorders, self-destructive behaviors, hypersexuality, sexual obsession and compulsivity, depression, anxiety, and negative states of mind (e.g., anger, pessimism) are associated with high-risk sexual behaviors with multiple partners (Kalichman, 1998). They are also associated with drug abuse and addiction, which can increase HIV risk through needle sharing and through decreasing the likelihood that safer-sex practices (such as condom use) will be used.

DEMOGRAPHIC RISK FACTORS FOR HIV

HIV risk behaviors are shaped in the context of demographic factors, such as gender, ethnicity, and age. By influencing social networks, these factors also make it more or less likely that individuals who engage in risky sexual or IV drug-using behavior will come into contact with persons who are themselves HIV+.

Gender

A person's biological *sex* classification (e.g., male, female), as well as the social roles associated with each biological sex category (*gender*), influence other risk factors for HIV/AIDS. For example, as was described earlier, men are less likely to acquire HIV from heterosexual sex than women are because of the anatomy of the penis. However, cultural norms in many parts of the world encourage men to demonstrate their masculinity by having multiple sex partners and coercing women into having sex, which increase HIV risk. Men are also much more likely than women to abuse alcohol and drugs, which increases the likelihood that they will engage in unprotected sex. Men are also more likely than women to inject drugs, exposing them to the risk of HIV from infected needles and syringes (Denny, 1995; UNAIDS, 2000).

Women, in contrast, are at greater risk of HIV infection from heterosexual sex than men are because of the anatomy of the vagina. In addition, although cultural norms in many parts of the world dictate that women should remain virgins until married (a factor that can reduce HIV risk), the denial of access to HIV education and the belief that women should be sexually passive decrease the likelihood that women will take steps to protect themselves from HIV in sexual relationships. Limited access to education, jobs, and bank credit makes women dependent on male partners, or forces them to exchange sex for food or money, thus limiting the control they have over the timing and circumstances of sex. Women are also far more likely than men to experience gender-based violence, including physical and sexual abuse, in which they do not have control over the safety of sexual intercourse (Clements-Nolle, Marx, Guzman, & Katz, 2001; Türmen, 2003; UNAIDS, 1999, 2005). (Further discussion of how gender norms and other sociocultural factors influence HIV/AIDS risk among both men and women may be found in Part 4.)

Transgender persons constitute a third (and often ignored) gender group that is at risk for HIV infection. Transgender individuals have a persistent and distressing discomfort with their birth sex, and so may assume the roles of the other sex through such behaviors as dress, occupation, or even sex-reassignment surgery (Denny, 1995). Although there is limited information about rates of HIV among transgender people, rates are expected to be higher because transgender people have more behavioral risks factors, such as substance abuse and use of shared needles (for injection of hormones as well as for illicit drugs), irregular condom use, and multiple sex partners (Department of Health and Human Services, n.d.; Quinn, 1993).

Sexual Orientation

In the United States, the group with the highest rates of HIV infection is men who have sex with men (CDC, 2005). This group has the highest rates of unprotected anal sex, which is a behavioral risk factor for HIV transmission. In most regions of the world, however, the group with the highest rates of HIV is people who have heterosexual intercourse.

Race/Ethnicity

In the United States, racial and ethnic minorities represent the majority of new AIDS cases, the majority of Americans living with AIDS, and the majority of deaths among persons with AIDS. Most of the excess risk of HIV/AIDS among African Americans and Latinos reflects discrimination in employment, housing, earning power, and educational opportunity (UNAIDS, 2002). This discrimination relegates minorities to lower levels of socioeconomic status (SES) and to the risks associated with lower SES, such as limited access to health care (see also later). Studies have shown that HIV-infected African Americans and Latinos are more likely than HIV-infected Whites to be uninsured, to have not received antiretroviral drugs, and to lack transportation for visiting doctors ("Multiple Barriers," 2003).

Socioeconomic Status (SES)

Socioeconomic status indicates people's standing in society and is usually measured by their income, occupation, or educational attainment. Socioeconomic status is one of the most powerful predictors of sickness and health. People with lower SES are more likely to contract and transmit HIV/AIDS, perhaps because they have less knowledge about HIV/AIDS, are surrounded by people who are more likely to have HIV/AIDS, and are more likely to use drugs and practice unsafe sex to escape from stress (Feldman, 1990; United Nations Population Fund [UNFPA], 2003). HIV+ people with lower SES also die sooner than HIV+ people with higher SES because of their lack of access to medical care, the high cost of antiretroviral drugs, and their lowered immunity from other illnesses.

Age

About half of all new HIV infections worldwide, or approximately 6,000 per day, occur among young people aged 15–24, the majority of them young women (UNFPA, 2003). In the United States, for men who have sex with men, younger age is strongly correlated with increased high-risk sexual behaviors (e.g., unprotected anal sex) (Kalichman, 1998). Despite high levels of sexual activity, young people often do not know the basic facts about HIV/AIDS, which puts them at risk (Feinstein & Prentice, 2001).

Place of Residence

HIV disease morbidity and mortality vary greatly within and between nations. In the United States, for example, annual number of deaths by HIV is highest in the South. U.S. regional differences continue to increase over time (CDC, n.d.). Limited access to health care, poverty, and discrimination all contribute to these regional disparities. Persons who live in geographic areas in which HIV is more prevalent and who engage in risky sex or drug use behaviors are more likely to do so with persons who are HIV+.

SOCIAL AND CULTURAL RISK FACTORS FOR HIV

HIV risk behaviors are shaped by a variety of social and cultural factors that influence one-on-one and small group interactions, as well as at the laws, policies, and practices of institutions. Examples of these social and cultural factors include the gender norms that were discussed earlier, inequality, discrimination, stigma, and violence. These factors, which are discussed in greater detail in Part 4, interact with biological, psychological, demographic, and behavioral factors to shape people's risks of giving and getting HIV.

BEHAVIORAL RISK FACTORS FOR HIV

HIV is transmitted through certain bodily fluids. Behaviors that increase a person's contact with the bodily fluids of others increase the likelihood of HIV transmission.

Unsafe Sexual Behaviors

Worldwide, unprotected sexual intercourse with an HIV-infected partner is the most common way of getting and giving HIV (Chin, 2000; Kalichman, 1998; NIAID, 2003). During sex, HIV can be transmitted through cuts and tears on the penis, vagina, or anus. Through these cuts and tears, infected blood, semen, vaginal fluids, and anal fluids may enter the uninfected person's body. Cuts and scrapes are more likely during anal sex, forced sex, dry sex, or when women are very young (because their cervixes are not fully developed and therefore more likely to rip or tear during intercourse).

Unsafe Drug Use Behaviors

Sharing injecting drug use paraphernalia, such as needles and syringes, increases the risk of HIV transmission and contraction because the paraphernalia are often tainted with blood. This risk is increased in areas where many drug users are also HIV+, as the chances that any given needle has infected blood on it are higher (Ostrow, 2000).

Mixing Sex and Drugs/Alcohol

Sex and drugs/alcohol interact in many ways to increase a person's risk of getting or giving HIV (Kalichman, 1998; Ostrow, 2000). When people use drugs or alcohol, their decision-making abilities, awareness of their surroundings and memories are altered, making them less likely to choose or remember to practice safer sex. In addition, use of these substances can increase sexual desire and enhance underlying personality characteristics, such as high sensation-seeking behavior and sexual compulsivity. Some people also may use drugs or alcohol to escape the awareness of sexual risk.

Drug use also can increase biological susceptibility to HIV transmission during sex by promoting local drying or irritation of vaginal or anal tissues, which can create tears and cuts through which HIV can enter the body. Cocaine and nitrite inhalants increase immune functioning, meaning that HIV becomes concentrated in bodily fluids and therefore easier to transmit. People who use drugs are also more likely to have STIs/STDs, which increase their risk for both contracting and transmitting HIV (Kalichman, 1998; Ostrow, 2000).

Not Taking Antiretroviral Drugs Properly

When taken on time and in the right dosages, antiretroviral drugs can decrease the amount of HIV in an HIV+ person's body. The less a person's viral load, the less likely he or she is to infect other people. However, when people do not take their antiretroviral drugs properly, they have more HIV in their systems, and are therefore more likely to infect other people through sexual transmission or through sharing needles. (For further discussion of antiretroviral therapy and its role in prevention of HIV transmission, see Part 3.)

REFERENCES

Centers for Disease Control and Prevention (CDC). (2005). *HIV/AIDS surveillance report, 2004.* Atlanta, GA: CDC.

Centers for Disease Control and Prevention (CDC). (2006). *Male circumcision and risk for HIV transmission: Implications for the United States.* Atlanta, GA: CDC.

Centers for Disease Control and Prevention (CDC). (n.d.). Trends in the percentage distribution of deaths due to HIV infection by geographic region, USA, 1987–1999. In *Mortality L285* [Slide series], slide 21. Atlanta, GA: CDC.

Chin, J. (Ed.). (2000). *Communicable diseases manual* (17th ed.). Washington, DC: American Public Health Association.

Clements-Nolle, K., Marx, R., Guzman, R., & Katz, M. (2001). HIV prevalence, risk behaviors, health care use, and mental health status of transgender persons: Implications for public health interventions. *American Journal of Public Health, 91*(6), 915–921.

Denny, D. (1995). *Transgendered youth at risk for exploitation, HIV, and hate crimes.* American Educational Gender Information Services, Inc.

Department of Health and Human Services (DHSS). (n.d.). *Fact sheet on AIDS and transgender persons.* Washington, DC: DHSS.

Farmer, P. E., Walton, D. A., & Furin, J. J. (2000). The changing face of AIDS: Implications for policy and practice. In K. H. Mayer & H. F. Pizer (Eds.), *The emergence of AIDS: The impact on immunology, microbiology, and public health* (pp. 139–161). Washington, DC: American Public Health Association.

Feinstein, N., & Prentice, B. (2001). *The UNAIDS gender and AIDS almanac.* Los Altos, CA: Sociometrics Corporation.

Feldman, D. A. (Ed.). (1990). *Culture and AIDS.* New York: Praeger.

Horn, T., & Sciola, A. (1998). Overview: Transmission and prevention. In R. A. Smith (Ed.), *The encyclopedia of AIDS: A social, political, cultural, and scientific record of the HIV epidemic.* Chicago: Fitzroy Dearborn.

Kalichman, S. C. (1998). *Preventing AIDS: A sourcebook for behavioral intervention.* Mahwah, NJ: Lawrence Erlbaum Associates.

Lawn, S. D., Butera, S. T., & Folks, T. M. (2001). Contribution of immune activation to the pathogenesis and transmission of human immunodeficiency virus type 1 infection. *Clinical Microbiology Review, 14*(4), 753–777.

Multiple barriers prevent minorities' early treatment, AIDS stigma, lack of transportation top list. (2003). *AIDS Alert, 18*(11), 137–138, 143.

National Institute of Allergy and Infectious Diseases (NIAID). (2003). *HIV infection and AIDS: An overview.* Bethesda, MD: NIAID.

Osmond, D. H. (1998). Sexual transmission of HIV. In L. Pieperl, S. Coffey, O. Bacon, & P. Volberding (Eds.), *HIV InSite knowledge base.* San Francisco: Center for HIV Information, University of California, San Francisco.

Ostrow, D. G. (2000). Sex and drugs and the virus. In K. H. Mayer & H. F. Pizer (Eds.), *The emergence of AIDS: The impact on immunology, microbiology, and public health* (pp. 63–76). Washington, DC: American Public Health Association.

Quinn, S. C. (1993). AIDS and the African American woman: The triple burden of race, class, and gender. *Health Education Quarterly, 20*(3), 305–320.

Szabo, R., & Short, R. V. (2000). How does male circumcision protect against HIV infection? *BMJ, 320,* 1592–1594.

Türmen, T. (2003). Gender and HIV/AIDS. *International Journal of Gynecology and Obstetrics, 82*(3), 411–418.

United Nations Population Fund (UNFPA). (2003). *State of world population 2003: Making 1 billion count: Investing in adolescents' health and rights.* New York: UNFPA.

United Nations Programme on HIV/AIDS (UNAIDS). (1999). Gender and HIV/AIDS: Taking stock of research and programmes. In *UNAIDS Best Practice Collection.* Geneva, Switzerland: UNAIDS.

United Nations Programme on HIV/AIDS (UNAIDS). (2000). *Men and AIDS: A gendered approach.* Geneva, Switzerland: UNAIDS.

United Nations Programme on HIV/AIDS (UNAIDS). (2002). *AIDS epidemic update: December 2002.* Geneva, Switzerland: UNAIDS.

United Nations Programme on HIV/AIDS (UNAIDS). (2005). *AIDS epidemic update: December 2005.* Geneva, Switzerland: UNAIDS.

Volberding, P. (Ed.). (1998). The most common opportunistic infections in women with HIV. *HIV Newsline, 4*(4).

World Health Organization (WHO). (2000). *Women and HIV/AIDS (Fact sheet no. 242).* Geneva, Switzerland: WHO.

Zierler, S., & Krieger, N. (2000). Social inequality and HIV infection in women. In K. H. Mayer & H. F. Pizer (Eds.), *The emergence of AIDS: The impact on immunology, microbiology, and public health* (pp. 76–97). Washington, DC: American Public Health Association.

Instructor Resources

LEARNING ACTIVITIES

ACTIVITY 1:

Group Activity: The Game
Developed by Donnovan Somera Yisrael and Carolyn Laub for the MidPeninsula YWCA, 1998. Used with permission.

Objective: To enable participants to see and critique the complex system of values and rules that regulate our sexual behavior.

Minimum Time: 45 minutes

View a detailed guide for this activity on the CD-ROM.

ACTIVITY 2:

Group Activity: Gender Role Play: What's Going On?
Adapted from Exercise 11 in Gender or Sex: Who Cares? Skills-building Resource Pack on Gender and Reproductive Health for Adolescents and Youth Workers (de Bruyn, 2001).

Objective: To guide participants through an analysis of situations involving gender norms, relationships, and sex, and to encourage them to think of ways to reduce possible risks.

Minimum Time: 30 minutes

View this activity at
www.genderandaids.org/modules.php?name=News&file=article&sid=173

ACTIVITY 3:

Assignment: The Face of HIV/AIDS

Objective: To understand how various regions or populations are affected by HIV/AIDS.

Pick a country or region of the world or an HIV/AIDS risk group.

Examples:

- sub-Saharan Africa
- Non-gay identifying African American men who have sex with men (i.e., men on the "down low")
- Migrant workers in the United States
- Injection drug-using women in U.S. cities
- Men and women in Jamaica

Write a two-page summary (using text and visuals) of the prevalence of HIV and AIDS, specific risk factors, and current HIV/AIDS prevention efforts in that country, region, or group.

DISCUSSION QUESTIONS

1. Why might low self-esteem be associated with a higher risk for HIV?
2. How do race/ethnicity and socioeconomic status (SES) impact HIV risk?
3. Which cultural norms increase men's risk of HIV? Which impact women's risk? Why?
4. How can alcohol and/or drug use increase risk of HIV?

QUIZ

1. The biological risk of contracting HIV through heterosexual sex is:
   a) Greater for men than women
   b) Greater for women than men
   c) Equal for men and women
   d) Unrelated to gender
2. At which stage of HIV disease is viral load highest?
   a) Primary infection
   b) Acute HIV syndrome
   c) Seroconversion
   d) Clinical latency
   e) Advanced HIV disease
3. True or False: In most regions of the world, the group with the highest rates of HIV is men who have sex with men.
4. Which factor is not a measurement of socioeconomic status (SES)?
   a) Income
   b) Gender
   c) Occupation
   d) Education level
5. How many new HIV infections per day occur among people aged 15–24?
   a) 1,000
   b) 3,000
   c) 6,000
   d) 9,000

ANSWERS

1. **B.** The biological risk of contracting HIV through heterosexual sex is greater for women than for men because the vagina has larger areas of exposed, sensitive skin than does the penis; HIV has an easier time surviving in the vagina than it does on the surface of the penis; and there are more copies of the virus in a man's semen than there are in the fluids of a woman's vagina.

2. **B.** Higher concentrations of HIV are found in the blood and semen during acute infection than during later stages of the disease.
3. **False.** Although men who have sex with men have the highest rates of HIV infection in the United States, in most regions of the world the group with the highest rates is those who have heterosexual intercourse.
4. **B.** SES is usually measured by income, occupation, or educational attainment.
5. **B.** About half of all new HIV infections worldwide, or approximately 6,000 per day, occur among young people aged 15–24.

RECOMMENDED READING

Biological Risk

Sexually Transmitted Infections and HIV/AIDS

Fleming, D. T., & Wasserheit, J. N. (1999). From epidemiological synergy to public health policy and practice: The contribution of other sexually transmitted diseases to sexual transmission of HIV infection. Sexually Transmitted Infections, *75(1):3–17.*

This article reviews the scientific data on the role of sexually transmitted diseases (STDs) in sexual transmission of HIV infection, and discusses the implications of these findings for HIV and STI/STD prevention policy and practice.

Behavioral Risk Factors

Sex and Drugs and the Virus

Ostrow, D. G. (2000). Sex and drugs and the virus. In K. H. Mayer & H. F. Pizer (Eds.), The emergence of AIDS: The impact on immunology, microbiology, and public health. *Washington, DC: American Public Health Association.*

In the early 1980s, the idea that drugs alone, apart from needle sharing, played a role in the transmission of HIV was not popularly accepted. Drug users and gay men were viewed as separate populations. Since then, nonintravenous "recreational" drug use has become well recognized as a significant factor in the homosexual transmission of HIV and other STDs. This chapter reviews the history of sex-drug research during the U.S. HIV/AIDS epidemic.

Psychological Risk Factors

Psychosocial Predictors of Risky Sexual Behaviors

Myers, H. F., Javanbakht, M., Martinez, M., & Obediah, S. (2003). Psychosocial predictors of risky sexual behaviors in African American men: Implications for prevention. AIDS Education and Prevention, 15*(1 Suppl A):66–79.*

Psychosocial predictors of sexual risk taking were investigated in a community sample of HIV+ and HIV– African American men enrolled in the African-American Health Project. HIV– men, men who have sex with men and women (MSM/W), and men who have sex with men (MSM) engaged in more high-risk sexual behaviors than heterosexuals and HIV+ men, but men who were HIV+ carried a heavier burden of psychosocial risk factors. High psychological distress, being HIV–, older age, low socioeconomic status (SES), and being an MSM/W were the best predictors of sexual risk. Results confirm previous findings of riskier sexual lifestyle among

MSM/W, men with low SES, and men who are experiencing significant psychological distress.

Demographic Risk Factors

The Triple Burden of Race, Class, and Gender

Quinn, S. C. (1993). AIDS and the African American woman: The triple burden of race, class, and gender. Health Education Quarterly, 20*:305–320.*

This article explores the interaction of race, gender, and social class as risk factors for HIV infection and addresses the need for health educators to overcome fear, class prejudice, and racial bias.

Social and Cultural Risk Factors

Social Inequality and HIV Infection in Women

Zierler, S., & Krieger, N. (2000). Social inequality and HIV infection in women. In K. H. Mayer & H. F. Pizer (Eds.), The emergence of AIDS: The impact on immunology, microbiology, and public health. *Washington, DC: American Public Health Association.*

Social inequality plays a significant role in HIV infection among U.S. women. To explain which women are at risk and why, this chapter reviews the epidemiology of HIV and AIDS among women in light of conceptual frameworks that link health with social justice.

POWERPOINT SLIDES

(Note: A full-color version of these slides, with graphics, is also available on the CD-ROM.)

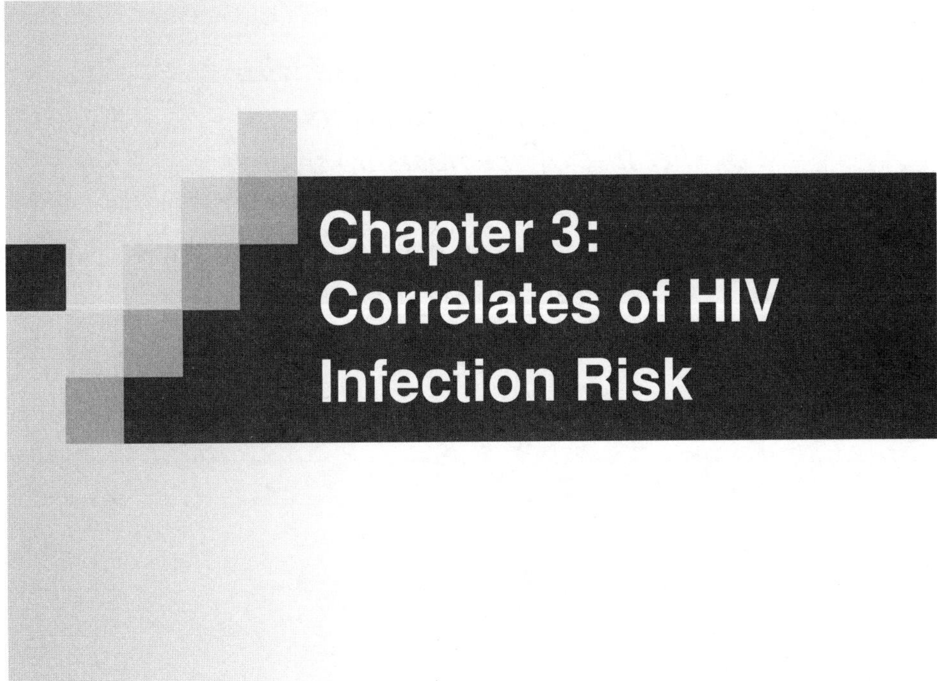

Correlates of HIV Infection Risk

- Unlike many viruses, HIV usually requires risky behaviors like sex and drug use for its transmission.
- Biological, psychological, demographic, and sociocultural factors affect both the likelihood and the consequences of these behaviors.

Overview of Risk Factors for HIV Infection

People become infected with HIV through behaviors, not because of membership in any particular "high risk group." HIV infection is a possibility for almost everyone, but an inevitability for almost no one.

Source: The Encyclopedia of AIDS: A Social, Political, Cultural, and Scientific Record of the HIV Epidemic (1)

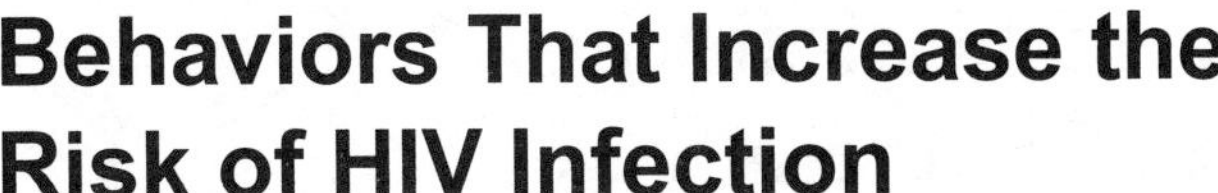

Behaviors That Increase the Risk of HIV Infection

- HIV is transmitted through bodily fluids.
- Behaviors that increase contact with infected body fluids increase the chance of contracting HIV.
- These behaviors include:
  - Unsafe sexual behaviors
  - Unsafe drug use
  - Mixing sex and drugs/alcohol
  - Not taking antiretroviral drugs properly

Overview of Risk Factors for HIV Infection

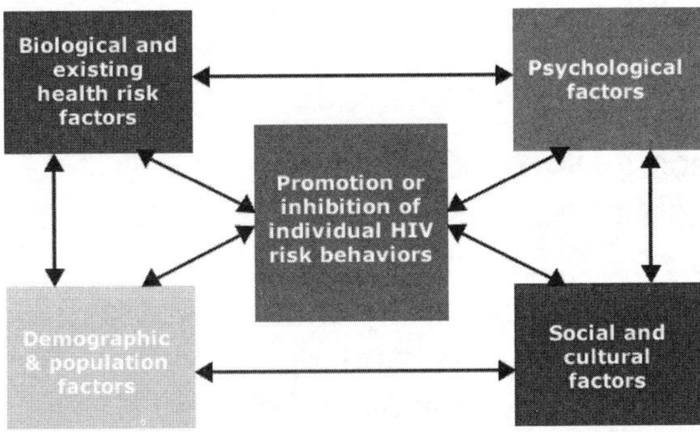

Biological and Existing Health Risk Factors

Many biological risk factors (both one's own and one's partners) make it easier for HIV to enter the body, including:

- presence of other STIs/STDs;
- structure of the vagina and of the anus;
- viral load;
- immune system health (self or partner);
- tissue/membrane vulnerability; and
- genetic character of the virus itself.

Psychological Factors

Individual psychological factors shape HIV risk behaviors. These include:

- personality;
- beliefs about HIV/AIDS;
- risk perception;
- coping styles;
- communication styles with sexual partners;
- mental health disorders; and
- depression and psychological distress.

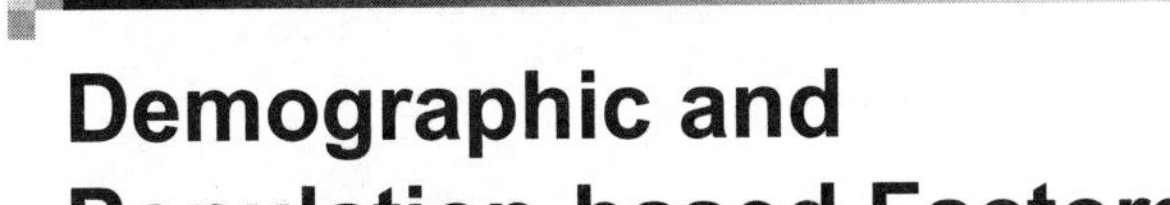

Demographic and Population-based Factors

HIV risk behaviors are shaped in the context of demographic factors and population-based factors. These include:

- race/ethnicity;
- age;
- sexual orientation;
- gender or transgender;
- migration;
- the number of HIV+ people in the population; and
- the frequency of risky behaviors in the population.

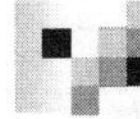

Social and Cultural Factors

HIV risk behaviors are shaped by social and cultural factors:

- Inequality
- Discrimination
- Stigma
- Gender roles and constraints
- Cultural rituals
- Values
- Norms
- Political unrest
- Economics
- Individual and social poverty
- Community transitions
- The availability and accessibility of medical and social services

Learning Objectives

- Review the processes and conditions for transmission of HIV infection
- Understand the falsehoods behind popular myths and misconceptions about HIV transmission
- Understand the sexual transmission of HIV
- Understand drug-associated transmission of HIV
- Understand vertical (parent-to-child) transmission of HIV
- Understand HIV transmission through transfusion, transplantation, and artificial insemination
- Understand HIV transmission in health care settings

Key Terms

CD4+
IDU
mucous membranes
perinatal transmission
vertical transmission

4

Transmission of HIV

People contract HIV when certain vulnerable cells are exposed to other people's HIV-infected body fluids. Chapter 4 describes how HIV is transmitted through sex and drug use; from parent to child; through transfusions, transplants, and artificial insemination; and in health care settings.

OVERVIEW OF TRANSMISSION OF HIV INFECTION

Transmission of HIV infection refers to the process by which the HIV virus invades a person's body. HIV is transmitted to an uninfected person when HIV-infected body fluids come in contact with the infectable cells (CD4+ cells) of an uninfected person. Body fluids that transmit HIV include blood and blood products, semen, preseminal fluid, vaginal and anal fluids, other body fluids that contain blood, breast milk, brain and spinal cord fluid, fluid around bone joints, and amniotic fluid (Chin, 2000; Mayer & Pizer, 2000; NIAID, 2003). These fluids may contain HIV particles and HIV-infected CD4+ cells, both of which can cause HIV infection.

HIV can reach the infectable cells of a person either through that person's blood or through his or her *mucous membranes*. Mucous membranes are the linings of certain cavities (such as the nose, mouth, vagina, and anus) that produce a protective layer of mucus. Blood and mucus are infectable because they contain the cells that HIV attacks—that is, CD4+ cells.

Unlike many other illnesses, HIV is not transmitted through routine casual contact, through the air, or through insect bites. This is because HIV does not survive well outside of people's bodies. HIV can be transmitted in the following ways:

- **Sexual activities:** As mentioned in chapter 1, HIV can be transmitted during sexual activities that involve direct contact between the HIV-infected person's bodily fluids (such as semen, vaginal secretions, and blood) and the uninfected person's blood or mucous membranes (such as in the vagina, rectum, and mouth). Two HIV+ people also can infect each other with different strains of HIV through sexual contact.
- **Injection drug use and other activities in which the skin is pierced:** HIV can be transmitted via skin-piercing instruments, such as needles for injecting drugs, razor blades, tattoo needles, piercing needles, or circumcision

instruments, that are used on more than one person. This is because some infected blood may be left on these instruments when they are used on others. In health care settings, HIV is sometimes transmitted by accidental stabs from contaminated needles or other sharp objects.

- **From parent to child:** HIV can be transmitted from mother to infant during pregnancy, childbirth, or breast-feeding. This is commonly referred to as *mother-to-child transmission*, *parent-to-child transmission*, or *vertical transmission*. There is strong evidence that use of antiviral medications during pregnancy markedly reduces the likelihood of vertical transmission of HIV (FHI, n.d.b).
- **Blood transfusions, transplants, and artificial insemination:** HIV can be transmitted from person to person through transfusions of blood and blood products, such as blood-clotting agents (platelets); organ, tissue, and bone transplants; and artificial insemination. Proper screening of these human products can reduce the risk of transmission through these routes to nearly zero (Donegan, 2003).
- **Other contacts with mucous membranes:** HIV can be transmitted by splashing mucous membranes (such as eyes) with infected blood or other HIV-infected body fluids (CDC, 2003).

Conditions for HIV Transmission

The following three conditions must be met for HIV to be transmitted (SFAF, n.d.):

HIV must be present.

HIV must be present in sufficient quantity.

HIV must get into the bloodstream.

1. HIV must be present. Infection can only happen if at least one of the people involved (e.g., a sexual partner, blood or organ donor, or user of injection drug use equipment) is infected with HIV. Certain behaviors alone, such as anal sex, do not cause HIV infection.

2. HIV must be present in sufficient quantity. The amount or concentration of HIV in the infected body fluid partly determines whether infection happens. The greater the concentration of HIV in the body fluid, the greater the chance that a person exposed to the body fluid will become HIV-infected. HIV is found in very low concentration—or is absent—in saliva, sweat, tears, and urine. It is found in medium concentration in anal secretions, and in high concentration in blood, semen, vaginal secretions, and breast milk. Thus, only a small amount of infected blood, semen, vaginal fluids, or breast milk is enough to infect someone, whereas much larger amounts of anal secretions are needed for HIV transmission. To date, there are no known cases of HIV transmission through saliva, tears, sweat, or urine.

Different people also have different concentrations of HIV, depending, in part, on their stage of HIV disease. In the first, primary stage of infection, people have much higher concentrations of HIV in their blood than they do in the middle, asymptomatic stage of infection. Concentrations of HIV rise during the late stage and full-blown AIDS (Hare, 2004; Lawn, Butera, & Folks, 2001). It is therefore more likely that an HIV+ person will transmit HIV to an uninfected sexual or injecting partner during the primary stages of infection and when the infection has progressed to advanced HIV disease (AIDS) than during the middle, asymptomatic stage, which can last several years.

3. HIV must get into the bloodstream. It is not enough just to touch HIV-infected fluid to become infected. Healthy, unbroken skin is an excellent barrier that prevents HIV from getting into the body. HIV can only enter through an open cut or sore, or through contact with the mucous membranes of the anus, rectum, genitals, mouth, or eyes.

Myths and Misconceptions About HIV Transmission

There have been many misconceptions and widespread myths over the years as to how HIV is transmitted (see Figure 4-1 for some examples). Unfortunately, these misconceptions and myths have often led to unfounded fears, stigma against people

"HIV can be transmitted through casual contact." Diverse studies have shown that HIV is not transmitted through casual, everyday contact, such as shaking hands or sharing eating utensils, even when people are living in close quarters (SFAF, n.d.).

"HIV can be transmitted through insect bites." Studies conducted by the U.S. Centers for Disease Control and Prevention (CDC) and others have shown no evidence of HIV transmission through bloodsucking or biting insects, including mosquitoes, flies, ticks, and fleas, perhaps because HIV cannot live and replicate in insects' bodies (CDC, 2003). If mosquitoes did indeed transmit HIV, children and the elderly—who are less likely to be exposed to HIV by sexual contact or intravenous drug use—would have higher rates of HIV infection than have been observed in areas with many mosquitoes and many AIDS cases (SFAF, n.d.).

"In the United States, donating blood or receiving donated blood is risky." According to the American Association of Blood Banks, many safeguards on our national blood supply help ensure safe blood for patients. When people volunteer to donate blood, they must answer a number of questions about their health and risk factors for disease. Only people with a clean bill of health are permitted to donate. Blood is drawn with sterilized needles that are used only once. The blood from each donor is type-tested and then subjected to nine separate screening tests that check for evidence of infection with HIV, hepatitis, syphilis, and other diseases (American Association of Blood Banks, n.d.; SFAF, n.d.).

"Pets and other animals can carry HIV and transmit it to people." Humans are the only animals that can harbor HIV. Some animals do carry viruses similar to HIV that cause immune deficiencies in their own species. For example, cats can get FIV (feline immunodeficiency virus) and some monkeys can get SIV (simian immunodeficiency virus). However, FIV and SIV cannot be transmitted to people, nor can people transmit HIV to their pets. An exception to this rule is chimpanzees that have been infected with HIV for research purposes. Contact with their blood could infect the researchers who work with them (SFAF, n.d.).

"HIV can be transmitted through contact with saliva, tears, or sweat." HIV can only be transmitted when a sufficient amount of HIV enters the body. Saliva, tears, sweat, and urine either contain no HIV or contain quantities too small to result in infection (SFAF, n.d.). To date, contact with saliva, tears, or sweat has never been shown to result in transmission of HIV (CDC, 2003). The only time these body fluids would pose a risk would be if they had blood in them.

Figure 4-1 Myths about HIV transmission.

living with HIV/AIDS, unnecessary and punitive restrictions, and discriminatory practices. These misconceptions and myths also may have diverted attention from the actual routes of HIV transmission and, as a consequence, may have increased the likelihood that some people would not follow established HIV prevention guidelines.

SEXUAL TRANSMISSION OF HIV

Unprotected Penile-Anal Intercourse (Male–Male or Male–Female)

Unprotected penile-anal intercourse, whether between two men or a man and a woman, exposes the anal and rectal mucous membranes of the receptive partner to semen, and exposes the penis (specifically, the mucous membrane in the opening of the penis) to anal mucus. Also, anal sex often causes tearing of the penis, anus, and rectum, so that both the receptive and the insertive partners may be exposed to blood. The anal and rectal tears, in turn, provide HIV with direct access to the bloodstream.

The receptive partner in anal sex (i.e., the person who is being penetrated) is at greater risk of HIV infection than the insertive partner for several reasons. First, the receptive partner is exposed to a larger amount of body fluids (semen,

FACT: Worldwide, unprotected sex with an infected partner is the most common way of spreading the HIV virus (Chin, 2000; Kalichman, 1998; NIAID, 2003).

possibly blood) than the insertive partner, who is only exposed to rectal mucus (possibly blood). In addition, the receptive partner is exposed to HIV-carrying fluids for longer than is the insertive partner, as the semen (and, perhaps blood) deposited into his or her rectum stays there longer than the fluids on the insertive partner's penis. HIV also has an easier time surviving in the rectum than on the penis. Finally, rectal and anal tissues tear more easily than do penile tissues, giving HIV a direct pathway to the bloodstream of the receptive partner (Osmond, 1998).

Unprotected Penile-Vaginal Intercourse

Unprotected penile-vaginal intercourse exposes the woman's vaginal and cervical mucous membranes to semen, and the man's penis (specifically, the mucous membrane at the penis's opening) to vaginal secretions. Moreover, if the sex is rough or dry, cuts and tears may expose the man and woman to blood, and may open delicate vaginal and penile mucous membranes for direct HIV transmission to the bloodstream.

Although both men and women are at risk of contracting HIV during heterosexual intercourse, the woman is at greater risk for several reasons. Usually, the woman is exposed to a larger amount of body fluids (semen and possibly blood) than is the man, who is only exposed to vaginal secretions (possibly blood as well). In addition, the vagina and cervix have larger areas of exposed mucous membranes than does the penis. The tissues of the vagina and cervix also tear more easily than those of the penis, and the virus has an easier time surviving in the vagina than it does on the surface of the penis. Finally, there are more copies of the virus in a man's semen than there are in the fluids of the vagina (United Nations Population Fund [UNPFA], 2002; Volberding, 1998; WHO, 2000).

Unprotected Oral-Genital and Oral-Anal Sex

Unprotected oral-genital and oral-anal sex can expose mucous membranes of the mouth to HIV-infected semen, vaginal fluids, or anal fluids. Although this is a biologically possible means of HIV transmission, very few cases of transmission through these routes have been documented, and the actual risk of infection is unknown. The risk of oral-penile and oral-anal transmission are thought to be low, and the risk of oral-vaginal contact is thought to be very low (Campo et al., 2006; Kalichman, 1998).

Factors That Increase the Risk of Sexual Transmission

Certain factors can increase the risk of sexual transmission of HIV. Multiple sexual partners is one significant factor in the spread of the disease. The more HIV+ people in a pool of sexual partners, the greater the chances that a person will encounter an HIV+ person and contract HIV himself or herself (Laumann, Gagnon, Michael, & Michaels, 1994). For this reason, the risk associated with having multiple sex partners varies significantly by geographic region and by the sexual mixing within a region (Osmond, 1998; Zierler & Krieger, 2000).

As was discussed in several previous sections, having another STI/STD greatly increases the risk of getting or giving HIV (Osmond, 1998). This is especially true of the STIs/STDs that cause sores on the genitalia, such as herpes and syphilis. Even if an STI/STD does not cause genital sores, it still increases the risk of HIV transmission and acquisition by increasing the number of CD4+ cells near the genitalia.

Sexual behavior that is accompanied by bleeding, such as whipping, cutting, or piercing skin during sex, also may increase transmission risk because of the possibility that HIV-infected body fluids will come into contact with another person's open cut or mucous membrane. However, so little data are available on such behaviors that it is difficult to know how much they increase the risk of HIV transmission (Osmond, 1998).

DRUG-ASSOCIATED TRANSMISSION OF HIV

When a person with HIV infection uses a syringe to inject drugs, the needle is contaminated with a small amount of infected blood. If the needle is shared, the next person to use it may inject the infected blood directly into his or her own bloodstream (Chin, 2000; NIAID, 2003).

Sharing needles greatly increases the spread of HIV.

Injection drug use (IDU) accounts for only 5–10% of worldwide HIV infections since the beginning of the HIV/AIDS epidemic. Nevertheless, in some parts of the world, IDU is the major mode of HIV transmission. For example, it is estimated that in China, Malaysia, and Vietnam at least half of HIV infections have resulted from IDU. Rapid spread of HIV through shared use of contaminated IDU equipment also has been observed in parts of Central and Eastern Europe (FHI, n.d.a). Because injection drug users are often linked in tight social networks and commonly share their injecting equipment without properly cleaning it, HIV often spreads very quickly in these populations.

In the United States in 2004, IDU transmission accounted for 29% of all African American adults and adolescents estimated to be living with HIV/AIDS, and 31% of Hispanic adults and adolescents estimated to be living with HIV/AIDS. In contrast, only 20% of estimated cases among White adults/adolescents were IDU-associated (CDC, 2005).

Injection drug use contributes to the epidemic's spread far beyond the circle of those who inject because people who have sex with an injection drug user also are at risk for infection through the sexual transmission of HIV. Children born to mothers who contracted HIV through sharing needles or having sex with an IDU may become infected as well.

VERTICAL TRANSMISSION OF HIV

As mentioned earlier in this chapter, the terms commonly used to describe HIV transmission from parents to their children include mother-to-child transmission, parent-to-child transmission, perinatal transmission, and vertical transmission. Many advocates recommend abandoning the term "mother-to-child" transmission because this term implicitly blames women for infecting their unborn children (GENDER-AIDS eForum, 2003). Indeed, women and their unborn children are often infected by their own husband/fathers (Feinstein & Prentice, 2001).

FACT: Vertical transmission of HIV is the most significant source of HIV infection in children under the age of 10 (WHO, 2001).

HIV can be transmitted from an infected mother to her child during pregnancy, during labor and delivery, or through breastfeeding. Without intervention, such as antiretroviral therapy, the risk of transmission from an HIV+ mother to her child before or during birth is 15–25%. Breastfeeding by an HIV+ mother raises the risk by 5–20%, to a total risk of 20–45% (Newell, 2004).

Vertical transmission of HIV has been virtually eliminated in the developed world. But, rates remain high in resource-constrained countries, particularly sub-Saharan African countries, where the vast majority of HIV-infected women of childbearing age reside. These high rates are largely a result of these women's lack of access to existing prevention interventions (see Part 2, chapter 7).

HIV TRANSMISSION VIA TRANSFUSION, TRANSPLANTATION, AND ARTIFICIAL INSEMINATION

HIV Transmission Through Transfusions

HIV transmission through blood transfusions and blood products (such as platelets or plasma) has become rare in developed countries since they began screening all donated blood for HIV antibodies (CDC, 2003; Donegan, 2003; Kalichman, 1998). Outside of developed countries, however, blood safety is not as predictably guaranteed. Currently, 80% of the world's population has access to only 20% of the world's supply of safe blood (Donegan, 2003).

Among those who receive HIV-infected blood in a transfusion, 90% become HIV+ (Donegan, 2003).

Receiving HIV-infected blood or blood products through a transfusion is the surest way to get HIV. Among those who receive infected blood, 90% become HIV+ (Donegan, 2003).

HIV Transmission Through Transplants

A person also can be infected with HIV by receiving an organ, bone, or tissue transplant from an HIV+ person because these body parts have blood in them. HIV has been transmitted through transplantations of kidneys, livers, hearts, pancreases, bones, and skin (Donegan, 2003). The majority of HIV transmission through transplantation happened before 1985, when HIV antibody testing became available.

HIV Transmission Through Artificial Insemination

As of late 2003, 15 women worldwide were known to have been infected with HIV through artificial insemination using sperm from anonymous donors (Donegan, 2003). All but one of these instances of insemination-related infection happened before 1985, when HIV antibody testing became available. Six of those 15 cases occurred in the United States. Because an estimated 75,000 women are artificially inseminated annually in the United States, it seems that HIV transmission from unrelated semen donors was an infrequent event before the availability of HIV testing (CDC, 1994).

Currently, the U.S. Centers for Disease Control and Prevention (CDC) recommends screening semen donors for HIV antibodies two times: first on the day the semen is collected, and then 6 months later. The semen is frozen in the interim. If the donor is HIV+ 6 months after the donation or if the donor does not return for his 6-month checkup, his semen is not used (CDC, 1994).

HIV TRANSMISSION IN HEALTH CARE SETTINGS

Patients Transmitting HIV to Health Care Workers

In health care settings, such as hospitals and doctors' offices, workers have been infected with HIV after being stuck with needles containing HIV-infected blood. Less frequently, workers also have contracted HIV after infected blood gets into an open cut or comes in contact with a mucous membrane (such as the eyes or inside of the nose) (CDC, 2003). Research suggests that infection after a needle stick injury is rare, happening about 3 times per 1,000 injuries involving HIV-infected blood (Noble, 2003).

Health Care Workers Transmitting HIV to Patients

As of 2003, there has been only one documented case of a health care worker giving HIV to patients in the United States. In this case, an HIV-infected dentist gave HIV to six patients. Investigations of 63 HIV+ physicians, surgeons, and dentists and their more than 22,000 patients found no other cases of this type of transmission in the United States (CDC, 2003).

REFERENCES

American Association of Blood Banks. (n.d.). *Receiving a blood transfusion: What every patient should know*. Retrieved October 13, 2004, from http://www.aabb.org/All_About_Blood/Receiving_Blood/receive.org

Campo, J., Perea, M. A., del Romero, J., Cano, J., Hernando, V., & Bascones, A. (2006). Oral transmission of HIV, reality or fiction? An update. *Oral Diseases, 12*(3), 219–228.

Centers for Disease Control and Prevention (CDC). (1994). Guidelines for preventing transmission of human immunodeficiency virus through transplantation of human tissue and organs. *Morbidity and Mortality Weekly Report, 43*(Suppl RR-8), 1–17.

Centers for Disease Control and Prevention (CDC). (2003). *Fact sheet: HIV and its transmission*. Atlanta, GA: CDC.

Centers for Disease Control and Prevention (CDC). (2005). *HIV/AIDS surveillance report, 2004*. Atlanta, GA: CDC.

Chin, J. (Ed.). (2000). *Communicable diseases manual* (17th ed.). Washington, DC: American Public Health Association.

Donegan, E. (2003). Transmission of HIV by blood, blood products, tissue transplantation, and artificial insemination. In L. Pieperl, S. Coffey, O. Bacon, & P. Volberding (Eds.), *HIV InSite knowledge base*. San Francisco: Center for HIV Information, University of California, San Francisco.

Family Health International (FHI). (n.d.a). *Fact sheet: Reducing HIV in injecting drug users (IDUs)*. Arlington, VA: FHI.

Family Health International (FHI). (n.d.b). *Reducing mother-to-child transmission (MTCT) of HIV*. Arlington, VA: FHI.

Feinstein, N., & Prentice, B. (2001). Fact sheet: The female condom. In *The UNAIDS gender and AIDS almanac*. Los Altos, CA: Sociometrics Corporation.

GENDER-AIDS eForum. (2003). Women "often blamed" for virus. *AEGiS Digest, 1159*(7). Retrieved October 10, 2003, from http://www.aegis.com/news/bp/2003/BP031003.html

Hare, C. B. (2004). Clinical overview of HIV disease. In L. Pieperl, S. Coffey, O. Bacon, & P. Volberding (Eds.), *HIV InSite knowledge base*. San Francisco: Center for HIV Information, University of California, San Francisco.

Kalichman, S. C. (1998). *Preventing AIDS: A sourcebook for behavioral intervention*. Mahwah, NJ: Lawrence Erlbaum Associates.

Laumann, E. O., Gagnon, J. H., Michael, R. T., & Michaels, S. (1994). *The social organization of sexuality: Sexual practices in the United States*. Chicago: University of Chicago Press.

Lawn, S. D., Butera, S. T., & Folks, T. M. (2001). Contribution of immune activation to the pathogenesis and transmission of human immunodeficiency virus type 1 infection. *Clinical Microbiology Review, 14*(4), 753–777.

Mayer, K. H., & Pizer, H. F. (Eds.). (2000). *The emergence of AIDS: The impact on immunology, microbiology, and public health*. Washington, DC: American Public Health Association.

National Institutes of Allergy and Infectious Diseases (NIAID). (2003). *HIV infection and AIDS: An overview*. Bethesda, MD: NIAID.

Newell, M. L. (2004). *HIV transmission through breastfeeding: A review of the available evidence*. Geneva, Switzerland: World Health Organization.

Noble, B. (2003). *Healthcare workers, AIDS and prevention*. Horsham, UK: AVERT.org. Retrieved December 22, 2003, from http://www.avert.org/needlestick.htm

Osmond, D. H. (1998). Sexual transmission of HIV. In L. Pieperl, S. Coffey, O. Bacon, & P. Volberding (Eds.), *HIV InSite knowledge base*. San Francisco: Center for HIV Information, University of California, San Francisco.

San Francisco AIDS Foundation (SFAF). (n.d.). How HIV is spread. In *AIDS 101: Guide to HIV basics*. Retrieved January 15, 2004, from http://www.sfaf.org/aids101/transmission.html

United Nations Population Fund (UNFPA). (2002). Addressing gender perspectives in HIV prevention. *HIV Prevention Now Programme Briefs, No. 4*. New York: UNFPA.

Volberding, P. (Ed.). (1998). The most common opportunistic infections in women with HIV. *HIV Newsline, 4*(4).

World Health Organization (WHO). (2000). *Women and HIV/AIDS (Fact sheet no. 242)*. Geneva, Switzerland: WHO.

World Health Organization (WHO). (2001). New data on the prevention of mother-to-child transmission of HIV and their policy implications: Conclusions and recommendations. In *WHO technical consultation on behalf of the UNFPA/UNICEF/WHO/UNAIDS Inter-Agency Task Team on mother-to-child transmission of HIV*. Geneva, Switzerland: WHO.

Zierler, S., & Krieger, N. (2000). Social inequality and HIV infection in women. In K. H. Mayer & H. F. Pizer (Eds.), *The emergence of AIDS: The impact on immunology, microbiology, and public health* (pp. 76–97). Washington, DC: American Public Health Association.

Instructor Resources

LEARNING ACTIVITIES

ACTIVITY 1:

Group Activity: The Sexual Transmission Risk Continuum

Adapted from The HIV and STD Risk Continuum activity in The Practicing Safer Sex Today (PSST!) Education Program developed and implemented by the Department of Health Services Research at the Palo Alto Medical Foundation Research Institute (PAMFRI). Used with permission.

Objective: To educate participants to be able to identify what are high-risk, safe, and safer activities with different types of partners.

View a detailed guide for this activity on the CD-ROM.

ACTIVITY 2:

Assignment: Modes of Transmission

Objective: To understand and explain how HIV is transmitted.

Think about the modes of transmission for HIV. In a three- to five-page paper, describe how different groups are affected in different ways by the means of infection. Explore the reasons that account for these differences, and explain how this might impact prevention strategies.

ACTIVITY 3:

Group Activity: Transmission Case Studies: Scenarios of Risk

Adapted from San Francisco AIDS Foundation, AIDS 101: How HIV Is Spread. http://www.sfaf.org/aids101/transmission.html

Objective: To educate participants in assessing their risk for acquiring HIV infection.

View a detailed guide for this activity on the CD-ROM.

DISCUSSION QUESTIONS

1. Given all that we know about the ways HIV is transmitted and how transmission can be prevented, why do you think there were still 4.9 million new infections worldwide in 2005?

QUIZ

1. Blood and mucus are infectable by HIV because they contain:
   a) Platelets
   b) Lymphocytes
   c) RNA
   d) CD4+ cells
2. In which of the following ways can HIV *not* be transmitted?
   a) From mother to infant during pregnancy
   b) Through blood transfusions
   c) Through insect bites
   d) Through sexual activity
   e) By donating blood
   f) Through contact with sweat
   g) Through injection drug use
   h) Through contact with animals
3. Which of the following fluids contain high concentrations of HIV?
   a) Saliva
   b) Breast milk
   c) Anal secretions
   d) Blood
   e) Vaginal secretions
   f) Tears
   g) Semen
   h) Sweat
   i) Urine
4. List the three conditions that must be present for HIV to be transmitted.
5. List any two factors that increase the risk of sexual transmission.
6. Injection drug use accounts for what percentage of HIV infections worldwide?
   a) Less than 1%
   b) 5–10%
   c) 15–20%
   d) More than 20%
7. Without intervention, the risk of transmission from an HIV+ mother to her child before or during birth is:
   a) Less than 10%
   b) 15–25%
   c) 35–45%
   d) 55–65%
8. True or False: HIV transmission through blood transfusions has become rare.
9. True or False: HIV+ health care workers frequently transmit HIV to their patients.

ANSWERS

1. **D.** CD4+ are the cells that HIV attacks.
2. **C, E, F, and H.** HIV is not transmitted through routine casual contact. It can be transmitted through sexual activity, injection drug use, other activi-

ties in which skin is pierced, from an infected mother to child, through blood transfusions, transplants, artificial insemination, or other contact with mucous membranes.

3. **B, D, E, and G.** HIV is found in high concentration in blood, semen, vaginal secretion, and breast milk. It is found in very low concentration, or is absent, from saliva, sweat, tears, and urine. It is found in medium concentration in anal secretions.
4. HIV must be present; it must be present in sufficient quantity; and it must get into the bloodstream.
5. Multiple sexual partners, the presence of another STI/STD, or sexual behavior that is accompanied by bleeding all may increase transmission risk.
6. **B.** Injection drug use accounts for only 5–10% of worldwide HIV infections since the beginning of the HIV/AIDS epidemic. However, in some parts of the world, it is the major mode of HIV transmission.
7. **B.** Without intervention, such as antiretroviral therapy, the risk of transmission from an HIV+ mother to her child before or during birth is 15–25%. Breast-feeding by an HIV+ mother raises the risk by 5–20%, to a total risk of 20–45%.
8. This statement is true in developed countries, since they began screening all donated blood for HIV antibodies. Outside of developed countries, however, blood safety is not as predictably guaranteed.
9. **False.** As of 2003, there has been only one documented case of a health care worker giving HIV to patients.

WEB RESOURCES

Overview of Transmission

AIDS 101: How HIV Is Spread (San Francisco AIDS Foundation)

http://www.sfaf.org/aids101/transmission.html

An indexed overview of activities that do and do not allow HIV transmission.

Prevention of Infection Through Sexual Contact

Safer Sex Resources (UCSF HIV InSite)

http://www.hivinsite.com/InSite?page=li-07-11

Provides links to research articles and additional resources relating to preventing the sexual transmission of HIV.

Instructions for Using a Male Condom

http://www.engenderhealth.org/res/onc/hiv/preventing/miw/hiv6miw3.html

Instructions for Using a Female Condom

http://www.engenderhealth.org/res/onc/hiv/preventing/miw/hiv6miw4.html

Female-Controlled Prevention Technologies: Related Resources (UCSF HIV InSite, 2003)

http://hivinsite.ucsf.edu/InSite.jsp?page=kbr-07-02-04

A series of links to research-based fact sheets, guidelines, FAQs, reports, discussions, interviews, articles, presentations, conference Web sites, conference reports, and additional resources for female-controlled prevention technologies.

Preventing Infection Through Injection Drug Use

Epidemiology and HIV Transmission in Injection Drug Users: Related Resources (UCSF HIV InSite)

http://www.hivinsite.com/InSite?page=kbr-07-04-01

Provides links to research articles and additional resources relating to injection drug use and HIV/AIDS.

Preventing Parent-to-Child Transmission

Women, Children, and HIV

http://www.womenchildrenhiv.org/

Contains a library of practical, applicable materials on mother and child HIV infection including preventing mother-to-child HIV transmission, infant feeding, clinical care of women, children, and orphans, plus up-to-date news on HIV/AIDS. The goal of this site is to contribute to an improvement in the scale and quality of international HIV/AIDS prevention, care, and treatment programs for women and children by increasing access to authoritative HIV/AIDS information.

RECOMMENDED READING

Preventing Infection Through Sexual Contact

Safer-Sex Methods (Lane & Palacio, 2003)

Lane, T., & Palacio, H. (2003). Safer-sex methods. In L. Pieperl, S. Coffey, O. Bacon, & P. Volberding (Eds.), HIV InSite knowledge base. *San Francisco: Center for HIV Information, University of California San Francisco.*
This chapter reviews the evidence that has led to the development of safer-sex guidelines, and concludes with specific recommendations for safer-sex practices. Available online at http://www.hivinsite.com/InSite?page=kb-07-02-02

Preventing Parent-to-Child Transmission

An International Perspective on Preventing Vertical Transmission (Etiebet et al., 2004)

Etiebet, M. A., Fransman, D., Forsyth, B., Coetzee, N., & Hussey, G. (2004). Integrating prevention of mother-to-child HIV transmission into antenatal care: Learning from the experiences of women in South Africa. AIDS Care, 16*(1):37–46.*

In 1999, for the first time in South Africa, a Mother-to-Child HIV Transmission (MTCT) prevention program was implemented at the routine primary care level and not as part of a research protocol. A total of 264 women attending prenatal care in these clinics were interviewed in Xhosa using a standardized questionnaire. All had been offered HIV testing, and 95% had accepted. Women who had not been tested were 4 times more likely to believe that in the community families reject HIV+ women. Of women who tested, 19% were HIV positive and 83% had told their partner that they had taken the test. HIV+ women who had not disclosed testing to their partners were 3 times more likely to believe that, in the community, partners are violent toward HIV+ women, and 86% stated that they would have taken AZT if found to be HIV+. Only 11% considered that the use of formula feeding indicated that a woman was HIV positive. In conclusion, routine prenatal HIV testing and interventions to reduce perinatal HIV transmission are acceptable to the majority of women in a South African urban township, despite an awareness of discrimination in the community toward HIV+ women.

Myths and Misconceptions About HIV Transmission and Infection

The Connection Between Accurate and Inaccurate Transmission Beliefs and Stigmatization (Boer & Emons, 2004)

Boer, H., & Emons, P. A. A. (2004). Accurate and inaccurate HIV transmission beliefs, stigmatizing and HIV protection motivation in northern Thailand. AIDS Care *16(2): 167–176.*

The authors of this article assessed the relationship between accurate beliefs about HIV transmission and inaccurate beliefs about HIV transmission and emotional reactions to people with AIDS (PWAs) and AIDS risk groups, stigmatizing attitudes and motivation to protect from HIV. Results of their study suggest that inaccurate beliefs about HIV transmission are related to fear and stigmatizing and undermine HIV prevention behavior.

POWERPOINT SLIDES

(Note: A full-color version of these slides, with graphics, is also available on the CD-ROM.)

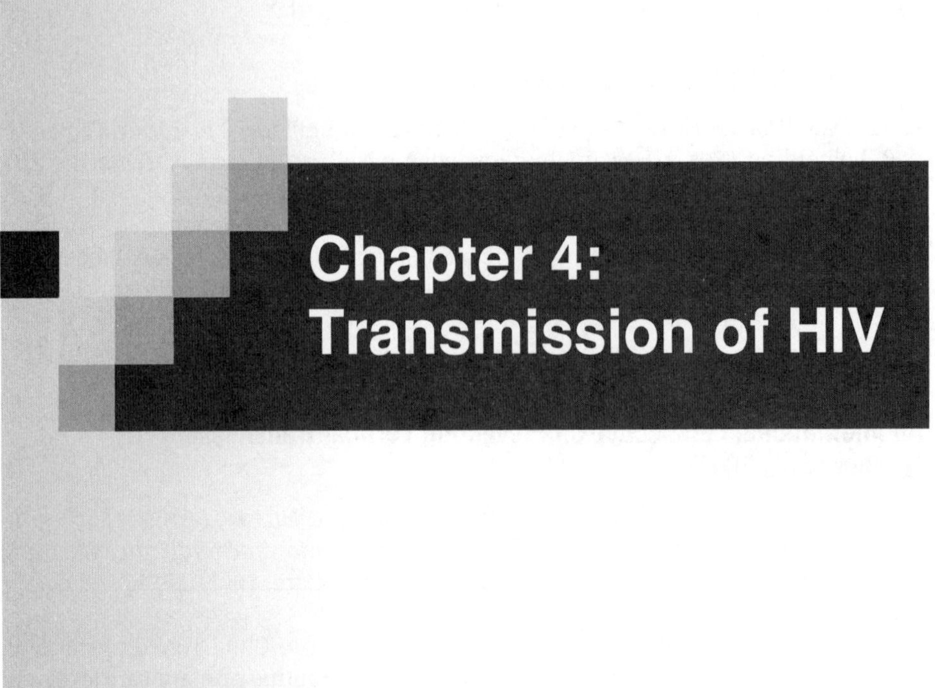

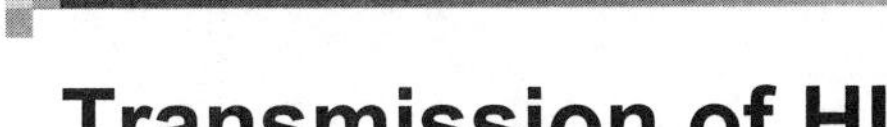

Transmission of HIV

- Transmission of HIV infection is the process by which HIV invades a person's body.
- HIV can reach the infectable cells of an uninfected person through that person's blood or mucous membranes.
- HIV is not transmitted through routine casual contact, through the air, or through insect bites.

Conditions for HIV Transmission

1. **HIV must be present.**
2. **HIV must be present in sufficient quantity.**
3. **HIV must get into the bloodstream.**

Sexual Transmission of HIV

HIV can be transmitted during sexual activities that involve direct contact between the HIV-infected person's bodily fluids and the uninfected person's blood or mucous membranes, including:

- unprotected penile-anal intercourse;
- unprotected penile-vaginal intercourse; and
- unprotected oral-genital sex.

Factors That Increase the Risk of Sexual Transmission of HIV

- Sexual behavior that is accompanied by bleeding, such as whipping, cutting, or piercing skin during sex
- Multiple sexual partners
- Other sexually transmitted infections

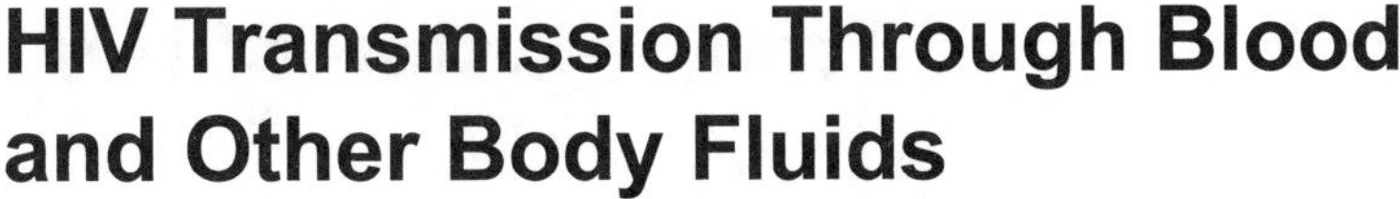

HIV Transmission Through Blood and Other Body Fluids

HIV can be transmitted via:

- skin-piercing instruments that are used on more than one person;
- transfusions of blood and blood products;
- organ, tissue, and bone transplants;
- splashing mucous membranes with infected blood or other body fluids; and
- accidental stabs from contaminated needles or other sharp objects.

Other Modes of Transmission of HIV

HIV Transmission Through Transfusions

- Is rare in developed countries since they began screening blood for HIV antibodies
- Is more likely outside of developed countries, where blood is less safe

HIV Transmission Through Transplants

- Including through transplantations of kidneys, livers, hearts, pancreases, bones, and skin
- Most transmission happened before 1985

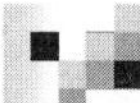

Other Modes of Transmission of HIV
(continued)

HIV Transmission Through Artificial Insemination

- As of late 2003, 15 women worldwide have been infected with HIV through artificial insemination.
- All but one of these cases happened before 1985.

HIV Transmission in Health Care Settings

- Workers have been infected after being stuck with needles containing HIV-infected blood.
- Such infections are rare, happening about 3 times per 1,000 needle stick injuries.
- As of 2003, there has been only one documented case of a health care worker giving HIV to patients in the United States.

PART II

Preventing HIV

HIV is deadly, but it is also preventable. This means that it is possible to stop the chain of events that leads to infection. HIV prevention efforts have slowed the spread of HIV both in the United States and worldwide and have saved countless lives. According to the CDC (2001), for example:

HIV prevention efforts have saved countless lives in the United States and worldwide.

- Prevention efforts have helped to slow the rate of new infections in the United States, from over 150,000 per year in the late 1980s to 40,000 per year since 2001.
- HIV prevalence among young White men in the United States declined by 50% between 1988 and 1993. Prevention efforts in New York City have contributed to a drop in HIV prevalence among injection drug users who are in drug treatment from almost 34% in 1990 to just over 4% in 1998.
- Between 1992 and 1998, the number of U.S. infants who acquired HIV through parent-to-child transmission declined 73%.
- Prevention efforts dramatically reduced the number of AIDS cases in Thailand and Uganda (where AIDS cases in urban areas fell by 50% between 1996 and 2001) and have prevented an expected epidemic in Senegal.

Until an effective vaccine is developed, preventing transmission requires the deployment of effective, culturally competent prevention strategies that address each route of transmission, including sex, injection drug use, parent-to-child transmission, and transmission in health care settings. These efforts must change behaviors—among both HIV– and HIV+ persons—that lead to HIV. They also must increase access to and use of tools—such as barrier methods, sterile syringes, and antiretroviral therapy—that can reduce the risk of getting or giving the virus.

In the past decade and a half, many interventions aimed at preventing the spread of HIV have been put into practice:

- *Individual-level* and *small group-level interventions* seek to directly influence the knowledge, attitudes, skills, and behaviors of persons who participate in intervention activities.

- *Community-level interventions* influence the knowledge, attitudes, skills, and behaviors of an entire community both directly and indirectly, often through a focus on changing social norms.
- *Structural interventions* indirectly influence risk behavior by effecting changes to policies, laws, organizational practices, or other structures that are related either to risk behaviors or to access to prevention information, tools, or services (CDC, 2006).

Part 2 first provides information on HIV prevention intervention basics and on theories of behavior that underlie effective interventions. It then goes on to discuss prevention approaches for each route of HIV transmission. Finally, it discusses the strategies and issues involved in each level of prevention, from individual level to structural level. There are also broader societal issues—issues of human rights and gender inequality—that must be addressed in global HIV prevention efforts. These issues will be covered in Part 4.

Learning Objectives

- Understand the need for effective HIV prevention interventions
- Identify goals and strategies for intervention programs
- Describe the different ways to evaluate an intervention program
- Assess the cost-effectiveness of an intervention program
- Understand the importance of cultural competence in intervention programs
- Define the concept of technology transfer

Key Terms

adapt
core components
cost-effectiveness
cultural competence
economic evaluation
formative evaluation
impact evaluation
long-term goals
needs and assets assessment
outcome evaluation
process evaluation
replicate
short-term objectives
technology transfer

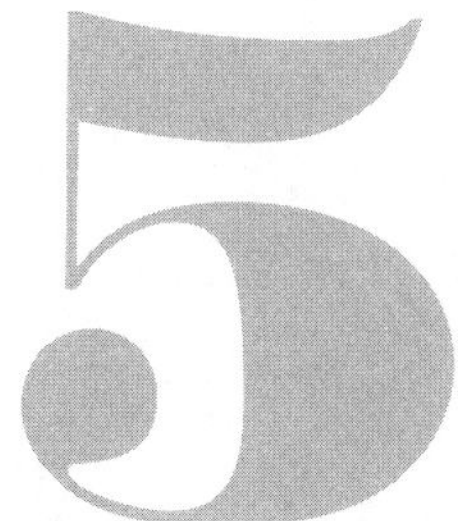

HIV Prevention Intervention Basics

PLANNING AN EFFECTIVE PREVENTION INTERVENTION

Prevention interventions should focus on "high-risk" people and behaviors. High-risk individuals include those who engage in unprotected sexual intercourse, have multiple sex partners, or use injection drugs. Often, these are also the individuals who have the most limited access to prevention and treatment services. For example:

- Men who have sex with men face discrimination and marginalization in both developing countries and industrialized nations, and have little access to care and prevention services.
- Injection drug users often find it difficult to seek information on HIV/AIDS or obtain prevention supplies (such as sterile syringes), as injection drug use is illegal in most countries.
- Lack of information and social pressures add to the vulnerability of youth. Girls are especially vulnerable to coerced sex, and may be forced to exchange sexual favors for money, food, or shelter.
- Women in many cultures have little control over the timing and context of intercourse, putting them at risk for HIV infection from their husbands and partners.

Prevention interventions also should be delivered in a variety of settings to reach a broad audience. Settings for prevention interventions should include neighborhoods, schools, workplaces, health care facilities, social gathering places, family planning centers, reproductive health service providers, and places where sex is sold or traded.

Planning an effective HIV prevention program that will meet the needs of a population, in a specific setting, first requires an understanding of that population's specific HIV-related needs and assets. Goals, objectives, and program strategies should be defined in ways that address the particular factors that put the target population at risk of HIV infection (see Figure 5-1).

Identify needs & assets ⟹ Identify goals & objectives ⟹ Identify strategies

Figure 5-1

Identifying HIV-Related Needs and Assets

Needs and assets assessment can be defined as the process of collecting and assessing data that describe the nature and magnitude of a community's needs, as well as its resources or assets (e.g., financial, organizational, intellectual, institutional, and human) (Card, Brindis, Peterson, & Niego, 2001). An HIV prevention–related needs and assets assessment should describe the extent, magnitude, and scope of the problem in the community, as well as current efforts and resources to address the problem. It also should identify gaps in existing services. In addition, it should gather information on causes of and potential solutions to the problem, both from research- and community-based perspectives. It is particularly important that information be gathered on the target population's HIV-related knowledge, attitudes, beliefs, skills, motivations, intentions, and access to preventive tools and services.

Program planners can sometimes get needs and assets data from existing sources, such as vital statistics records, ongoing national and regional surveys, needs and assets assessment reports, and journal articles. New data also may be collected through surveys, focus groups, individual interviews, and community forum meetings.

Identifying Goals, Objectives, and Strategies

Once the HIV-related needs and assets of the target community have been defined, program planners should identify specific long-term goals and short-term objectives for the intervention. *Long-term goals* are the changes in behaviors and health status (e.g., sexual risk-taking behavior, injection drug use behavior, HIV status, viral load) that the program will seek to achieve over a long period of time (perhaps 6 months to a year or more after completion of the intervention). *Short-term objectives* are the immediate changes in knowledge, attitudes, beliefs, skills, intentions, behaviors, and other factors that the intervention will seek to achieve on completion of the intervention or shortly thereafter. The short-term objectives should be logically linked to the long-term goals. For example, a particular intervention may have a short-term objective of increasing condom-related knowledge and skills, in service of the long-term goal of program participants using condoms at every act of intercourse.

The strategies that the intervention uses should be based on past research on "what works" to achieve the desired objectives and goals with similar populations. When possible, interventions that have already been rigorously evaluated and shown positive findings with similar groups and in similar settings should be *replicated* (reimplemented) (Kelly et al., 2000; Kirby, 2001). If these programs need to be *adapted* (changed) to better address the needs of the new population or setting, they should not be changed in ways that undermine what the original developer and/or research on the program has defined as the *core components* (Solomon, Card, & Malow, 2006). Core components are the basic elements of the intervention that are believed to be responsible for its effectiveness. Most effective interventions are based on one or more theories of behavior or behavior change (see chapter 6). The goals, objectives, and strategies of any prevention intervention, whether developed from scratch or adapted from an existing program, should reflect the elements of one or more such theories.

EVALUATING A PREVENTION INTERVENTION

Several types of evaluation can help to assess the effects of prevention interventions, as well as provide input to their improvement (Hotgrave, Gilliam, Gentry, & Sy, 2002). For example:

- *Formative evaluation* involves the collection of data concerning a population's needs and assets, as well as the pilot testing of an initial version of an intervention that addresses those needs and assets.
- *Process evaluation* addresses who was served by an intervention, with what activities or services, as compared to what was planned. It also can assess satisfaction among program staff and clients with the intervention as delivered.
- *Outcome evaluation* assesses whether or not an intervention achieved its intended objectives and goals—that is, whether it achieved the desired changes in the target population. Outcome evaluation that is conducted over an extended period, to assess the very long-term impacts of an intervention, is sometimes referred to as *impact evaluation*.
- *Economic evaluation* addresses the costs and consequences of HIV prevention programs through techniques such as assessing the resources consumed by the intervention and balancing the costs of the interventions with the economic and public health effects of the intervention activities. These assessment activities are sometimes referred to as *cost-effectiveness* or *cost-benefit* analysis.

COST-EFFECTIVENESS

Some interventions cost a lot of money to implement but prevent only minimally the spread of HIV. Others cost little to implement and are quite effective in changing the behaviors that spread HIV. In the age of limited resources and competing priorities, it is important to consider both the cost of implementing an HIV prevention program and the *effectiveness* of the program in changing human sexual or drug-related behaviors that cause the spread of HIV.

The Importance of Assessing Cost-Effectiveness

Sexually transmitted infections and diseases (STIs/STDs), including HIV/AIDS, cost the United States $17 billion annually (Eng & Butler, 1997). Beyond its monetary impact, HIV/AIDS exacts an immeasurable toll on the friends, family, and loved ones of HIV+ people. Despite the widely acknowledged severity of the global HIV/AIDS crisis, resources for combating the epidemic are severely limited. As a result, these scarce resources must be spent wisely, on highly effective HIV/AIDS prevention interventions.

Cost-effectiveness analyses evaluate how well interventions are meeting their goals in light of how much they cost. Goals vary by intervention and may include changing HIV-associated sexual and drug use risk behaviors, reducing HIV incidence, or increasing community involvement in prevention (Center for AIDS Prevention Studies [CAPS], 2002). For example, a cost-effectiveness analysis may compare the cost and impact of several different programs aimed at reducing unprotected sex among teenagers. The most cost-effective program is the one that causes the greatest reduction in unprotected sex for the least amount of money. Note that if a program greatly reduces unprotected sex but also costs a lot, it is not necessarily the most cost-effective one. Likewise, a program that is very cheap, but has limited impact, is usually not the most cost-effective.

Cost-effectiveness analyses of HIV/AIDS prevention interventions help people in the following ways (Marseille, 2002):

- ***Cost-effectiveness analyses help people see all the prevention options.*** Cost-effectiveness analyses require clear descriptions of the goals, costs, and effectiveness of all prevention options. Describing these programs can help people crystallize what their own goals are, as well as choose solutions that are most likely to achieve those goals.
- ***Cost-effectiveness analyses take many perspectives into account.*** A program that may not be cost-effective to a particular governmental agency may nonetheless be desirable from a societal perspective. In defining goals, the terms of the policy debate may shift from money to a broader assessment of the social good.
- ***Cost-effectiveness analyses inform rational resource allocation.*** In a world of limited resources and dire need, cost-effectiveness analyses prevent the overspending of scarce prevention dollars on less effective programs, as well as underspending on more effective ones.

Results of Cost-Effectiveness Studies

Studies have shown that, all other things being equal, *interventions targeted to areas with high HIV prevalence tend to be more cost-effective than interventions targeted to low HIV prevalence areas* (Marseille, 2002). In addition, *low cost does not mean cost-effective*. Spending money on a more expensive, more intensive intervention may be most cost-effective in the long run (Marseille, 2002). Finally, *reaching more people for the same amount of money is not always the best thing to do*; for example, passing out brochures to a lot of people produces little behavior change. By contrast, teaching a few, high-risk people to use condoms correctly, to negotiate safer sex, or to recognize and avoid high-risk situations can result in pronounced behavior change that may, as a consequence, translate into substantial reductions in HIV transmission (Marseille, 2002). Prevention interventions that have proved highly cost-effective in resource-poor settings include: sex worker interventions, male and female condom promotion, STI/STD control, voluntary counseling and testing, blood supply safety measures, and parent-to-child transmission prevention.

CULTURAL COMPETENCE IN PREVENTION

HIV prevention practitioners, researchers, and funding agencies have long recognized the importance of tailoring HIV/AIDS-related services to better meet the needs of diverse populations at risk for acquiring HIV. Behavior change cannot be promoted successfully without understanding the cultural as well as structural determinants of HIV (e.g., poverty, poor housing, low levels of educational achievement, acculturation pressures, racism, sexism) and their influence on gendered behavior, sexuality, drug use, and health service access (Worth, 1990).

Recent literature on racial/ethnic disparities in HIV/AIDS and effective HIV/AIDS prevention programs underscores the importance of *cultural competence* in the delivery of HIV/AIDS-related services (Auerbach & Coates, 2000; Betancourt et al., 2003; Bok & Morales, 2001; Vinh-Thomas et al., 2003). Cultural competence may be defined as set of congruent behaviors, attitudes, and policies—including a consideration of linguistic, socioeconomic, and functional concerns that influence behavior—that come together in a system, agency, or among professionals, thus: (1) enabling that system, agency, or those professionals to work effectively with the target population and (2) resulting in services that are accepted by the target

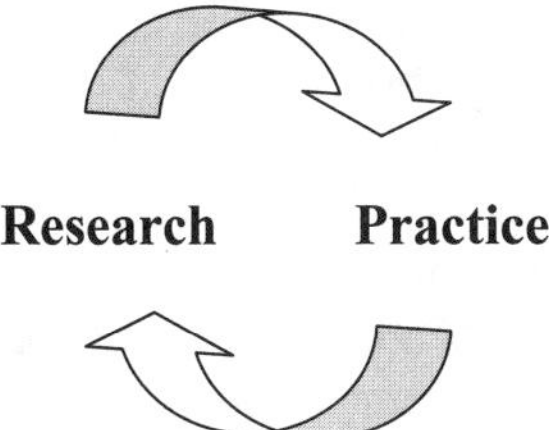

Figure 5-2 The research-to-practice feedback loop.

population (Cross, Bazron, Dennis, & Isaacs, 1989; Dana, Behn, & Gonwa, 1992; Like, Steiner, & Rubel, 1996). Culturally competent programs:

- Look inward at agency and staff beliefs, norms, and assumptions;
- Look outward at the cultural factors that influence the HIV-related behaviors and health and social service access of their clients;
- Apply an understanding of agency, client, and community needs and assets to the development and ongoing refinement of tailored client services and staff training programs; and
- Involve members of the target population and community actively and respectfully in planning, implementation, and evaluation efforts.

For a complete guide to implementing and evaluating culturally competent HIV prevention programs, see Card, Solomon, and Berman, *Tools for Building Culturally Competent HIV Prevention Programs with CD-ROM*, published by Springer Publishing Company (ISBN: 978-0-8261-1517-1) and available September 2007 at http://www.springerpub.com or through all major booksellers.

RESEARCH TO PRACTICE, AND PRACTICE TO RESEARCH

For HIV prevention efforts to advance, it is important that prevention research and prevention practice inform each other in cyclical fashion. This is represented in Figure 5-2.

Building Bridges From Research to Practice

Scientific research has documented that many prevention interventions work, and should therefore be used by many people. Unfortunately, research findings are often only published in hard-to-read research reports, theoretical papers, and literature reviews, which prevention providers seldom read. As a result, there is a gap between research and practice.

To realize the benefits of prevention research, it is imperative that effective, science-based prevention interventions be put into the hands of more prevention practitioners for widespread use. Transferring the best science-based prevention interventions to prevention providers involves identifying them, putting them in a format that can be readily used in service settings, disseminating these materials widely, and supporting their use. This process of transferal is sometimes called *technology transfer*.

Technology Transfer Tools

A number of tools and services are available to help get effective programs into the hands of service providers. The Centers for Disease Control and Prevention's (CDC's) Replicating Effective Prevention Programs (REP) initiative has developed program packages for a number of effective interventions (see http://www.cdc.gov/

hiv/projects/rep), and it provides training and technical assistance in use of these programs through the Diffusion of Effective Behavioral Interventions (DEBI) project (see http://www.effectiveinterventions.org).

Other vehicles for distributing effective HIV/AIDS prevention interventions are Sociometrics' HIV/AIDS Prevention Program Archive (HAPPA) and Program Archive on Sexuality, Health, and Adolescence (PASHA) (see http://www.socio.com/program.htm). HAPPA and PASHA each contain ready-made intervention kits that have everything needed to implement and reevaluate effective HIV/AIDS prevention programs. Each of these programs has effectively reduced risky behaviors (like unprotected sex or injection drug use) in at least one subpopulation of the United States (Card, 2001; Card, Benner, Shields, & Feinstein, 2001; Feinstein, Card, Shields, Benner, & Hamner, 2001).

The Importance of Practice Informing Research

For HIV prevention efforts to advance, it is also important for practice to inform research. The experiences of health and social service providers as they plan, adapt, and implement HIV prevention interventions in "real-world" settings are crucial to the advancement of research on the factors that influence HIV risk, the key characteristics of effective interventions, and how interventions can be made more cost-effective.

REFERENCES

Auerbach, J. D., & Coates, T. J. (2000). Commentaries–HIV prevention research: Accomplishments and challenges for the third decade of AIDS. *American Journal of Public Health, 90*(7), 1029–1032.

Betancourt, J. R., Green, A. R., Carrillo, J. E., & Ananeh-Firempong, O. (2003). Defining cultural competence: A practical framework for addressing racial/ethnic disparities in health and health care. *Public Health Reports, 118*, 293–302.

Bok, M., & Morales, J. (2001). Latino communities in the U.S. and HIV/AIDS. *Journal of HIV/AIDS Prevention and Education for Adolescents and Children, 4*(1), 61–70.

Card, J. J. (2001). The Sociometrics program archives: Promoting the dissemination of evidence-based practices through replication kits. *Research on Social Work Practice, 11*(4), 521–526.

Card, J. J., Benner, T., Shields, J. P., & Feinstein, N. (2001). The HIV/AIDS Prevention Program Archive (HAPPA): A collection of promising prevention programs in a box. *AIDS Education and Prevention, 13*(1), 1–28.

Card, J. J., Brindis, C., Peterson, J. L., & Niego, S. (2001). *Guidebook: Evaluating teen pregnancy prevention programs* (2nd ed.). Los Altos, CA: Sociometrics Corporation.

Center for AIDS Prevention Studies (CAPS). (2002). *CAPS fact sheet #12ER: Can cost-effectiveness analysis help in HIV prevention?* San Francisco: CAPS, University of California, San Francisco.

Centers for Disease Control and Prevention (CDC). (2006). Evolution of HIV/AIDS prevention programs—United States, 1981–2006. *Morbidity and Mortality Weekly Report, 55*(21), 597–603.

Centers for Disease Control and Prevention (CDC), Divisions of HIV/AIDS Prevention. (2001). *Prevention saves lives*. Atlanta, GA: CDC.

Cross, T. L., Bazron, B. J., Dennis, K. W., & Isaacs, M. R. (1989). *Towards a culturally competent system of care: A monograph on effective services for minority children who are severely emotionally disturbed*. Washington, DC: CASSP Technical Assistance Center, Georgetown University Child Development Center.

Dana, R. H., Behn, J. D., & Gonwa, T. (1992). A checklist for the examination of cultural competence in social service agencies. *Research on Social Work Practice, 2*(2), 220–233.

Eng, T. R., & Butler, W. T. (Eds.). (1997). *The hidden epidemic: Confronting sexually transmitted diseases*. Washington, DC: National Academy of Sciences.

Feinstein, N., Card, J. J., Shields, J. P., Benner, T., & Hamner, K. (2001). *Case studies in effective AIDS prevention*. Los Altos, CA: Sociometrics Corporation.

Hotgrave, D. R., Gilliam, A., Gentry, D., & Sy, F. S. (2002). Evaluating HIV prevention efforts to reduce new infections and ensure accountability. *AIDS Education and Prevention, 14*(Suppl A), 1–4.

Kelly, J. A., Heckman, T. G., Stevenson, L. Y., Williams, P. N., Ertl, T., Hays, R. B., et al. (2000). Transfer of research-based HIV prevention interventions to community service providers: Fidelity and adaptation. *AIDS Education and Prevention*, *12*(Suppl A), 87–98.

Kirby, D. (2001). *Emerging answers: Research findings on programs to reduce teen pregnancy.* Washington, DC: National Campaign to Prevent Teen Pregnancy.

Like, R. C., Steiner, R. P., & Rubel, A. J. (1996). STFM core curriculum guidelines: Recommended core curriculum guidelines on culturally sensitive and competent health care. *Family Medicine*, *28*, 291–297.

Marseille, E., Morin, S. F., Collins, C., Summers, T., Coates, T. J., & Kahn, J. G. (2002). Cost-effectiveness of HIV prevention in developing countries. In L. Pieperl, S. Coffey, O. Bacon, & P. Volberding (Eds.), *HIV InSite knowledge base.* San Francisco: Center for HIV Information, University of California, San Francisco.

Solomon, J., Card, J. J., & Malow, R. M. (2006). Adapting efficacious interventions: Advancing translational research in HIV prevention. *Evaluation and the Health Professions*, *29*(2), 162–194.

Vinh-Thomas, P., Bunch, M. M., & Card, J. J. (2003). A research-based tool for identifying and strengthening culturally competent and evaluation-ready HIV/AIDS prevention programs. *AIDS Education and Prevention*, *15*(6), 481–498.

Worth, D. (1990). Minority women and AIDS: Culture, race, and gender. In D. A. Feldman (Ed.), *Culture and AIDS* (pp. 111–135). Westport, CT: Praeger.

Instructor Resources

LEARNING ACTIVITIES

ACTIVITY 1:

Assignment: Primary, Secondary, and Tertiary Prevention

Objective: To understand different ways of preventing HIV/AIDS.

Minimum time: 15 minutes

Preventive measures are classified according to when they occur in the progression of injury or illness:

Primary Prevention strategies attempt to stop the occurrence of injury or illness.

Secondary Prevention strategies attempt to decrease any further development of the injury or disease once it happens.

Tertiary Prevention strategies attempt to alleviate the effects of injury, disease, and disability.

- What are some examples of primary prevention of HIV/AIDS?
- What are some examples of secondary prevention of HIV/AIDS?
- What are some examples of tertiary prevention of HIV/AIDS?

ACTIVITY 2:

Assignment: Most Effective Level of Prevention

Objective: To understand levels of HIV/AIDS prevention.

Write a three- to five-page paper in response to the following question:

In your opinion, which is the most effective level of prevention for HIV/AIDS?

Defend your opinion with evidence from actual prevention interventions.

ACTIVITY 3:

Assignment: Tracking Teen Activities for HIV/AIDS Prevention

Objective: To understand how to alter HIV prevention strategies to address new social trends.

Findings reported by Child Trends (http://childtrendsdatabank.org) show that the percentage of 10th graders for whom religion is very important increased in 2002 (from 32 to 35%), as did the percentage who regularly attend religious services (from

40 to 42%). By contrast, school-based activities such as participation in athletics, music, and other performing arts declined modestly during that time.

Write a three- to five-page paper on how HIV/AIDS prevention activities aimed at American youth could change to reflect these trends.

DISCUSSION QUESTIONS

1. The individuals at highest risk of HIV infection also often face the most limited access to prevention and treatment programs. Discuss why each of the following groups might have difficulty accessing resources: men who have sex with men, injection drug users, young people, and women.
2. Why is it important for an HIV prevention program to have both long-term goals and short-term objectives?
3. Describe any HIV prevention programs in your community of which you are aware (public service announcements on television or radio, health education programs offered in school or community groups, etc.). How would you rate their effectiveness? Why?
4. Why do you think cultural competence is an important factor in the overall effectiveness of an HIV prevention program?

QUIZ

1. Define individuals at high risk of HIV infection.
2. Which setting would be an appropriate place for HIV prevention interventions?
   a) Schools
   b) Workplaces
   c) Churches and religious institutions
   d) Bars, clubs, and other social settings
   e) All of the above
   f) None of the above
3. _____ are basic elements of an intervention that are believed to be responsible for its effectiveness.
   a) Short-term objectives
   b) Long-term goals
   c) Needs and assets
   d) Core components
4. Match the evaluation method with its definition:

a) Formative evaluation	1) Assesses the long-term effects of an intervention
b) Process evaluation	2) Assesses whether an intervention achieved its objectives
c) Outcome evaluation	3) Pilot testing of an intervention
d) Economic evaluation	4) Assesses who the intervention served and with what activities
e) Impact evaluation	5) Addresses the intervention costs and consequences

5. STIs/STDs, including HIV/AIDS, cost the United States how much every year?

6. True or False: In any given community, the least expensive HIV prevention program is, by definition, the most cost-effective one.
7. True or False: In any given community, the HIV prevention program that reaches the most people will be the most effective.
8. A culturally competent program would consider which of the following factors of its clients?
   a) Language
   b) Socioeconomic status
   c) Education level
   d) Race and ethnicity
   e) Cultural mores
   f) All of the above
   g) None of the above

ANSWERS

1. "High-risk" individuals include those who engage in unprotected sexual intercourse, have multiple sex partners, or use injection drugs.
2. **E.** Prevention interventions should be delivered in a wide variety of settings to reach a broad audience.
3. **D.** Core components are the basic elements of the intervention that are believed to be responsible for its effectiveness.
4. **A–3; B–4; C–2; D–5; E–1.** *Formative evaluation* involves the collection of data concerning a population's needs and assets, as well as the pilot testing of an initial version of an intervention that addresses those needs and assets. *Process evaluation* addresses who was served by an intervention, with what activities or services, as compared to what was planned. It also can assess satisfaction among program staff and clients with the intervention as delivered. *Outcome evaluation* assesses whether or not an intervention achieved its intended objectives and goals—that is, whether it achieved the desired changes in the target population. Outcome evaluation that is conducted over an extended period, to assess the very long-term impacts of an interventions, is sometimes referred to as *impact evaluation*. *Economic evaluation* addresses the costs and consequences of HIV prevention programs through techniques such as assessing the resources consumed by the intervention and balancing the costs of the interventions with the economic and public health effects of the intervention activities.
5. STIs/STDs, including HIV/AIDS, cost the United States $17 billion annually.
6. **False.** The most cost-effective program is one that causes the greatest impact for the least amount of money.
7. **False.** Reaching more people may not necessarily create the most impact. Handing out brochures to a lot of people will likely produce little behavior change; teaching high-risk individuals to practice safer sex, by contrast, may have a much greater impact in overall HIV reduction.
8. **F.** Cultural competence may be defined as a set of congruent behaviors, attitudes, and policies that come together to ensure successful work with a target population.

WEB RESOURCES

HIV/AIDS Prevention Information

CDC's National Center for HIV, STD, and TB Prevention

http://www.cdc.gov/nchstp/od/nchstp.html

Includes information on prevention media campaigns, publications, and a collection of slides and graphics.

The Body's Safe Sex and Prevention Section

http://www.thebody.com/safesex/safer.html

Features a risk assessment survey and a collection of articles from media sources on a variety of prevention issues. Topics range from the general to specific concerns of gay men, drug users, women, and youth. The site also offers information about STDs and vaccines.

California AIDS Clearinghouse

http://www.hivinfo.org

Offers a variety of HIV educational and prevention materials, in both English and Spanish. A primary source of the California AIDS Hotline's printed materials.

Resources for Best Practices in HIV/AIDS Prevention

The Centers for Disease Control: Replicating Effective Programs Plus

http://www.cdc.gov/hiv/projects/rep/default.htm

Helps service providers identify and implement HIV/AIDS prevention programs that have been shown to work.

Diffusion of Effective Behavioral Interventions for HIV

http://www.effectiveinterventions.org/

Provides high-quality training and technical assistance for selected evidence-based HIV/STD prevention interventions to state and community program staff.

Sociometrics Corporation: Program Archives

http://www.socio.com/program.htm

Effective HIV/AIDS prevention programs can be found in the "HIV/AIDS Prevention Program Archive" (HAPPA) and the "Program Archive on Sexuality, Health, and Adolescence" (PASHA).

Center for AIDS Prevention Services (CAPS) Model Prevention Programs

http://www.caps.ucsf.edu/projects/

Describes HIV prevention programs that were designed by CAPS researchers and that have either been evaluated or are in the process of being evaluated.

HIV/AIDS Prevention Fact Sheet Compilations

Fact Sheets From Centers for Disease Control and Prevention

http://www.cdc.gov/hiv/pubs/facts.htm

Topics include transmission (populations affected/risk behaviors), vaccine research, virology, and CDC prevention programs. Some fact sheets are available in Spanish.

Center for AIDS Prevention (CAPS) HIV Prevention Fact Sheets

http://www.caps.ucsf.edu/pubs/FS/

Include information about condom use, the role of HIV testing in prevention, and the prevention needs of women, adolescents, homeless people, African Americans, Latinos, sex workers, and substance users. Fact sheets are available in English and Spanish. Select fact sheets are available in Kiswahili.

University of California, San Francisco: HIV Insite

http://hivinsite.ucsf.edu/InSite?page=Prevention

Discusses a variety of prevention issues, with links to basic fact sheets from a variety of reputable sources.

Resources for Program Evaluation

Sociometrics' Program Evaluation Resources

http://www.socio.com/eval.htm

Offers a wide variety of evaluation products and services to professionals across the world. The evaluation workshops and training services, technical publications, evaluation tools, and data sets are all designed to assist practitioners, administrators, evaluators, and funders to design and implement successful evaluation systems.

Centers for Disease Control and Prevention Evaluation Working Group

http://www.cdc.gov/eval/index.htm

Provides an overall framework for evaluation and program planning, and additional resources that may help when applying the framework.

Resources for Cultural Competence in HIV Prevention

Sociometrics' Cultural Competence Resources

Provides toolkits for developing, implementing, evaluating, and replicating culturally competent HIV prevention interventions.

http://www.socio.com/srch/summary/misc/ccsub.htm

RECOMMENDED READING

Overview of HIV/AIDS Prevention

Preventing AIDS: Theories and Methods of Behavioral Interventions (DiClemente & Peterson, 1994)

DiClemente, R. J., & Peterson, J. L. (Eds.). (1994). Preventing AIDS: Theories and methods of behavioral interventions. *New York: Plenum.*

This book describes the principal theories and methods employed in behavioral change interventions, and examines their impact in a variety of populations. Chapters are written by behavioral researchers who have conducted major research on HIV primary prevention interventions.

Handbook of HIV Prevention (Peterson & DiClemente, 2000)

Peterson, J. L., & DiClemente, R. J. (Eds.). (2000). Handbook of HIV prevention. *New York: Kluwer Academic/Plenum.*

This book provides a broad and comprehensive assessment of HIV prevention research mainly conducted in the United States. The volume is divided into a number of chapters, each addressing a particular at-risk population. Each chapter describes the scope of the HIV threat for this specific population, epidemiology information about risk and preventive practices, intervention efficacy with this population, and unmet research and policy needs. It is a good source of information about effective intervention approaches and how the field may enhance the efficacy of these intervention strategies.

Evaluating HIV/AIDS Prevention

Evaluating HIV Prevention Programs (Holtgrave, Gilliam, & Gentry, 2002)

Special Supplement to AIDS Education and Prevention:
Holtgrave, D. R., Gilliam, A., & Gentry, D. (Eds.). (2002). Evaluating HIV prevention programs. AIDS Education and Prevention, 14*(3 Suppl A).*

These articles discuss formative, process, outcome, and impact evaluations in HIV prevention, as well as their policy implications.

Replicating Best Practices in HIV/AIDS Prevention

Turning HIV Prevention Research Into Practice (Neumann, Sogolow, & Kelly, 2000)

Special Supplement to AIDS Education and Prevention:
Neumann, M. S., Sogolow, E. D., & Kelly, J. A. (Eds.). (2000). Turning HIV prevention research into practice. AIDS Education and Prevention, 12 *(5 Suppl A).*

These articles discuss access to and use of effective HIV prevention interventions.

POWERPOINT SLIDES

(Note: A full-color version of these slides, with graphics, is also available on the CD-ROM.)

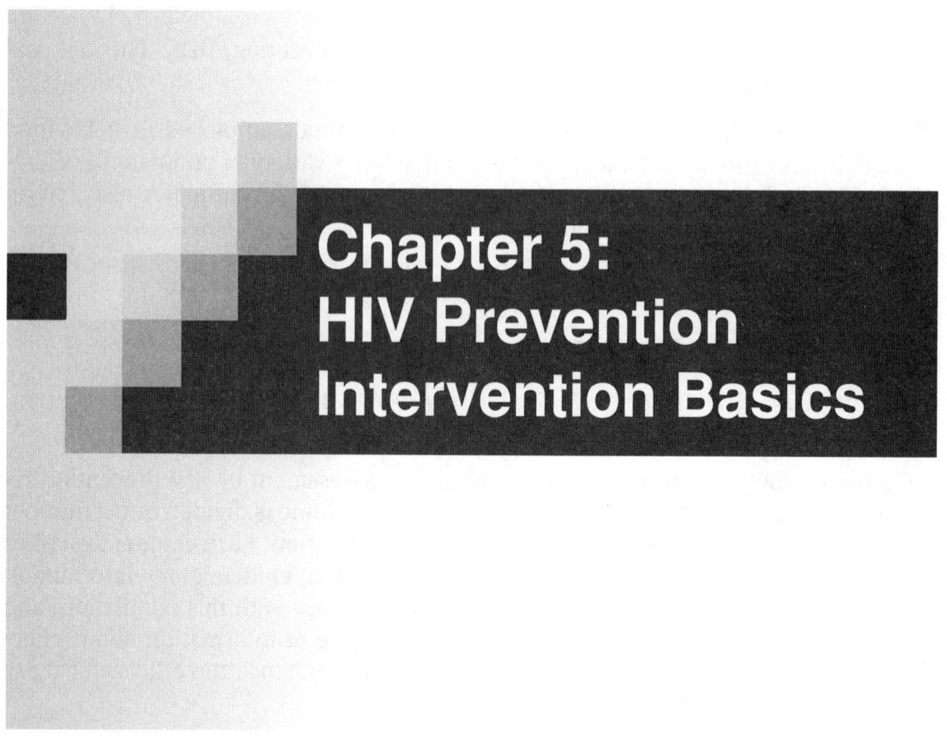

HIV Prevention Intervention Basics

- PREVENTION: Scientifically based, strategic interventions into the natural evolution of causal chain of events leading to injury or illness
- Primary prevention: Attempts to stop the occurrence of injury or illness
- Secondary prevention: Attempts to decrease any further development of the injury or disease once it has happened
- Tertiary prevention: Attempts to alleviate the effects of injury, disease, and disability

HIV/AIDS Prevention Works

- Rates of new HIV infections in the United States have slowed from 150,000+/year (late 1980s) to 40,000 in 2001.
- In New York City, prevalence among injection drug users in drug treatment has dropped from 34% in 1990 to approximately 4% in 1998.
- Between 1992 and 1998, the number of U.S. infants who acquired HIV through parent-to-child transmission declined by 73%.
- Prevention efforts dramatically reduced the number of AIDS cases in Thailand and Uganda.

Advances in Primary Prevention of HIV/AIDS

- Primary prevention entails *stopping the behaviors through which HIV is transmitted.*
- Effective prevention interventions are theory-based, culturally tailored, and designed to enhance people's cognitive, social, and risk reduction skills.

Advances in Primary Prevention of HIV/AIDS (continued)

- In the United States, prevention interventions have reduced unsafe sex and drug use among:
  - the general population,
  - men who have sex with men,
  - injection drug users,
  - young people,
  - heterosexual men and women,
  - HIV+ people, and
  - other high-risk groups.

Best Practices in HIV/AIDS Prevention

Effective HIV prevention programs:

- Take into account sociocultural factors and recognize the needs of traditionally disempowered groups
- Combine scientific theory with awareness of social norms, gender inequalities, stigma, discrimination, and poverty
- Focus on *"high-risk" people* and are given in a *variety of settings*
  - "High-risk" individuals include: people who engage in unprotected sex, have multiple sex partners, or use injection drugs
  - Settings should include: neighborhoods, schools, health care settings, etc.

Cost-Effectiveness of HIV/AIDS Prevention

- Sexually transmitted infections and diseases including HIV/AIDS cost the United States **$17 billion annually.**
- Beyond the monetary impact, HIV/AIDS exacts an immeasurable toll on the friends, family, and loved ones of HIV+ people.
- Resources to combat the epidemic are severely limited and must be spent on interventions that avert HIV transmission in cost-efficient ways.

Why Is Cost-Effectiveness Important?

- Cost-effectiveness analyses evaluate how well interventions meet their goals, in light of how much they cost.
- Cost-effectiveness analyses of HIV/AIDS prevention interventions:
  - help people see all prevention options;
  - take many perspectives into account; and
  - inform rational resource allocation.
- Results of cost-effectiveness studies suggest:
  - interventions targeted to areas with high HIV prevalence are most cost-effective;
  - low cost does not mean cost-effectiveness; and
  - reaching more people for the same amount of money isn't always the best thing to do.

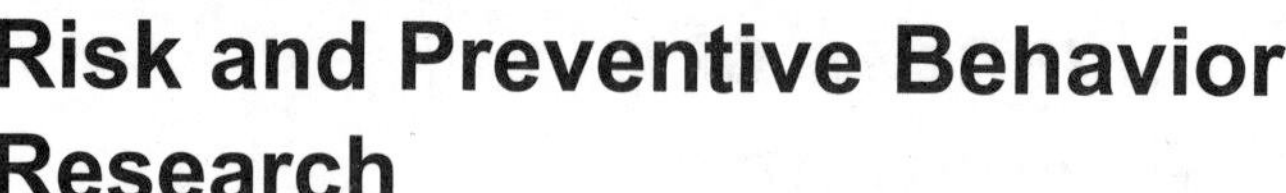

Risk and Preventive Behavior Research

National U.S. surveys have taught us what we know:

- The National Longitudinal Survey of Adolescent Health (Add Health)
- National Health and Social Life Survey (NHSLS)
- Youth Risk Behavior Survey (YRBS)
- National Health Interview Survey (NHIS)

Evaluating HIV/AIDS Prevention Efforts

Formative Evaluation: understanding a population's needs and assets, and pilot testing the interventions based on those needs and assets

Process Evaluation: answers who was served, with what HIV prevention intervention, where, and when

Outcome Evaluation: assesses whether or not an intervention achieved its intended short-term objectives

Impact Evaluation: assesses the long-term consequences of a prevention program

Economic Evaluation: addresses the costs and consequences of HIV prevention programs

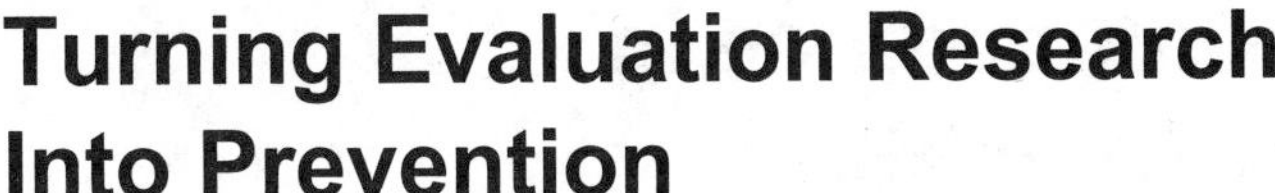

Turning Evaluation Research Into Prevention

It is imperative to put effective, science-based prevention interventions in the hands of prevention practitioners.

- Building bridges from research to practice is necessary.
- Research findings are often published in sources prevention providers rarely read.
- Transferring the best science-based prevention interventions to prevention providers involves identifying, translating, disseminating, and supporting the use of these programs.
- This process of transferal is called "technology transfer."

Best Practices in Program Replication

Some key issues in successful prevention program replication include:

- quality and attractiveness of the intervention;
- attention to local context;
- investment of the implementing agency;
- leadership;
- partnership and collaborations;
- fidelity of the implementation; and
- plans and resources for evaluation.

Cultural Competence in HIV/AIDS Prevention

- HIV/AIDS prevention practitioners, researchers, and funding agencies have long recognized the importance of tailored HIV/AIDS prevention programs to meet the needs of diverse populations.
- Racial disparities in HIV/AIDS morbidity, mortality, and prevention underscore the importance of cultural congruency in the delivery of services and care.
- Culturally congruent prevention programs are developed for and implemented by a defined, specific target population, usually with the participation of that population.
- Cultural congruence throughout the prevention program life cycle can greatly magnify the program's effectiveness.

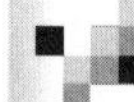

Prevention Program Life Cycle

1. Program Development

The prevention intervention is created and designed. Culturally congruent program development includes:

- ☐ encouraging community involvement;
- ☐ assessing community needs and assets;
- ☐ defining an intervention based on community needs and assets;
- ☐ describing program goals and objectives;
- ☐ developing a program model, often with community input; and
- ☐ creating program materials, often with community input.

The Program Life Cycle

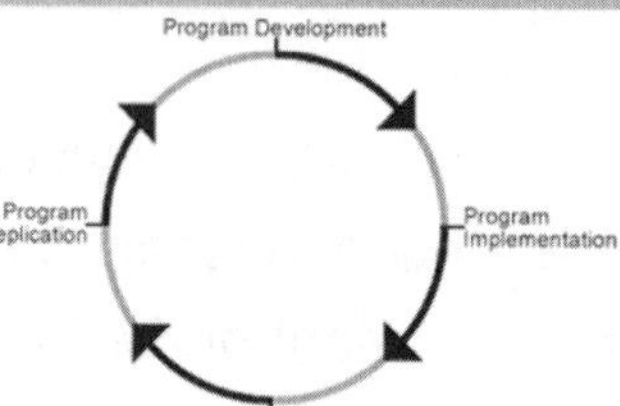

Prevention Program Life Cycle (continued)

2. Program Implementation

The program is given to clients. Culturally competent program implementation includes:

- □ staff recruitment (from the target community or those who know the community well);
- □ training of staff, using culturally meaningful and appropriate strategies;
- □ recruitment of participants, using strategies that are sensitive to the population;
- □ delivery of services;
- □ monitoring of the program;
- □ soliciting feedback; and
- □ adapting the program to the feedback.

The Program Life Cycle

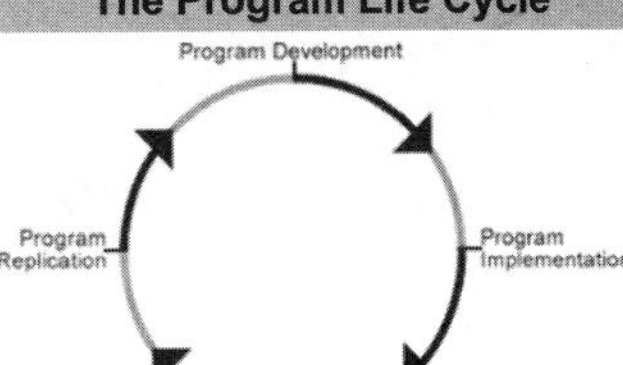

Prevention Program Life Cycle (continued)

3. Program Evaluation

Program performance is compared to objectives so prevention providers can gauge success, as well as decide what changes are needed.

4. Program Replication

Transferring an effective program from one context to another. Through program replication, a successful program can be shared, and practitioners can be saved from "reinventing the wheel."

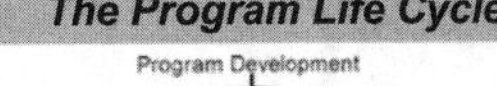

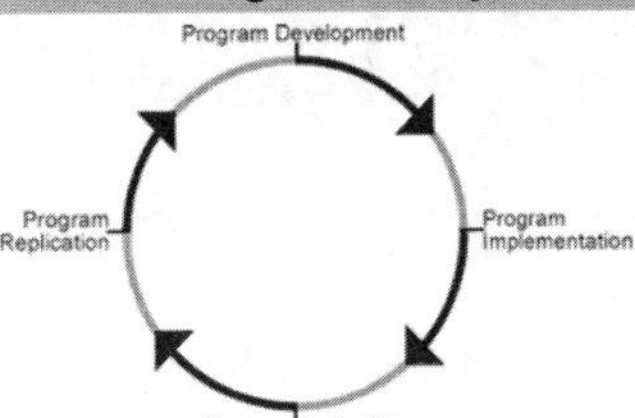

Learning Objectives

- Define, compare, and contrast the intrapersonal behavioral models: the health belief model, the theory of reasoned action, the theory of planned behavior, the transtheoretical model, and the harm reduction model
- Define, compare, and contrast the interpersonal behavioral models: AIDS risk reduction model, social cognitive theory, and the information-motivation-behavioral skills model
- Define, compare, and contrast the community behavioral models: diffusion of innovation, leadership-focused model, social movement theory, and the theory of gender and power

Key Terms

AIDS risk reduction model
behavior
diffusion of innovations theory
formal theory
harm reduction model
health belief model
information-motivation-behavioral skills model
interpersonal
intrapersonal
leadership-focused models
perceived behavioral control
self-efficacy
social cognitive theory
social movement theory
stages of change model
theory of gender and power
theory of planned behavior
theory of reasoned action
transtheoretical model

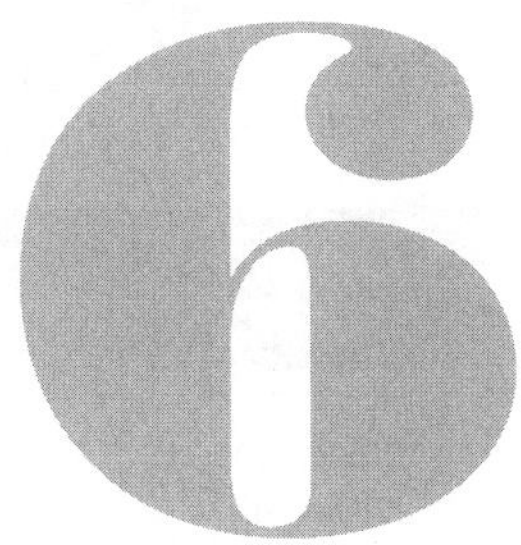

Behavioral Theories and Models

HIV transmission is dependent on people's behavior. Behavior is shaped by what is in individuals' minds, including knowledge, attitudes, beliefs, motivation, past experience, and skills. Behavior is also shaped by people's interpersonal experiences—the opinions, advice, support, and behavior of their friends, family, coworkers, and others. In addition, behavior is influenced by the social structures, movements, and policies of communities and their institutions (Friedman, Des Jarlais, & Ward, 1994; National Cancer Institute, 2005).

A variety of theories and models (often called *formal theories*) about how these factors interact to influence behavior and behavior change have been useful to the development, implementation, evaluation, and subsequent adaptation of HIV prevention interventions (CDC, 2001; Kalichman, 1998). According to one analysis (Fishbein et al., 2001), the theories that most commonly underlie effective HIV prevention interventions collectively indicate that eight factors must be in place for positive behavior change (such as consistent use of condoms with sexual partners) to take place:

1. The person has formed a positive intention to perform the behavior.
2. There are no environmental constraints that make it impossible for the behavior to be performed.
3. The person has the skills necessary to perform the behavior.
4. The person has a positive attitude toward the behavior.
5. The person perceives more social pressure to perform the behavior than to not perform it.
6. The person perceives behavior to be more consistent than inconsistent with his or her self-image (e.g., the person believes him- or herself to be the "kind of person" who would use condoms).
7. The person's emotional reaction to performing the behavior is more positive than negative.
8. The person perceives *self-efficacy* to perform the behavior—that is, he or she believes that he or she is capable of performing the behavior under different circumstances.

This suggests that a prevention effort will be most likely to reduce HIV risk behavior if it can successfully address all or most of these factors.

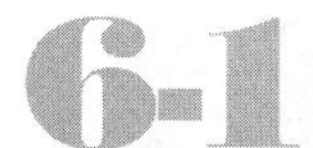

Formal Theories and Models of Behavior and Behavior Change (Herlocher, Hoff, & DeCarlo, 1996; Kalichman, 1998; National Cancer Institute, 2005)

LEVEL OF INFLUENCE	THEORY	BRIEF DESCRIPTION
Intrapersonal (Individual)	Health Belief Model	Behavior is influenced by perception of the threat of a health problem, and assessment of the benefits vs. costs of engaging in behavior to prevent it.
	Theory of Reasoned Action	Behavior is influenced by beliefs about the behavior's consequences, perception of social pressure, and intentions.
	Theory of Planned Behavior	Behavior is influenced by beliefs about the behavior's consequences, perception of social pressure, perceived control over the behaviors, and intentions.
	Transtheoretical Model (Stages of Change)	A person moves through stages of readiness to action that include: no risk perception, risk perception, preparation for action, action, and maintenance; relapses into prior behavior may occur.
	Harm Reduction Model	The negative consequences of harmful behaviors can be reduced, taking into consideration current attitudes and beliefs.
Interpersonal	Social Cognitive Theory	Behavior interacts with and is influenced by personal factors (self-efficacy, skills, motivation) and environmental factors (observational learning, reinforcement).
	AIDS Risk Reduction Model (ARRM)	People progress through different levels toward behavior change, including labeling themselves as at risk, committing to change, and enacting new behaviors, often with the help of others.
	Information-Motivation-Behavioral Skills (IMB) Model	Information and motivation influence behavior directly; they also influence it indirectly by influencing behavioral skills. Support from others is an important aspect of motivation to change.
Community	Diffusion of Innovation	New ideas, products, and social practices spread within a community or from one community to another; the pattern of spread depends on the social group and the nature of the innovation.
	Leadership-Focused Models	For behavior change to take place, group leaders must make innovations acceptable or "cool" to their group members.
	Social Movement Theory	Behavior change takes place when large groups of people unite to address the behavioral problem.
	Theory of Gender and Power	Economic iniquities, social norms, and power inequities lead to socioeconomic circumstances, interpersonal conditions, and behaviors that put women at risk of adverse health outcomes.

Twelve formal theories that focus on intrapersonal (individual), interpersonal, and community influences on behavior are summarized in Table 6-1 and discussed in the remainder of this chapter. Most HIV prevention interventions that have been effective in changing behavior are based on one or a combination of several of these theories.

HEALTH BELIEF MODEL

The *health belief model* (Rosenstock, Strecher, & Becker, 1994), represented in Figure 6-1, is based on the premise that a person must perceive a threat to him- or herself before he or she will take preventive action. According to this model (see Figure 6-1), whether people change their risky behaviors (like unsafe sex or drug-use) depends on (Kalichman, 1998):

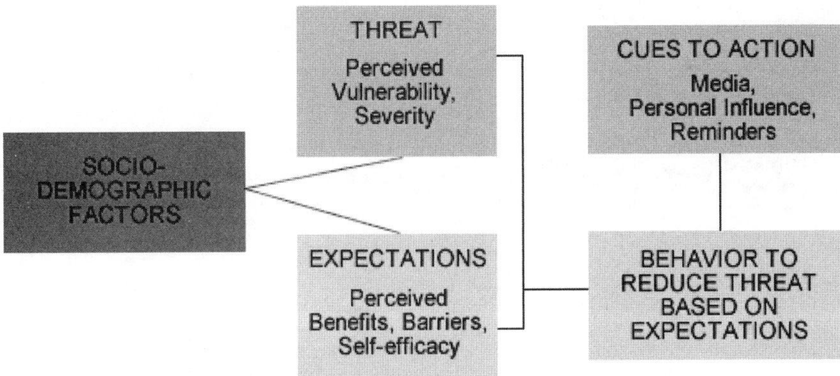

Figure 6-1 Health belief model (Kalichman, 1998, p. 40, Figure 2.2).

1. Sociodemographic factors (such as age, sex, gender, race, ethnicity, and socioeconomic status).
2. The threat posed by the illness, including people's perceived vulnerability to the illness, as well as the perceived severity of the illness.
3. Their expectations about the benefits of and barriers to changing behaviors, as well as their expectations about their own ability to change behavior.
4. Cues to action in the environment, like easy-access condom dispensers, mentions and depictions of safe sex in movies and music, posters and fliers, etc.

When applied to HIV prevention, the health belief model theorizes that people's willingness to change their risky behaviors corresponds to their perceived vulnerability to HIV/AIDS, their beliefs about the severity of HIV/AIDS, their expectations about their ability to perform less risky behaviors and the benefits of performing these behaviors, and their exposure to environmental cues that either encourage or discourage behavior change.

THEORY OF REASONED ACTION

According to the *theory of reasoned action* (Fishbein & Ajzen, 1975), represented in Figure 6-2, changing risky behaviors is not just a matter of translating knowledge into action. Instead, behavior change is the last link in a causal chain that also involves beliefs, attitudes, norms, and intentions. The chain begins with two kinds of beliefs: people's beliefs about the consequences of a given risky behavior, and their beliefs about other people's opinions of the risky behavior. Beliefs about the

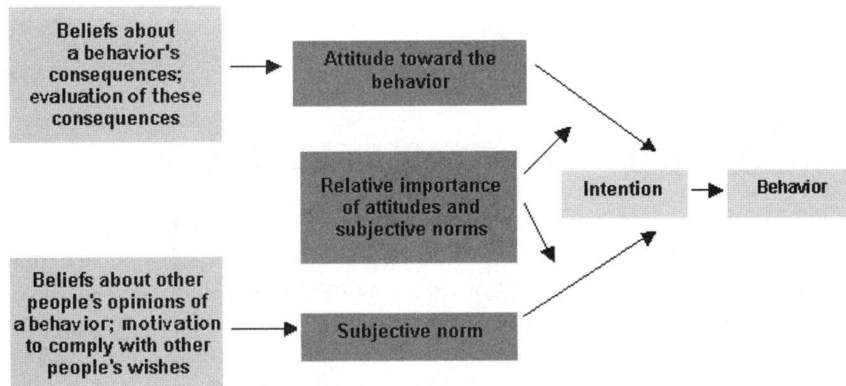

Figure 6-2 Theory of reasoned action (Kalichman, 1998, p. 31, Figure 2.3).

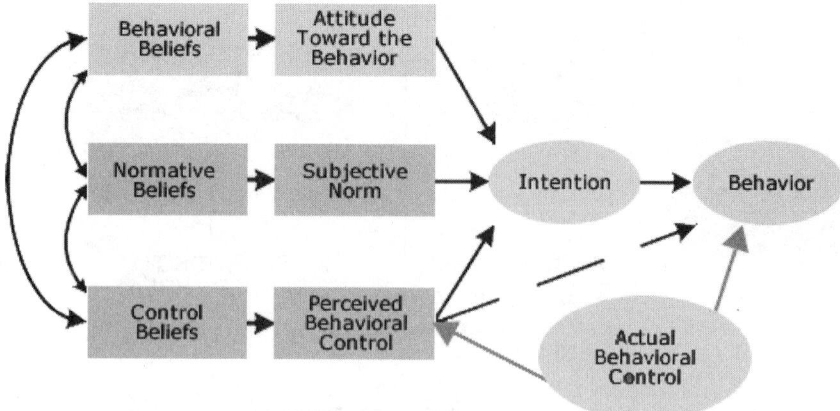

Figure 6-3 Theory of planned behavior (Ajzen, 1991).

consequences of the act combine with evaluations of those consequences to form an attitude toward the behavior. Similarly, beliefs about other people's opinions combine with motivations to comply with others' expectations to form subjective social norms. If a person's attitudes and subjective norms regarding the risky behavior are sufficiently negative, he or she may develop the intention to change the risky behavior. The intention to change behavior, in turn, is necessary for behavior change (Ajzen & Fishbein, 1980; Kalichman, 1998).

In the context of HIV prevention, the theory of reason action assumes that to reduce risk, people must perceive that particular sexual or drug use behaviors bring serious health consequences, and they must also perceive that others who are important to them hold negative views of those risky behaviors. These beliefs lead to negative attitudes toward the behaviors and motivation to change them, which in turn leads to intention to change and ultimately to behavior change itself.

THEORY OF PLANNED BEHAVIOR

One limitation of the theory of reasoned action is that it does not account for the fact that some behaviors are easier to control than others. To address this limitation, the theory's creators added a new component—*perceived behavioral control*—to their model. Perceived behavioral control, much like self-efficacy, refers to how much control a person thinks he or she has over performing a certain behavior, such as using a condom or cleaning injection drug paraphernalia. Figure 6-3 illustrates the new model, which the authors named the *theory of planned behavior* (Ajzen, 1991). Both the theory of reasoned action and the theory of planned behavior have been used to predict and explain why people do or do not perform a variety of sexual health-related behaviors, including contraceptive and condom use (Fishbein, Middlestadt, & Hitchcock, 1994).

TRANSTHEORETICAL MODEL (STAGES OF CHANGE)

The *transtheoretical model* (Prochaska, DiClemente, & Norcross, 1992), represented in Figure 6-4, is sometimes referred to as the *stages of change* model, as it says that people move through a series of stages toward behavior change. A person's advancement to a higher stage marks an increase in her or his motivation for, confidence about, and commitment to a change in behavior. People do not always advance straight through the stages, however. Because changing complex, intimate behaviors can be difficult, people often relapse to previous stages (Prochaska et al., 1992).

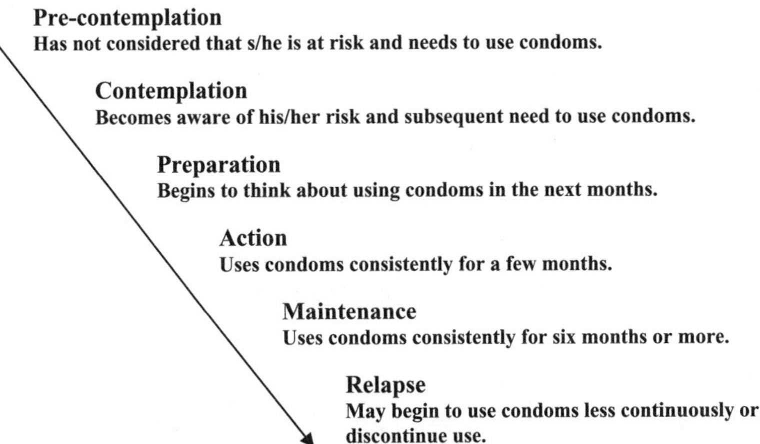

Figure 6-4 Transtheoretical model (stages of change) (Kalichman, 1998, p. 44, Figure 2.5).

One of the strengths of the transtheoretical model is that it allows HIV prevention practitioners and health care providers to tailor their interventions to the client's stage. Interventions then help the person advance to the next stage, until the behavior change is achieved and maintained (Prochaska et al., 1992).

HARM REDUCTION MODEL

Many interventions aim for complete abstinence from risky behavior. The *harm reduction model*, in contrast, aims to lessen the negative consequences of these behaviors, both for the people performing them and for the general public, while taking into consideration current attitudes, beliefs, and abilities (Herlocher, Hoff, & DeCarlo, 1996; Marlatt, 1998).

For example, needle-exchange programs accept that most injection drug users (IDUs) will have a difficult time in stopping their use of drugs. Therefore, harm reduction approaches attempt to protect the IDUs and their sex partners from HIV by providing IDUs with clean needles as a strategy to avoid their becoming infected with HIV and transmitting it to others. Studies show that needle-exchange programs reduce HIV transmission (Des Jarlais, Friedman, & Ward, 1993). Other examples of effective harm reduction strategies include:

- Methadone treatment (in which injectable opioids such as heroine and morphine are replaced with methadone, which is taken by mouth and does not cause the same level of cognitive impairment as do injectable opioids).
- "Safe-use" education campaigns, which show IDUs how to sterilize their injection equipment with bleach and water.
- Offering drug treatment instead of imprisonment to drug offenders.
- Decriminalizing sex work, so that sex workers can have access to the same legal, social, and medical protections as other people.
- Teaching safer sex practices to adolescents and young adults.
- Making condoms readily available to adolescents and young adults.

Despite their proven ability to reduce HIV transmission, many harm reduction approaches are quite controversial in the United States, where they clash with prevailing emphases on abstinence from extramarital intercourse and "zero tolerance" of drug use. Despite evidence to the contrary, people fear that making extramarital sex and drug use safer will make these activities more socially acceptable

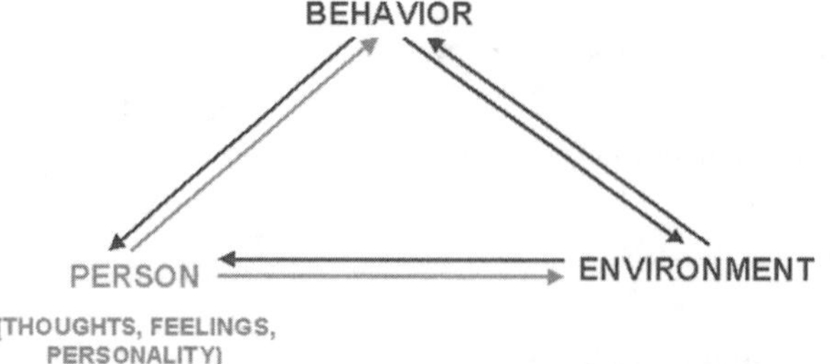

Figure 6-5 Social cognitive theory (Kalichman, 1998, p. 43, Figure 2.4).

and commonplace (MacCoun, 1998). There is no empirical evidence to indicate that this fear is justified.

SOCIAL COGNITIVE THEORY

Social cognitive theory (Bandura, 1986), represented in Figure 6-5, views people's lives as made up of interactions between their internal state and events, which are their thoughts, feelings, and personality (P); their behaviors (B); and their external social and physical environments (E). Because these three components interact with one another, changes to each component are essential to achieving behavior change. In the context of HIV prevention, to reduce risk in the psychological component, people need to know about HIV/AIDS and to believe in their own ability to perform risk-reducing behaviors (that is, they must have *self-efficacy*). To reduce risk in the behavior component, people need to practice the safer behaviors. Finally, risk-reduction in the external component involves increasing social support

Drs. Gina Wingood and Ralph DiClemente of Emory University and their colleagues have developed several interventions for African American women that have shown positive effects on sexual risk behaviors:

- SiSTA was designed for African American women ages 18–29 (DiClemente & Wingood, 1995).
- SiHLE was developed for African American adolescent females ages 14–18 (DiClemente et al., 2004).
- WiLLOW was designed for HIV+ women ages 18–50 and was originally tested with a sample that was largely African American (Wingood et al., 2004).

All three of these programs are based on social cognitive theory and the theory of gender and power. *Social cognitive theory* informed the common focus in SiSTA, SiHLE, and WiLLOW on increasing participants' knowledge, positive attitudes, self-efficacy, and skills pertaining to safer sex behaviors, particularly consistent and correct condom use. This theory also informed these interventions' emphasis on modeling of safer sex behaviors for participants, including proper application of condoms and the use of culturally appropriate assertive communication skills to negotiate condom use.

The *theory of gender and power* (see Figure 6.9) informed the common focus in SiSTA, SiHLE, and WiLLOW on fostering partner norms that support consistent condom use within the context of a male-female relationship in which women tend to feel subordinated to men. It also informed the intervention's treatment of the impact of gender-based violence and abuse on HIV risk and its provision of follow-up referrals to counseling and shelters to women in unhealthy relationships.

Figure 6-6 Three effective interventions based on social cognitive theory and the theory of gender and power.

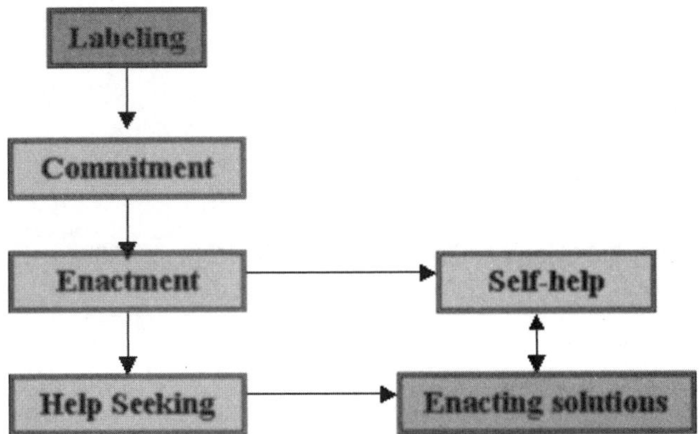

Figure 6-7 AIDS risk reduction model (Catania, Kegeles, & Coates, 1990).

for the new and improved behaviors (Kalichman, 1998). For examples of effective HIV prevention interventions based on social cognitive theory, see Figure 6-6.

AIDS RISK REDUCTION MODEL (ARRM)

AIDS risk reduction model, or ARRM (Catania, Kegeles, & Coates, 1990), represented in Figure 6-7, was developed specifically to organize the many factors that influence whether people change their HIV risk behaviors.

ARRM is a stage model, which means that people progress through different levels toward behavior change. According to ARRM, people must first label themselves as vulnerable to HIV infection (stage 1). People label themselves as "at risk" based on knowledge of how HIV is transmitted, recognition of their personal susceptibility, a belief that having HIV/AIDS is undesirable, and a perception of social norms against risky behaviors. Next, people commit to changing their behaviors (stage 2). They do this based on the conclusion that the benefits of changing outweigh the costs, a perception that behavior change does not interfere with enjoyment of sex (or drugs), a belief that behavior change will lower risk of getting HIV/AIDS, a belief in their own ability to change the behavior, and the presence of social support for the behavior change. Finally, people enact the new, less risky behaviors, in part by seeking other people's help (stage 3). Successful behavior change is more likely when self-help and social support resources are available and when a person can communicate effectively with sex and drug-use partners.

INFORMATION-MOTIVATION-BEHAVIORAL SKILLS (IMB) MODEL

According to the *information-motivation-behavioral skills (IMB) model* of behavioral risk reduction, which is represented in Figure 6-8, three factors contribute to HIV risk-related behavioral change. First, information regarding HIV/AIDS transmission and prevention must be relevant and easy to apply in the person's environment. Second, motivation to change HIV/AIDS-risk behavior must come from both from the person's own attitudes toward the change and from other people's support. Third, the person must have behavioral skills for performing specific HIV/AIDS-preventive acts and believe in his or her ability to perform the acts (Fisher & Fisher, 1992).

As the figure shows, information and motivation can either act through behavioral skills to result in preventive behavior, or they can directly influence people's

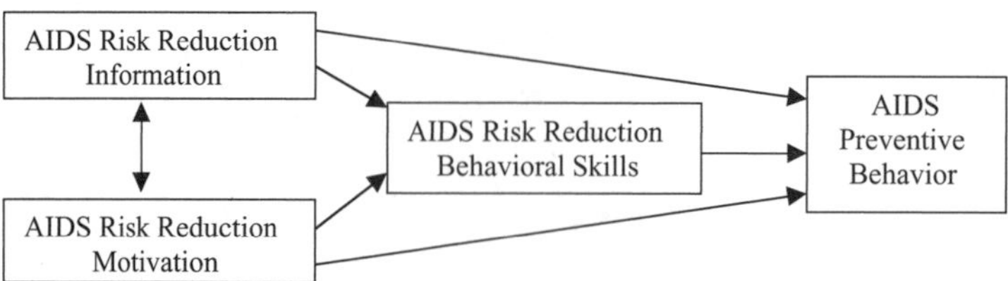

Figure 6-8 Information-motivation-behavioral skills (IMB) model (Kalichman, 1998, p. 47, Figure 2.7).

behavior. For example, information about how condoms can prevent HIV transmission may induce relatively easy-to-perform behaviors, such as buying condoms. However, more difficult behaviors, such as actually using condoms, may require not only information but also the motivation to use condoms and the skills required to use them properly.

DIFFUSION OF INNOVATIONS THEORY

Diffusion of innovations theory explains how an *innovation* (a new idea, object, or behavior practice) *diffuses* (spreads) among members of a social group (Rogers, 1983). According to this theory, as social groups are unique, the origins, speed, and channels of innovation-spread are also unique to each group. The theory also emphasizes that innovations themselves have properties that make them more or less likely to be adopted by different groups (see Figure 6-9). For example, a San Francisco program for reducing HIV transmission among injection drug users spread two innovations: the fact that bleach decontaminates needles, which was communicated by word-or-mouth, and the bleach itself. The fact and the bleach were quickly diffused among injection drug users, in part because people trusted the information, and in part because bleach is cheap, widely available, and easy to use (Newmeyer, Feldman, Biernacki, & Watters, 1989).

LEADERSHIP-FOCUSED MODELS

Leadership-focused models emphasize the role of leaders in changing the behaviors of their groups. Innovations such as behavior change often run counter to a group's established norms. For behavior change to take place, group leaders therefore must make these innovations acceptable or "cool" to their group members.

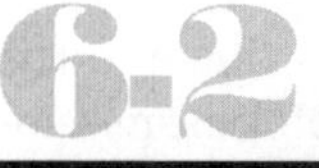

Key Attributes Affecting the Speech and Extent of Diffusion of an Innovation (National Cancer Institute, 2005, p. 28, Figure 8)

ATTRIBUTE	KEY QUESTION
Relative advantage	Is the innovation better than what it will replace?
Compatibility	Does the innovation fit with the intended audience?
Complexity	Is the innovation easy to use?
Trialability	Can the innovation be tried before making a decision to adopt?
Observability	Are the results of the innovation observable and easily measurable?

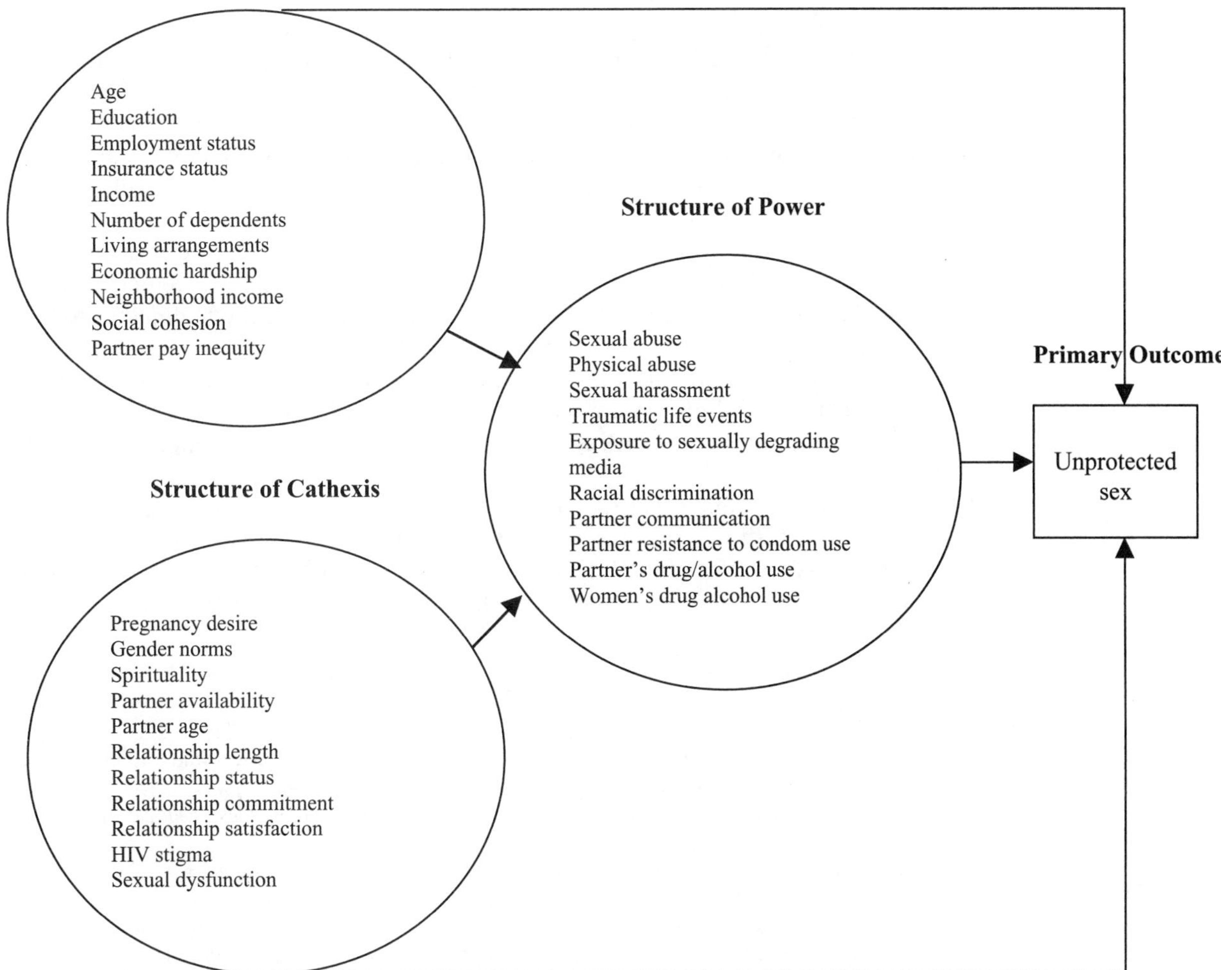

Figure 6-9 Theory of gender and power, as applied to HIV risk behavior (based on Wingood & DiClemente, 2000, 2002).

Leadership-focused models work best in groups that do not have powerful pockets of resistance to the change, that have been in existence for a while, and that have relatively stable leadership (Middlestadt, Hoffman, Madden D'Andrea, & Ruscavage, 1996).

SOCIAL MOVEMENT THEORY

Social movement theory proposes that behavior change takes place when large groups of people unite to address the behavioral problem. Often, these social movements are in opposition to local leaders or common practices. One of the best examples of a public health social movement is the mobilization of lesbians and gays to combat HIV/AIDS. Drawing on networks and methods that had already been established to fight discrimination, gays and lesbians were quickly able to amplify concern about the HIV/AIDS crisis among governments and the medical establishment (Brown et al., 2004). Raising awareness about HIV/AIDS helped all people be able to discuss sex, drug use, and condoms more openly.

THEORY OF GENDER AND POWER

According to the *theory of gender and power* (Connell, 1987), which is represented in Figure 6-9 (as applied to HIV sexual risk behavior), three major structures characterize the gendered relationships between men and women. These structures are: the sexual division of labor, which concerns economic inequities favoring males; the sexual division of power, which concerns inequities and abuses of authority and control in relationships and institutions favoring males; and cathexis, which concerns social norms and affective attachments (e.g., societal expectations about women's sexuality; connections between women's sexuality and other social concerns, such as immorality). The three structures are overlapping but distinct, and serve to explain the gender roles assumed by men and women. Together, they constrain women's daily practices by producing gender-based inequalities in earning potential, control of resources, and expectations of roles. These factors, in turn, lead to socioeconomic circumstances (e.g., economic dependence on a male partner), interpersonal conditions (e.g., inability to negotiate safer sex practices), and behaviors (e.g., unprotected sex) that increase the likelihood of HIV infection (see also Part 4).

Public health and social/behavioral interventions at the individual, small group, community, institutional, and societal levels that target these factors can reduce women's risk of infection (Wingood & DiClemente, 2000). (For examples of effective interventions based on the theory of gender and power, see Figure 6-6.)

REFERENCES

Ajzen, I. (1991). The theory of planned behavior. *Organizational Behavior and Human Decision Processes, 50*, 179–211.

Ajzen, I., & Fishbein, M. (1980). *Understanding attitudes and predicting social behavior*. Englewood Cliffs, NJ: Prentice Hall.

Bandura, A. (1986). *Social foundations of thought and action: A social cognitive theory*. Englewood Cliffs, NJ: Prentice Hall.

Brown, P., Zavestoski, S., McCormick, S., Mayer, B., Morello-Frosch, R., & Gasior Altman, R. (2004). Embodied health movements: New approaches to social movements in health. *Sociology of Health and Illness, 26*(1), 50–80.

Catania, J. A., Kegeles, S. D., & Coates, T. S. (1990). Toward an understanding of risk behavior: An AIDS risk reduction model (ARRM). *Health Education Quarterly, 17*(1), 53–72.

Centers for Disease Control and Prevention (CDC). (2001). *Compendium of HIV prevention interventions with evidence of success*. Atlanta, GA: CDC.

Connell, R. W. (1987). *Gender and power*. Stanford, CA: Stanford University Press.

Des Jarlais, D. C., Friedman, S. R., & Ward, T. P. (1993). Harm reduction: A public health response to the AIDS epidemic among injecting drug users. *Annual Review of Public Health, 14*, 413–450.

DiClemente, R. J., & Wingood, G. M. (1995). A randomized controlled trial of an HIV sexual risk-reduction intervention for African-American women. *Journal of the American Medical Association, 274*(16), 1271–1276.

DiClemente, R. J., Wingood, G. M., Harrington, K. F., Lang, D. L., Davies, S. L., Hook, E. W., et al. (2004). Efficacy of an HIV prevention intervention for African American adolescent girls. *Journal of the American Medical Association, 292*(2), 171–179.

Fishbein, M., & Ajzen, I. (1975). *Belief, attitude, intention and behavior: An introduction to theory and research*. Reading, MA: Addison-Wesley.

Fishbein, M., Middlestadt, S. E., & Hitchcock, P. J. (1994). Using information to change sexually transmitted disease-related behaviors: An analysis based on the theory of reasoned action. In R. J. DiClemente & J. L. Peterson (Eds.), *Preventing AIDS: Theories and methods of behavioral interventions* (pp. 61–78). New York: Plenum.

Fishbein, M., Triandis, H. C., Kanfer, F. H., Becker, M., Middlestadt, S. E., & Eichler, A. (2001). Factors influencing behavior and behavior change. In A. Baum, T. A. Revenson, & J. E. Singer (Eds.), *Handbook of health psychology* (pp. 3–17). Mahwah, NJ: Lawrence Erlbaum Associates.

Fisher, J. D., & Fisher, W. A. (1992). Changing AIDS-risk behavior. *Psychological Bulletin, 111*(3), 455–474.

Friedman, S. R., Des Jarlais, D. C., & Ward, T. P. (1994). Social models for changing health-relevant behavior. In R. J. DiClemente & J. L. Peterson (Eds.), *Preventing AIDS: Theories and methods of behavioral interventions* (pp. 95–116). New York: Plenum.

Herlocher, T., Hoff, C., & DeCarlo, P. (1996). *Can theory help in HIV prevention?* San Francisco: Center for AIDS Prevention Studies (CAPS), University of California, San Francisco.

Kalichman, S. C. (1998). *Preventing AIDS: A sourcebook for behavioral interventions*. Mahwah, NJ: Lawrence Erlbaum Associates.

MacCoun, R. J. (1998). Toward a psychology of harm reduction. *American Psychologist, 53*, 1199–1208.

Marlatt, G. A. (Ed.). (1998). *Harm reduction: Pragmatic strategies for managing high-risk behaviors*. New York: Guilford.

Middlestadt, S., Hoffman, C., Madden D'Andrea, E., & Ruscavage, D. (1996). Appendix B: Quick guide to key behavioral and social-level theories in HIV prevention. In *What intervention studies say about effectiveness: A resource for HIV prevention community planning groups*. Washington, DC: The Academy for Educational Development.

National Cancer Institute. (2005). *Theory at a glance: A guide for health promotion practice*. Bethesda, MD: National Institutes of Health.

Newmeyer, J. A., Feldman, H. W., Biernacki, P., & Watters, J. K. (1989). Preventing AIDS contagion among intravenous drug users. *Medical Anthropology, 10*, 167–175.

Prochaska, J. O., DiClemente, C. C., & Norcross, J. C. (1992). In search of how people change: Applications to addictive behaviors. *American Psychologist, 47*(9), 1102–1114.

Rogers, E. M. (1983). *Diffusion of innovations* (3rd ed.). London: The Free Press.

Rosenstock, I. M., Strecher, V. J., & Becker, M. H. (1994). The health belief model and HIV risk behavior change. In R. J. DiClemente & J. L. Peterson (Eds.), *Preventing AIDS: Theories and methods of behavioral interventions* (pp. 5–24). New York: Plenum.

Wingood, G. M., & DiClemente, R. J. (2000). Application of the theory of gender and power to examine HIV-related exposures, risk factors, and effective interventions for women. *Health Education and Behavior, 27*(5), 539–565.

Wingood, G. M., & DiClemente, R. J. (2002). The theory of gender and power: A social structural theory for guiding the design and implementation of public health interventions to reduce women's risk of HIV. In R. J. DiClemente, R. A. Crosby, & M. Kegler (Eds.), *Emerging theories in health promotion practice and research: Strategies for enhancing public health* (pp. 313–347). San Francisco: Jossey-Bass.

Wingood, G. M., DiClemente, R. J., Mikhail, I., Lang, D. L., McCree, D. H., Davies, S. L., et al., (2004). A randomized controlled trial to reduce HIV transmission risk behaviors and sexually transmitted diseases among women living with HIV: The WiLLOW Program. *Journal of Acquired Immune Deficiency Syndromes, 37*(Suppl 2), 58–67.

Instructor Resources

LEARNING ACTIVITIES

ACTIVITY 1:

Assignment: Theory-Based Prevention

Objective: To understand how behavior change theory underlies HIV/AIDS prevention programs.

Identify a prevention program that has been researched and evaluated in the HIV/AIDS prevention literature. (See, for example, the peer-reviewed journal *AIDS Education and Prevention.*) Write a summary of the prevention program's approaches and activities, define what is the behavior change theory that drives the intervention, and report on the efficacy of this approach.

ACTIVITY 2:

Assignment: Theories in Action

Objective: To utilize a behavior change theory to create an HIV/AIDS prevention program.

Select a population or a community in which you would like to implement a HIV/AIDS prevention program and write a two-page proposal describing your intended population, the theory behind your intervention, and the strategies your program will undertake to change HIV/AIDS risk behavior(s). Use the questions below to help organize your thoughts.

1. Which communities/populations are targeted for services?
2. What are the specific behaviors that put them at risk for HIV/AIDS?
3. What are the factors that impact risk-taking behaviors?
4. Which factors are the most important and can be realistically addressed?
5. What theory(ies) or models best address the identified factors?
6. What kind of intervention can best address these factors?

DISCUSSION QUESTIONS

1. Describe any HIV prevention program in your community of which you are aware (public service announcements on television or radio, health education programs offered in school or community groups, etc.). Which behavioral change model(s) does it use?
2. Programs based on the harm reduction model (i.e., safe sex campaigns or needle exchanges) are controversial in the United States, where they clash with abstinence-only or "zero-tolerance" approaches. What are the relative positives or negatives about each approach?
3. Leadership focused models emphasize the role of leaders in changing the behaviors of their groups. Can you think of any leaders who have encouraged behavior change regarding HIV/AIDS?

QUIZ

1. Name any three influences that shape a person's behavior, and identify whether they are intrapersonal, interpersonal, or community-based.
2. Name any three of the eight factors that must be present for positive behavior change.
3. Believing yourself capable to perform a given behavior under different circumstances is known as:
   a) Self-efficacy
   b) Self-esteem
   c) Self-control
   d) Self-confidence
4. Easy-access condom dispensers and depictions of safe sex in television and movies are important positive action cues, according to which model?
   a) Harm reduction model
   b) AIDS risk reduction model
   c) Information-motivation-behavioral skills model
   d) Health belief model
5. Needle-exchange programs follow which theory or model?
   a) AIDS risk reduction model
   b) Information-motivation-behavioral skills model
   c) Harm reduction model
   d) Health belief model
6. The theory of planned behavior added which additional element to the theory of reasoned action?
   a) Cultural influences
   b) Perceived self-control
   c) Perceived behavioral control
   d) Interpersonal influences
7. Which is an advantage of the transtheoretical model?
   a) It takes into account the person's stage of behavior change.
   b) It addresses both information and motivation.
   c) It includes a person's perceived behavioral control.
   d) It mobilizes an entire community to endorse behavior change.

8. True or False: According to the information-motivation-behavioral skills model, providing information about how condoms can prevent HIV is enough to induce behavior change.

9. The mobilization of lesbians and gays to combat HIV/AIDS as a group is a good example of:
   a) Leadership-focused model
   b) Theory of gender and power
   c) Social cognitive theory
   d) Social movement theory

ANSWERS

1. Intrapersonal influences on behavior include knowledge, attitudes, beliefs, motivation, past experience, and skills. Interpersonal influences include the opinions, advice, support, and behavior of friends, family, coworkers, and others. Community influences include social structures, movements, and policies of communities and their institutions.

2. The person has formed a positive intention to perform the behavior; there are no environmental constraints that make it impossible for the behavior to be performed; the person has the skills necessary to perform the behavior; the person has a positive attitude toward the behavior; the person perceives more social pressure to perform the behavior than to not perform it; the person perceives behavior to be more consistent than inconsistent with his or her self-image; the person's emotional reaction to performing the behavior is more positive than negative; and the person perceives self-efficacy to perform the behavior.

3. **A.** Self-efficacy is the belief in one's own ability to perform risk-reducing behaviors.

4. **D.** The health belief model suggests that whether people change their risky behaviors depends on sociodemographic factors; the threat posed by the risky behavior; their expectations about the benefits and barriers to changing behaviors; and cues to action in the environment.

5. **C.** Many interventions aim for complete abstinence from risky behavior. Harm reduction model, in contrast, aims to lessen the negative consequences of these behaviors.

6. **C.** One limitation of the theory of reasoned action is that it did not account for the fact that some behaviors are easier to control than others. To address this limitation, the theory's creators added perceived behavioral control to their model. Perceived behavioral control refers to how much control a person thinks he or she has over performing a certain behavior, such as using a condom or cleaning injection drug paraphernalia.

7. **A.** The transtheoretical model is sometimes referred to as the stages of change model, as it says that people move through a series of stages toward behavior change. One of the strengths of the transtheoretical model is that it allows HIV prevention practitioners and health care providers to tailor their interventions to the client's stage.

8. **False.** According to the IMB model of behavioral risk reduction, three factors contribute to HIV risk-related behavioral change. First, information regarding HIV/AIDS transmission and prevention must be relevant to HIV/AIDS and easy to

apply in the person's environment. Second, motivation to change HIV/AIDS-risk behavior must come from both from the person's own attitudes toward the change and from other people's support. Third, the person must have behavioral skills for performing specific HIV/AIDS-preventive acts and believe in his or her ability to perform the act. So for example, information about how condoms can prevent HIV transmission may induce relatively easy-to-perform behaviors, such as buying condoms. However, more difficult behaviors, such as actually using condoms, may require not only information but also the motivation to use condoms and the skills required to use them properly.

9. **D.** Social movement theory proposes that behavior change takes place when large groups of people unite to address the behavioral problem.

WEB RESOURCES

Behavior Change Theories and Models

http://www.csupomona.edu/~jvgrizzell/best_practices/bctheory.html

Because theories and models of human behavior can guide the development and refinement of health promotion and education efforts, this page reviews elements of behavioral and social science theories and models.

The Communication Initiative's Change Theories

http://www.comminit.com/changetheories.html

Summarizes theories and assumptions about the nature of change and how best change can be encouraged and facilitated to inform strategy development and evaluation initiatives.

RECOMMENDED READING

Preventing AIDS: Theories and Methods of Behavioral Interventions (DiClemente & Peterson, 1994)

DiClemente, R. J. & Peterson, J. L. (Eds.). (1994). Preventing AIDS: Theories and methods of behavioral interventions. *New York: Plenum.*

This well-organized textbook brings together a multidisciplinary group of behavioral researchers who have conducted major research on in HIV primary prevention interventions. This publication identifies the principal theories and methods utilized in behavioral change interventions, and examines their impact in a variety of populations.

Handbook of HIV Prevention (Peterson & DiClemente, 2000)

Peterson, J. L., & DiClemente, R. J. (Eds.). (2000). Handbook of HIV prevention. *New York: Kluwer Academic/Plenum.*

Emerging Theories in Health Promotion Research and Practice: Strategies for Enhancing Public Health (DiClemente, Crosby, & Kegler, 2002)

DiClemente, R. J., Crosby, R., & Kegler, M. (Eds.). (2002). Emerging theories in health promotion research and practice: Strategies for enhancing public health. *San Francisco: Jossey-Bass.*

Using a Combination of Behavior Change Theories and Models (CDC, 1996)

Centers for Disease Control and Prevention (CDC). (1996). Community-level prevention of human immunodeficiency virus infection among high-risk populations. Morbidity and Mortality Weekly Report, 45*(RR-6):1–16.*

The AIDS Community Demonstration Projects (ACDPs) were community-level HIV prevention programs targeting high-risk populations in five U.S. cities. For the intervention design, researchers developed a common study protocol based on behavior-change theories and models. This report describes the common study protocol used in the ACDPs, the preliminary findings, and the conclusions regarding the design, implementation, and evaluation of a community-level intervention; specific case studies from each project site are also described.
Available online at http://www.cdc.gov/mmwr/preview/mmwrhtml/00041336.htm

Health Belief Model (Maes & Louis, 2003)

Maes, C. A., & Louis, M. (2003). Knowledge of AIDS, perceived risk of AIDS, and at-risk sexual behaviors among older adults. Journal of American Academic Nurse Practitioners, 15*(11):509–516.*

The purpose of this study was to identify older adults' knowledge of acquired immune deficiency syndrome (AIDS), perceptions of their risk of AIDS, and risk behaviors by using a questionnaire derived from the health belief model. Five hypotheses based on the health belief model were tested. Statistical analyses showed significant predictors of the likelihood of using recommended safe sexual practices were gender, knowledge of AIDS, perceived susceptibility to AIDS, and perceived threat of AIDS. The results indicated the respondents were knowledgeable about HIV transmission through casual contact and medical aspects of AIDS. Although the respondents recognized the seriousness of AIDS, they generally did not believe that they were susceptible to this disease, even though about 10% indicated sexual activity outside of a long-term relationship.

Theory of Reasoned Action (Albarracin et al., 2001)

Albarracin, D., Johnson, B. T., Fishbein, M., & Muellerleile, P. A. (2001). Theories of reasoned action and planned behavior as models of condom use: A meta-analysis. Psychological Bulletin, 127*(1), 142–161.*

To examine how well the theories of reasoned action and planned behavior predict condom use, the authors synthesized 96 data sets containing associations between the models' key variables. Consistent with the theory of reasoned action's predictions, (a) condom use was related to intentions, (b) intentions were based on attitudes and subjective norms, and (c) attitudes were associated with behavioral beliefs, and norms were associated with normative beliefs. Consistent with the theory of planned behavior's predictions, perceived behavioral control was related to condom use intentions and condom use, but, in contrast to the theory, it did not contribute significantly to condom use. The strength of these associations, however, was influenced by the consideration of past behavior. Implications of these results for HIV prevention efforts are discussed.

Social Cognitive Theory (Norr et al., 2004)

Norr, K. F., Norr, J. L., McElmurry, B. J., Tlou, S., & Moeti, M. R. (2004). Impact of peer group education on HIV prevention among women in Botswana. Health Care for Women International, *25(3), 210–226.*

A peer group HIV prevention intervention based on social-cognitive learning theory, gender inequality, and the primary health care model for community-based health promotion was developed for more than 300 urban employed women in Botswana. All women volunteered to participate in the intervention. To control for self-selection, matched workplaces were assigned to the intervention group or to the delayed control group. Compared with women in the delayed control group, women in the intervention group had significantly higher post-intervention levels of knowledge of HIV transmission, sexually transmitted diseases, and HIV prevention behaviors; positive condom attitudes and confidence in condom use; personal safer-sex behaviors; and positive attitudes toward persons living with HIV/AIDS and community HIV/AIDS-related activities. The peer group leaders have sustained the program for more than 5 years after the end of research funding. Peer groups are a low-cost and sustainable intervention that can change HIV prevention knowledge, attitudes, and behaviors for ordinary urban employed women in sub-Saharan Africa.

Transtheoretical Model (Cabral et al., 2004)

Cabral, R. J., Cotton, D., Semaan, S., & Gielen, A. C. (2004). Application of the transtheoretical model for HIV prevention in a facility-based and a community-level behavioral intervention research study. Health Promotion Practice, *5(2), 199–207.*

This article describes the application of the transtheoretical model of behavior change to prevention programs for women at risk for or infected with HIV. The focus of these multisite demonstration projects was to increase condom and contraceptive use. The model was operationalized for use in the following two different intervention approaches: facility-based interventions (individual counseling for women in clinics, shelters, and drug treatment centers) and community-level interventions (including production of small media materials, street outreach, and community mobilization). The authors found that interventions derived from a complex theory can be disseminated to frontline providers who have little prior HIV education experience or academic training. They suggest that the transtheoretical model has value for the design and implementation of HIV prevention programs.

AIDS Risk Reduction Model (Malow & Ireland, 1996)

Malow, R. M., & Ireland, S. J. (1996). HIV risk correlates among non-injection cocaine dependent men in treatment. AIDS Education and Prevention, *8(3), 226–235.*

Guided by the AIDS risk reduction model (ARRM), psychosocial correlates of HIV risk behavior were examined among noninjection cocaine dependent, heterosexual men (NI-CD-HM) in treatment. Subjects completed a structured interview to measure ARRM mediating variables and HIV risk behaviors. The results indicated that greater perceived susceptibility to contracting HIV, lower sexual self-efficacy, higher lifetime incidence of sexually transmitted diseases, and being under the influence of alcohol or other drugs during sex predicted having more sexual partners in the month before admission. Despite adequate knowledge of safer sex guidelines, subjects remained misinformed regarding certain aspects of HIV transmission. Men who perceived that their partners viewed condoms more positively and who exchanged drugs for sex were more likely to use condoms, yet condom use skills were typically inadequate to ensure effective prevention.

Information-Motivation-Behavioral Skills (IMB) Model (Fisher & Fisher, 1992)

Fisher, J. D., & Fisher, W. A. (1992). Changing AIDS-risk behavior. Psychological Bulletin, 111*(3), 455–474.*

This article contains a comprehensive, critical review of the literature on interventions that have targeted risky sexual behavior and intravenous drug use practices. A conceptually based, highly generalizable model for promoting and evaluating AIDS-risk behavior change in any population of interest is then proposed. The model holds that AIDS-risk reduction is a function of people's information about AIDS transmission and prevention, their motivation to reduce AIDS risk, and their behavioral skills for performing the specific acts involved in risk reduction. Supportive tests of this model, using structural equation modeling techniques, are then reported for populations of university students and gay male affinity group members.

Social Models for Behavior Change (Fernandez et al., 2003)

Fernandez, M. I., Gowen, G. S., Gay, C. L., Mattson, T. R., Bital, E., & Kelly, J. A. (2003). HIV, sex, and social change: Applying ESID principles to HIV prevention research. American Journal of Community Psychology, 32*(3–4), 333–344.*

The HIV epidemic has been the most significant public health crisis of the last 2 decades. Although Experimental Social Innovation and Dissemination (ESID) principles have been used by many HIV prevention researchers, the clearest application is the series of model-building and replication experiments conducted by Kelly and colleagues. The model mobilized, trained, and engaged key opinion leaders to serve as behavior change and safe-sex endorsers in their social networks. This article illustrates how ESID principles were used to develop, test, and disseminate an innovative social model and discusses the challenges of applying ESID methodology in the midst of a public health emergency.

POWERPOINT SLIDES

(Note: A full-color version of these slides, with graphics, is also available on the CD-ROM.)

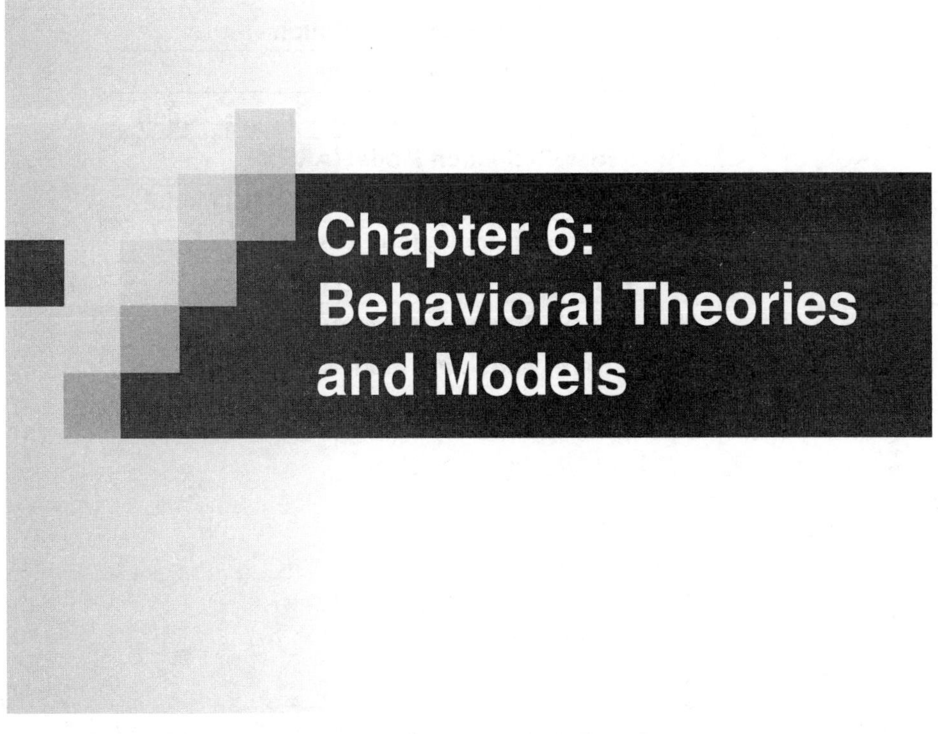

Behavioral Theories and Models

For the most part, people get and give HIV through their behaviors. Because the HIV epidemic is driven by individuals' behaviors, researchers and prevention providers use scientific theories of behavior change to design their interventions.

Behavioral Theories and Models
(continued)

The Health Belief Model
The Theory of Reasoned Action
Social Cognitive Theory
The Transtheoretical Model (Stages of Change Model)
AIDS Risk Reduction Model (ARRM)
Information-Motivation-Behavioral Skills (IMB) Model
Diffusion of Innovations Theory
Leadership-Focused Model
Social Movement Theory
Harm Reduction Model
Theory of Gender and Power

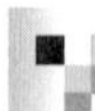

Examples of Theory-Based Prevention Interventions

- Many prevention interventions borrow from several theories. For example, one program could work on all of the following:
    - **heightening clients' perceptions of own risk (Health Belief Model)**
    - **strengthening clients' intention to change risk behaviors (Theory of Reasoned Action)**
    - **fortifying clients' belief in ability to change behavior (Social Cognitive Theory)**

Examples of Theory-Based Prevention Interventions (continued)

- Many prevention interventions borrow from several theories. For example, one program could work on all of the following:
  - **increasing clients' readiness to change behavior (Transtheoretical Model)**
  - **augmenting clients' commitment to behavior change (ARRM)**
  - **teaching clients how to perform safer behaviors, like using condoms or sterilizing needles (IMB)**
  - **spreading new ideas and behaviors through a social network (Diffusion of Innovations Theory)**

Examples of Theory-Based Prevention Interventions (continued)

- Many prevention interventions borrow from several theories. For example, one program could work on all of the following:
  - **encouraging group leaders to adopt safer behaviors (Leadership-Focused Model)**
  - **building an HIV/AIDS awareness-raising campaign (Social Movement Theory)**
  - **creating a condom-distribution or needle-exchange program (Harm Reduction Model)**

The Health Belief Model

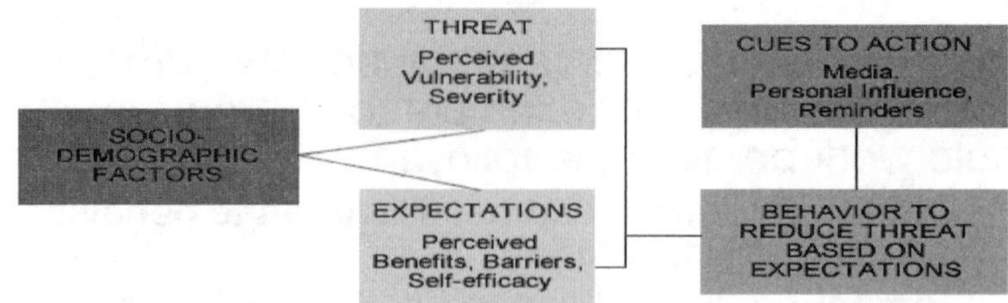

- According to this model, whether people change their risky behaviors (like unsafe sex) depends on:
  - sociodemographic factors
  - the threat posed by the illness
  - their expectations about change
  - cues to action in the environment

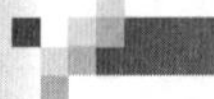

The Theory of Reasoned Action

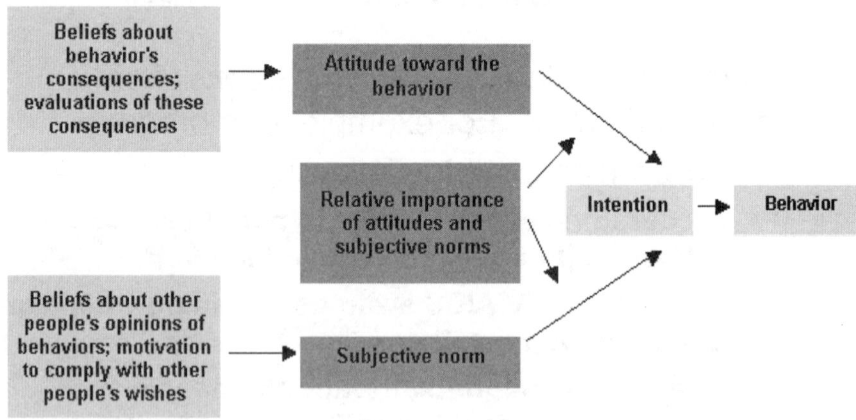

- According to this theory, behavioral change is the last link in a causal chain that involves beliefs, attitudes, norms, and intentions.

The Theory of Planned Action

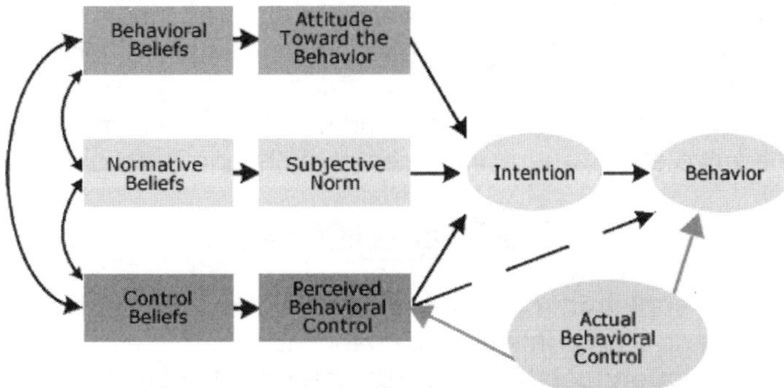

- This theory is a modified version of the theory of reasoned action, because of an added component—perceived behavioral control.

Social Cognitive Theory

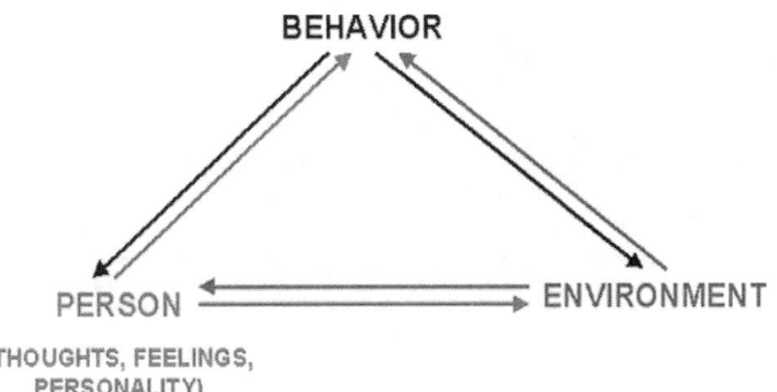

- This theory views people's lives as made up of three components (Person, Behavior, and Environment). Behavior change requires change to each component.

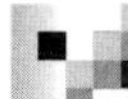

The Transtheoretical Model

- Sometimes referred to as the "stages of change" model
- Says people move through a series of stages toward behavior change
- Advancement to a higher stage marks an increase in motivation for, confidence about, and commitment to a change in behavior

The Stages of Change

- **Pre-contemplation:** person is not aware that a behavior is not healthy, and has no intention to change it
- **Contemplation:** person recognizes need to change
- **Preparation:** person begins plan of action
- **Action:** person takes steps to change behavior
- **Maintenance:** person tries to sustain behavior changes
- **Relapse:** person falls back into old, unhealthy behavior patterns

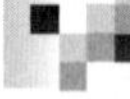

AIDS Risk Reduction Model (ARRM)

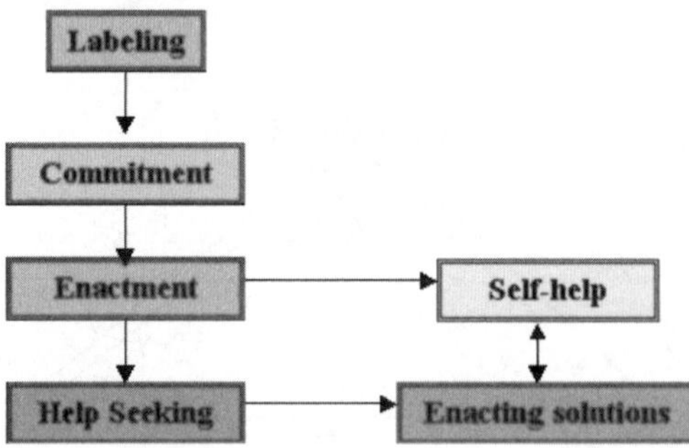

- This model organizes the many factors that influence whether people successfully change their risky behaviors.
- It is a stage model, which means that people progress through different levels toward behavior change.

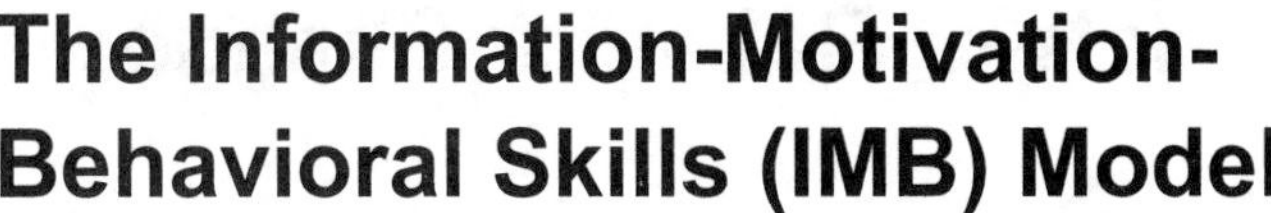

The Information-Motivation-Behavioral Skills (IMB) Model

Says three factors contribute to HIV risk-related behavioral change:

1) Information regarding HIV/AIDS transmission and prevention: this information must be easy to apply
2) Motivation to change HIV/AIDS-risk behavior: comes both from the person's own attitudes and from other people's support
3) Behavioral skills for performing a specific HIV/AIDS-preventive act: both the objective ability to perform the act and the belief that one has the ability to perform the act (self-efficacy)

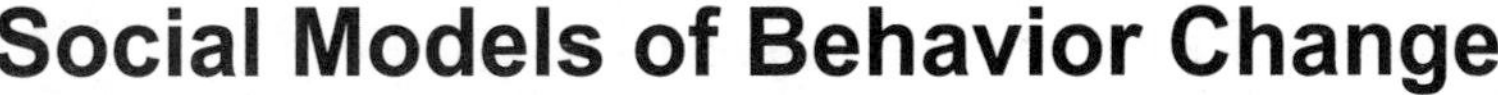

Social Models of Behavior Change

Diffusion of Innovations Theory

- Diffusion happens when an innovation (an idea, object, or behavior practice) spreads among members of a social group.
- Diffusion of Innovations Theory says that since social groups are unique, the catalysts, speed, and channels of innovation spread are also unique to each group.

Leadership-Focused Models

- These models emphasize the role of leaders in changing the behaviors of their groups.
- For behavior change to take place, group leaders must therefore make innovations acceptable or “cool” to their group members.

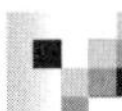

Social Models of Behavior Change
(continued)

Social Movement Theory

- This theory proposes that behavior change takes place when larger groups of people unite to address the behavioral problem.
- Often, these movements are in opposition to local leaders or common practices.
- The best example of a public-health social movement is the mobilization of lesbians and gays to combat HIV/AIDS.

Theory of Gender and Power

- According to this theory, there are three structures that characterize the gendered relationships between men and women: the sexual division of labor, the sexual division of power, and cathexis.
- The theory argues that the gender-based disparities in expectations that arise from each structure generate different "exposures" or "risk factors" that influence women's risk for disease.

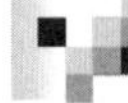

Harm Reduction Model

- Aims to lessen the negative consequences of these behaviors, both for the people performing them and for the general public.
- Many harm reduction approaches are controversial in the United States, where they clash with prevailing emphasis on abstinence from extramarital sex and "zero tolerance" toward illegal drug use.
- Effective harm reduction approaches include:
  - needle-exchange programs, and
  - making condoms readily available to adolescents and young adults.

Learning Objectives

- Define the "ABCs" and "DEFs" of HIV prevention
- Understand how male and female barrier methods, microbicides, and STI/STD prevention impact HIV transmission
- Describe methods by which injection drug-related transmission can be prevented
- Understand how parent-to-child transmission can be prevented
- List measures that prevent transmission in health care settings
- Discuss issues relevant to HIV-positives

Key Terms

abstinence
barrier method
dental dam
disclosure
female-controlled prevention method
microbicides
pathogen
postexposure prophylaxis
primary prevention
safer sex
secondary prevention
serostatus
vaccine

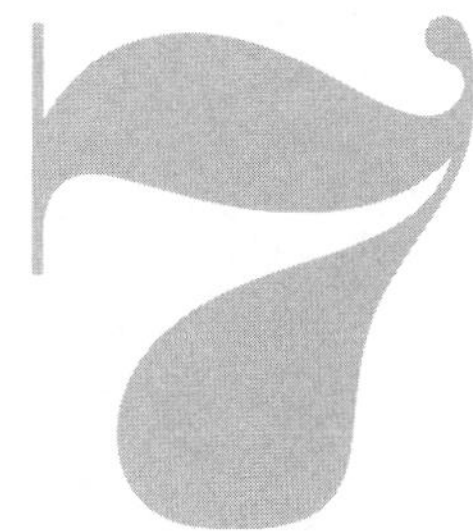

Routes of Transmission: Prevention Strategies

This chapter addresses how the transmission of HIV through sexual contact, through drug use, from parents to children, and in health care settings may be prevented. It also provides an overview of advances in research to develop a vaccine to prevent HIV infection.

PREVENTING SEXUAL TRANSMISSION

Worldwide, HIV infection most commonly results from sexual transmission of the virus (see chapter 4). Abstaining from (not engaging in) sex or having sex with only one, uninfected partner will prevent the sexual transmission of HIV. Aside from these methods, engaging in *safer sex*—that is, using condoms, dental dams, or other barriers that prevent or reduce contact with partners' blood, semen, and other body fluids—is the most effective way to prevent sexual transmission. Communication about sex among partners is often essential to safer sex practices, but is not always possible, particularly when partners do not have equal power in sexual relationships. The development of female-controlled barrier methods and microbicides that kill or disable the HIV virus promises to reduce sexual transmission of HIV further by empowering people to protect themselves. Finally, treating other sexually transmitted diseases and infections (STDs/STIs) is essential to preventing sexual transmission of HIV, since these infections make it easier to both give and acquire the virus.

The ABCs of HIV Prevention

The "ABC" approach to HIV prevention (Figure 7-1) refers to a combination of three behavioral strategies: *abstinence* (particularly delayed sexual initiation among youth); *being faithful* (mutual monogamy to reduce the number of sexual partners); and using *condoms* correctly and consistently, especially for casual sexual activity and other high-risk situations.

The "ABC" strategies can be highly effective, as shown by declines in HIV prevalence in Uganda, Zambia, and Thailand after these strategies were adopted

Abstinence (delayed sexual initiation among youth)

Being faithful (mutual monogamy to reduce the number of sexual partners)

Condoms used correctly and consistently (especially for casual sexual activity and other high-risk situations)

Figure 7-1 The ABCs of HIV prevention.

(U.S. Agency for International Development [USAID], 2003). However, the ABCs are sometimes hard to implement. Communication about sex is needed for people to judge their own risks of getting and giving HIV, and to make responsible decisions about condom use and other risk-reduction strategies. However, sex is a taboo topic among many cultural groups, and talking about sex makes most people feel at least slightly embarrassed, uncomfortable, or awkward. Moreover, being sexually intimate implies a high level of trust between two people. When one person insists on safer sex, the other person may feel that he or she is not trusted. Similarly, one person may not insist on safer sex out of fear of offending his or her partner. Partners also may equate a request for safer sex as a sign of unfaithfulness, and may react by being angry, withdrawing financial support, or terminating the relationship.

Women in particular may find it difficult to negotiate safer sex, since women often have less power and control in their relationships (Commonwealth Secretariat, 2001; Fleischman, 2004; Türmen, 2003; Wingood & DiClemente, 2002). For example, many women have little power to refuse sex or to insist that condoms be used because of their social and economic dependency on men. Gay and bisexual men who are in subordinate roles in intimate relationships also may experience coercion to engage in unprotected anal intercourse (Kalichman & Rompa, 1995; Kippax, Crawford, Davis, Rodden, & Dowsett, 1993). Some activists therefore suggest the "DEF" approach (Fleischman, 2004).

The DEFs of Prevention (USAID, 2003)

The "DEF" approach (Figure 7-2) includes disclosure, education, and female-controlled prevention methods.

Disclosure means telling other people of one's own serostatus—that is, whether one is HIV+. Women living with HIV/AIDS, in particular, are often afraid to disclose their serostatus, as they risk violence, abandonment, and blame for bringing the virus into the household—even though they are often themselves infected by their husbands. It is imperative that all HIV+ people be helped to disclose their status with appropriate social and economic support structures, including legal recourse in cases of violence. Training police and law enforcement officials on the links between gender-based violence and HIV/AIDS, establishing safe shelters and referral services for HIV+ people, and providing support to people living with HIV/AIDS are examples of programs that would help people to disclose safely.

Vulnerability to infection is linked to lack of access to *education*. Not only does lack of education make it difficult for people to find out about HIV/AIDS, but it also

Disclosure

Education

Female-controlled methods

Figure 7-2 The DEFs of prevention.

makes it more difficult for them to secure safe economic resources. Addressing educational needs requires teaching about HIV/AIDS in schools, providing scholarships and skills training for women and youth, and keeping schools safe for girls.

In the absence of a vaccine, some prevention scientists believe that the best ways that women have of protecting themselves from HIV/AIDS are *female-controlled prevention methods*. These include microbicides, which kill or disable HIV, and female condoms (see later). Putting these tools in women's hands requires increased funding for microbicide research, wider distribution of female condoms, and the integration of HIV/AIDS prevention services into reproductive health and family planning clinics.

Barrier Methods

Barrier methods, particularly male and female condoms, are an important component of both the ABC and DEF approaches to preventing sexual transmission of HIV. When used consistently and correctly, *male condoms* made of latex (rubber) have been shown to be highly effective in preventing sexual transmission of HIV. In a study of couples in which one partner had HIV, all 123 couples who used condoms for every sexual act over 4 years prevented HIV transmission. Among the 122 couples who did not use condoms for every sexual act, 12 partners became infected (Saracco et al., 1993). Condoms are also effective in reducing transmission of a number of STIs/STDs.

Male condoms do have some drawbacks, however. They must be used consistently and correctly, every time a person has sex, to be effective in preventing the spread of HIV. Some people object to condom use because applying them may interrupt sexual activity or reduce sexual pleasure. Women (and gay men who are the receptive partners in male-male anal intercourse) cannot use male condoms unless their male partners agree to do so. Latex condoms must also be stored away from sun, excessive heat, and dampness, and they cannot be used with oil-based lubricants, which break down rubber and can cause breakages. Also, male condoms will not prevent skin-to-skin transmission of STIs/STDs between uncovered areas.

In 1993, a new barrier method, the *female condom*, was introduced on the market in the United States. The female condom is a thin, soft, loose-fitting polyurethane (plastic) pouch that lines the vagina. It has two flexible rings: a smaller inner ring at the closed end, used to insert the device inside the vagina and to hold it in place, and a larger, outer ring which remains outside the vagina and covers the woman's external genitalia. Studies of contraceptive effectiveness and disease transmission for female condoms show similar rates to those of male condoms (Farr, Babelnick, Sturgen, & Dorflinger, 1994; Trussell, 1994).

Female condoms offer a number of advantages over male condoms. They are a female-controlled method, affording greater power to women to reduce their risk of HIV. They also have been reported to be more comfortable for men, affording less decrease in sensation than with the male latex condom, and (unlike male condoms) they can be inserted before sexual activity begins. Female condoms are also stronger than male condoms (polyurethane is 40% stronger than latex), and they have no special storage requirements, because polyurethane is not affected by changes in temperature and dampness. Female condoms can be used with any type of lubricant, even oil-based ones. This is advantageous in countries where personal, water-based lubricants are hard to find or nonexistent. Additionally, because female condoms provide more coverage of body surfaces than do male condoms, female condoms may offer additional protection against infections that can be transmitted through skin-to-skin contact (e.g., herpes).

Female condoms do have some drawbacks, however (FHI, 2003b, 2003c; Feinstein, 2001). They are more expensive and less widely available than male condoms. Some women also find the female condom difficult to insert and to remove.

In addition, once inserted, the outer ring is visible outside the vagina, which can make some women feel self-conscious. It is also possible for a man to "go around" the female condom during sex.

A third barrier method is the *dental dam*. A dental dam is a small sheet of latex that acts as a barrier between the vagina or anus and the mouth. Dental dams can be purchased at condom specialty stores and some drugstores, or can be made by cutting a latex condom or a latex glove. The effectiveness of dental dams in preventing HIV infection has not been studied (Sexual Health InfoCenter, n.d.). One challenge to studying their effectiveness is that the risk of HIV transmission from oral-genital and oral-anal contact is believed to be quite low (Campo et al., 2006).

Microbicides

Microbicides offer new possibilities for men and women to protect themselves from HIV and other sexually transmitted infections.

Currently under development, *microbicides* are creams, gels, and foams that can be inserted into the vagina or rectum to help prevent sexual transmission of HIV and other STIs/STDs (Farrington, 2002). They work by killing or immobilizing viruses and bacteria that cause disease, or by blocking viruses or bacteria from infecting the body (NIAID, 2003; Van de Wijgert & Coggins, 2002). When inserted in the body during childbirth, microbicides also may reduce transmission from mothers to infants (Padian, Shiboski, Glass, & Vittinghoff, 1997).

Microbicides would not eliminate the need for condoms. When used consistently and correctly, male and female condoms are likely to provide better protection against HIV and STIs/STDs than microbicides alone (Access Working Group, 2002). In addition, microbicides would not necessarily protect against all STIs/STDs. Because sexually transmitted diseases are caused by viruses and bacteria, a microbicide that works against one disease-causing agent would not necessarily protect against another (Access Working Group, 2002).

An advantage of microbicides is that they would afford men and women greater control over their sexual risk for HIV transmission. For example, women could insert microbicidal cream or gel before sex, without discussing it with their partner or needing his cooperation. However, there are some factors that might make people less likely to use microbicides, including nonsupportive cultural practices, such as a preference for dry sex; lack of discretion in packaging and application; lack of availability; difficulty in use or application; and an unacceptable odor or taste. In addition, microbicides that kill sperm (and are thus useful as contraception) may not be favored by women who want to protect themselves against HIV without inhibiting their ability to become pregnant (Access Working Group, 2002; Global Campaign for Microbicides, 2002; Morrow et al., 2003; Padian et al., 1997).

STI/STD Prevention and Treatment

People who are infected with another sexually transmitted infection or disease have up to 10 times the risk of getting and giving HIV through sexual intercourse than do people without STIs/STDs (Osmond, 1998; Wasserheit, 1992). This is true for both *ulcerative* infections (those that cause sores on the genitalia, such as syphilis and herpes), and *inflammatory* infections (those that do not cause sores, such as gonorrhea and chlamydia). The presence of STIs/STDs in an HIV-infected person also can speed up the development of AIDS (Wasserheit, 1992).

The same strategies discussed earlier for HIV prevention—ABC, DEF, the use of barrier methods, and the development of microbicides—also can prevent transmission of other STIs/STDs. In addition, early detection and treatment of STIs/STDs is crucial for reducing HIV risk (CDC, 1998). Testing and treatment efforts should include counseling to help patients adhere to their prescribed treatment and take steps to reduce the likelihood that they will transmit their infections to others.

Intervention protocols also should help patients to notify partners so that they can be tested and treated (CDC, 1998).

PREVENTING INJECTION DRUG-RELATED TRANSMISSION

Just as having unprotected sex with an HIV+ partner can result in the transmission of the HIV virus, so can sharing injection drug needles with an HIV+ person result in the transmission of the virus.

Injection Drug-Related Behaviors

The most effective way to prevent injection drug use–related transmission of HIV is to stop injection drug use. When complete abstinence from drugs is not possible, changing from injection to noninjection drugs can significantly reduce the risk of HIV transmission. For example, numerous studies have shown that programs administering methadone (an oral medication for heroin and morphine addicts) reduce injection drug users' (IDUs') use of injectable drugs and curb the spread of HIV and other diseases such as hepatitis (FHI, 2003a). (Switching from injection to noninjection drugs does not eliminate HIV transmission risk entirely because use of noninjection drugs can still affect the body and mind in ways that put people at risk—refer to chapter 3.)

For persons who continue to inject drugs, risk of HIV transmission can be reduced by:

- **Always using new (sterile) needles, syringes, and other injection equipment.** Needle and syringe exchange programs, at which IDUs can exchange old injecting equipment for new injecting equipment, effectively reduce the transmission of HIV and do not increase the use of illegal drugs.
- **Never sharing injecting equipment.** Most of the infections among IDUs are a result of sharing or reusing contaminated equipment, or of infecting drug preparations.
- **Sterilizing equipment between uses with clean water and bleach.** When sterile syringes are not available, injection equipment should be sterilized with bleach and clean water.

It is also important that used syringes be disposed of safely after use.

Barriers to Reducing IDU-Related Transmission

A number of factors hamper HIV prevention efforts with injection drug users. Illicit drug use, especially addiction to illicit drugs, is stigmatized in most societies. This stigma restricts effective HIV/AIDS prevention and treatment, since drug users often suffer social alienation and political disenfranchisement. As a result, it is very hard to target illicit drug users for prevention and treatment (Burack & Bangsberg, 1998; Metzger & Navaline, 2003).

Legal barriers are also present. In the United States, federal government funds may not be used to support domestic needle exchange programs, and most states continue to classify syringes as "drug paraphernalia," making it illegal to buy or own one without a prescription. This prevents public health professionals from providing HIV prevention services, such as needle exchange programs, to IDUs (Gostin, Lazzarini, Jones, & Flaherty, 1997). Despite the significant body of evidence on the effectiveness of needle exchange programs in reducing HIV transmission, they are considered by many political leaders to be too controversial to support (Public Broadcasting System [PBS], 2006a). Former President Clinton has stated that needle exchange programs did not receive federal funding during his presidency because "politically the country wasn't ready for it" (PBS, 2006b). Changing these laws may help reduce the transmission of HIV among IDUs. For example, after Connecticut partially deregulated the sale and possession of syringes, pharmacy sales of sterile syringes to IDUs increased, and the use of contaminated syringes fell (Groseclose et al., 1995).

PREVENTING PARENT-TO-CHILD TRANSMISSION

Parent-to-child transmission is how most children under 10 years of age get HIV (WHO, 2001). HIV can be transmitted from an infected mother to her child during pregnancy, labor, delivery, or breast-feeding. Parent-to-child transmission of HIV has been virtually eliminated in the developed world. However, rates remain high in resource-constrained countries, particularly in sub-Saharan African countries, where the majority of HIV-infected women of childbearing age reside. These high rates are a result of lack of access to the multiple strategies that can prevent perinatal transmission, including (FHI, n.d.; Kanabus & Noble, n.d.; United Nations Children's Fund [UNICEF], n.d.):

- Interventions to protect women of childbearing age against HIV infection.
- Interventions to help HIV+ women avoid unwanted pregnancies.
- Voluntary HIV counseling and testing (VCT) of women and their partners.
- Administration of antiretroviral therapy to HIV+ women during pregnancy and delivery.
- Adequate health care for women during the perinatal period.
- Selective Cesarean section for HIV+ women (which reduces the risk of transmission during labor and delivery).
- Breast-feeding alternatives, including use of formula instead of breast milk.

Even in places that do offer such interventions to protect children from HIV, the mothers often receive far from adequate or appropriate care. In many cases, no one explains to the mothers why they are being tested for HIV, and no one gives them information after the test. Women who are found to have HIV are sometimes stripped of their rights by being coerced into abortion or sterilization. They are also often not informed of the potential adverse effects of antiretroviral therapy or other therapies that are provided to them (GENDER-AIDS eForum, 2003; WHO, 2000).

PREVENTION OF HIV TRANSMISSION IN HEALTH CARE SETTINGS

The Centers for Disease Control and Prevention (CDC) developed universal precautions to prevent the transmission of blood-borne pathogens (e.g., HIV, hepatitis B) in health care settings (CDC, 1987a, 1987b, 2002). Specifically, CDC recommends that health care workers consider *all* patients to be potentially infected with HIV, especially those receiving emergency care, where the risk of blood exposure is increased and the patient's serostatus is unknown (CDC, 1987a). Recommended precautions for health care workers include (CDC, 2002):

- Wearing gloves, masks, protective eyewear, and gowns during all procedures that could expose them to blood, bloody body fluids, amniotic fluid, semen, vaginal fluid, or cerebrospinal fluid.
- Washing hands and other skin surfaces immediately after contact with blood or body fluids.

- Taking care in handling and disposing of sharp instruments during and after use.

Safer design and placement of disposal containers for needles and other sharp instruments is contributing to a decline in needle-stick injuries to workers in health care settings. CDC also has developed *postexposure prophylaxis (PEP)* guidelines for treating workers in health care settings who are occupationally exposed to bodily fluids that are or may be infected with HIV (Panlilio, 2005). These guidelines cover the circumstances under which antiretroviral therapy should be administered; the combinations of antiretroviral drugs that should be used; and procedures for monitoring and managing the side effects and toxicity of PEP.

HIV PREVENTION FOR HIV-POSITIVES

During the first decade of the HIV/AIDS epidemic, most HIV prevention efforts traditionally encouraged safer sex and safer drug use among people who were not infected with HIV (CDC, 2006). This focus on HIV– people is referred to as a *primary prevention* approach. Such prevention efforts were separate from the treatment and end-of-life care efforts targeted at HIV+ people.

However, since antiretroviral treatments became available in 1987, people with HIV have been living longer and healthier lives. Studies suggest that over 70% of HIV+ individuals are sexually active after learning they are infected (Crepaz & Marks, 2002). Although many engage in safer-sex practices, risk behaviors remain prevalent among a considerable percentage (DiClemente, Wingood, Del Rio, & Crosby, 2002; McGowan et al., 2004). Unprotected sex can transmit HIV to HIV-negative partners; infect HIV-positive persons with different strains of the virus; and increase the risk of spreading other STIs/STDs, which can further increase HIV transmission. These dynamics suggest that *secondary prevention* programs (prevention for positives) are vital to curbing the epidemic (CDC, 2006; Janssen & Valdiserri, 2004; Wolitski, Janssen, Onorato, Purcell, & Crepaz, 2005).

Those already living with HIV represent a growing focus of current HIV prevention efforts.

Secondary HIV prevention efforts strive to reduce barriers to HIV testing and provide access to quality medical care (including care for other STIs/STDs) and antiretroviral treatment (CDC, 2003). Effective treatment with antiretroviral therapy reduces the amount of active virus in HIV+ people's body fluids, and therefore decreases the chances of HIV transmission. Secondary prevention efforts also provide ongoing prevention services to people living with HIV/AIDS, so that they can reduce the likelihood that they will pass HIV to others through risky sexual and drug use practices.

HIV/AIDS VACCINES

Vaccines are medicines made of dead or weakened pathogens (viruses, bacteria) that, when injected or eaten, strengthen the body's immune system against a particular disease. Vaccines are among the most powerful and cost-effective disease prevention tools available. An HIV/AIDS vaccine would be better than other HIV prevention interventions because it could reach populations that have limited access to ongoing health care and prevention services, and it would work without consistent and sustained behavior change (Collins, 2001).

Research is currently being conducted on a variety of potential HIV/AIDS vaccines. However, once a vaccine is developed, it may only be partially effective, and may only stop or delay progression of the disease or reduce infectiousness among people already infected, rather than prevent transmission of the virus (EngenderHealth, n.d.). Moreover, the possibility of vaccination may cause people to resume risky drug use and sexual behaviors.

In anticipation of the potential increased risk behaviors in response to future HIV vaccine availability, prevention messages and interventions should educate people about vaccines' partial efficacy. They also should combat people's belief in an HIV vaccine as a "magic bullet" that can cure HIV/AIDS (Newman, Duan, Rudy, & Johnston-Roberts, 2004).

REFERENCES

Access Working Group, Microbicide Initiative. (2002). *Preparing for microbicide access and use.* New York: The Rockefeller Foundation.

Burack, J. H., & Bangsberg, D. (1998) Epidemiology and HIV transmission in injection drug users. In L. Pieperl, S. Coffey, O. Bacon, & P. Volberding (Eds.), *HIV InSite knowledge base.* San Francisco: Center for HIV Information, University of California, San Francisco.

Campo, J., Perea, M. A., del Romero, J., Cano, J., Hernando, V., & Bascones, A. (2006). Oral transmission of HIV, reality or fiction? An update. *Oral Diseases, 12*(3), 219–228.

Centers for Disease Control and Prevention (CDC). (1987a). Recommendations for prevention of HIV transmission in health-care settings. *Morbidity and Mortality Weekly Report, 36*(Suppl 2), 1S-18S.

Centers for Disease Control and Prevention (CDC). (1987b). Update: Universal precautions for prevention of human immunodeficiency virus, hepatitis B virus, and other blood-borne pathogens in health-care settings. *Morbidity and Mortality Weekly Report, 37*(24), 377–382, 387–388.

Centers for Disease Control and Prevention (CDC). (1998). HIV prevention through early detection and treatment of other sexually transmitted diseases—United States recommendations of the Advisory Committee for HIV and STD Prevention. *Morbidity and Mortality Weekly Report, 47*(RR12), 1–24.

Centers for Disease Control and Prevention (CDC). (2002). *Preventing occupational HIV transmission to healthcare personnel.* Atlanta, GA: CDC.

Centers for Disease Control and Prevention (CDC). (2003). *Advancing HIV prevention: The science behind the new initiative.* Atlanta, GA: CDC.

Centers for Disease Control and Prevention. (2006). Evolution of HIV/AIDS prevention programs—United States, 1981–2006. *Morbidity and Mortality Weekly Report, 55*(21), 597–603.

Collins, C. (2001). Policy issues in vaccine development. In L. Pieperl, S. Coffey, O. Bacon, & P. Volberding (Eds.), *HIV InSite knowledge base.* San Francisco: Center for HIV Information, University of California, San Francisco.

Commonwealth Secretariat. (2001). *HIV/AIDS: An inherent gender issue.* London: The Commonwealth Secretariat/UNIFEM.

Crepaz, N., & Marks, G. (2002). Towards an understanding of sexual risk behavior in people living with HIV: A review of social, psychological, and medical findings. *AIDS, 16*(2), 135–149.

DiClemente, R. J., Wingood, G. M., Del Rio, C., & Crosby, R. A. (2002). Prevention interventions for HIV positive individuals. *Sexually Transmitted Infections, 78*(6), 393–395.

EngenderHealth. (n.d.). Preventing HIV infection. In *HIV and AIDS online minicourse.* New York: EngenderHealth. Retrieved December 18, 2003, from http://www.engenderhealth.org/res/onc/hiv/preventing/index.html

Family Health International (FHI). (2003a). *Fact sheet: Reducing HIV in injecting drug users (IDU).* Arlington, VA: FHI.

Family Health International (FHI). (2003b). *Female condoms.* Arlington, VA: FHI.

Family Health International (FHI). (2003c). *Male condoms FAQ.* Arlington, VA: FHI.

Family Health International (FHI). (n.d.) *Reducing mother-to-child transmission (MTCT) of HIV.* Arlington, VA: FHI.

Farr, G., Babelnick, H., Sturgen, K., & Dorflinger, L. (1994). Contraceptive efficacy and acceptability of the female condom. *American Journal of Public Health, 84*(12), 960–964.

Farrington, A. (2002). Microbicides: What they are and why we need them. *Health and Sexuality, 7*(3). Retrieved April 27, 2004, from http://www.arhp.org/healthcareproviders/onlinepublications/healthandsexuality/microbicides/whattheyare.cfm

Feinstein, N., & Prentice, B. (2001). Fact sheet: The female condom. In *The UNAIDS gender and AIDS almanac.* Los Altos, CA: Sociometrics Corporation.

Fleischman, J. (2004, June 30). Beyond "ABC": Helping women fight AIDS. *The Washington Post,* p. A23.

GENDER-AIDS eForum. (2003). Women "often blamed" for virus. *AEGiS Digest, 1159*(7). Retrieved October 10, 2003, from http://www.aegis.com/news/bp/2003/BP031003.html

Global Campaign for Microbicides. (2002, March). *Frequently asked questions about microbicides*. Washington, DC: Global Campaign for Microbicides.

Gostin, L. O., Lazzarini, Z., Jones, T. S., & Flaherty, K. (1997). Prevention of HIV/AIDS and other blood-borne diseases among injection drug users. A national survey on the regulation of syringes and needles. *Journal of the American Medical Association, 277*(1), 53–62.

Groseclose, S. L., Weinstein, B., Jones, T. S., Valleroy, L. A., Fehrs, L. J., & Kassler, W. J. (1995). Impact of increased legal access to needles and syringes on practices of injecting-drug users and police officers—Connecticut, 1992–1993. *Journal of Acquired Immune Deficiency Syndromes and Human Retrovirology, 10*(1), 82–89.

Janssen, R. S., & Valdiserri, R. O. (2004). HIV prevention in the United States: Increasing emphasis on working with those living with HIV. *Journal of Acquired Immune Deficiency Syndromes, 37*(Suppl 2), S119–S121.

Kalichman, S. C., & Rompa, D. (1995). Sexually coerced and noncoerced gay and bisexual men: Factors relevant to risk for human immunodeficiency virus (HIV) infection. *Journal of Sex Research, 32*, 45–50.

Kanabus, A., & Noble, R. (n.d.). *Preventing mother-to-child transmission of HIV*. Horsham,West Sussex, UK: AVERT.org. Retrieved December 1, 2003, from http://www.avert.org/motherchild.htm

Kippax, S., Crawford, J., Davis, M., Rodden, P., & Dowsett, G. (1993). Sustaining safe sex: A longitudinal sample of homosexual men. *AIDS, 7*, 257–263.

McGowan, J. P., Shah, S. S., Ganea, C. E., Blum, S., Ernst, J. A., Irwin, K. L., et al. (2004). Risk behavior for transmission of human immunodeficiency virus (HIV) among HIV-seropositive individuals in an urban setting. *Clinical Infectious Diseases, 38*(1), 122–127.

Metzger, D. S., & Navaline, H. J. (2003). HIV prevention among injection drug users: The need for integrated models. *Journal of Urban Health, 80*(4 Suppl 3), 59–66.

Morrow, K., Rosen, R., Richter, L., Emans, A., Forbes, A., Day, J., et al. (2003). The acceptability of an investigational vaginal microbicide, PRO 2000 Gel, among women in a phase 1 clinical trial. *Journal of Women's Health, 12*(17), 655–666.

National Institute of Allergy and Infectious Diseases (NIAID). (2003). *Topical microbicides: Preventing sexually transmitted diseases*. Bethesda, MD: NIAID, National Institutes of Health.

Newman, P. A., Duan, N., Rudy, E. T., & Johnston-Roberts, K. (2004). HIV risk and prevention in a post-vaccine context. *Vaccine, 22*(15–16), 1954–1963.

Osmond, D. H. (1998). Sexual transmission of HIV. In L. Pieperl, S. Coffey, O. Bacon, & P. Volberding (Eds.), *HIV InSite knowledge base*. San Francisco: Center for HIV Information, University of California, San Francisco.

Padian, N. S., Shiboski, S. C., Glass, S. O., & Vittinghoff, E. (1997). Heterosexual transmission of human immunodeficiency virus (HIV) in Northern California: Results from a ten-year study. *American Journal of Epidemiology, 146*, 350–357.

Panlilio, A. L., Cardo, D. M., Grohskopf, L. A., Heneine, W., & Ross, C. S. (2005). Updated U.S. Public Health Service guidelines for the management of occupational exposures to HIV and recommendations for postexposure prophylaxis. *Morbidity and Mortality Weekly Report, 54*(RR-9), 1–17.

Public Broadcasting System (PBS). (2006a, May 20). Needle exchange: A primer. In *Frontline: The Age of AIDS*.

Public Broadcasting System (PBS). (2006b, May 30). Interview with Bill Clinton. In *Frontline: The Age of AIDS*.

Saracco, A., Musicco, M., Nicilosi, A., Angarano, G., Arici, C., Gavazzeni, G., et al. (1993). Man-to-woman transmission of HIV: Longitudinal study of 343 steady partners of infected men. *Journal of Acquired Immune Deficiency Syndromes, 6*, 497–502.

Sexual Health InfoCenter. (n.d.). *Dental dams*. Retrieved January 13, 2004, from http://www.sexhealth.org/safersex/dentaldam.shtml

Trussell, J., Sturgen, K., Strickler, J., & Dominik, R. (1994). Comparative contraceptive efficacy of the female condom and other barrier methods. *Family Planning Perspectives, 26*(2), 66–72.

Türmen, T. (2003). Gender and HIV/AIDS. *International Journal of Gynecology and Obstetrics, 82*, 411–418.

United Nations Children's Fund (UNICEF). (n.d.). Mother-to-child transmission of HIV/AIDS. Retrieved December 3, 2003, from http://www.unicef.org/programme/hiv/focus/mtct/mtct_str.htm

U.S. Agency for International Development (USAID). (2003, August). *The ABCs of HIV prevention*. Washington, DC: USAID.

Van de Wijgert, J., & Coggins, C. (2002). Microbicides to prevent heterosexual transmission of HIV: Ten years down the road. *Bulletin of Experimental Treatments for AIDS, 15*(2), 23–28.

Wasserheit, J. N. (1992). Epidemiological synergy. Interrelationships between human immunodeficiency virus infection and other sexually transmitted diseases. *Sexually Transmitted Diseases, 19*, 61–77.

Wingood, G. M., & DiClemente, R. J. (2002). HIV/AIDS in women. In G. M. Wingood & R. J. DiClemente (Eds.), *Handbook of women's sexual and reproductive health* (pp. 281–301). New York: Kluwer Academic/Plenum.

Wolitski, R. J., Janssen, R. S., Onorato, I. M., Purcell, D. W., & Crepaz, N. (2005). An overview of prevention with people living with HIV. In S. C. Kalichman (Ed.), *Positive prevention: Reducing HIV transmission among people living with HIV/AIDS* (pp. 1–28). New York: Kluwer Academic/Plenum.

World Health Organization (WHO). (2000). *Human rights, women and HIV/AIDS. (Fact sheet no. 247)*. Geneva, Switzerland: WHO.

World Health Organization (WHO). (2001). *New data on the prevention of mother-to-child transmission of HIV and their policy implications: Conclusions and recommendations*. WHO Technical Consultation on behalf of the UNFPA/UNICEF/WHO/UNAIDS Inter-Agency Task Team on Mother-to-Child Transmission of HIV. Geneva, Switzerland: WHO.

Instructor Resources

LEARNING ACTIVITIES

ACTIVITY 1:

Group Activity: Transmission Myths and Facts

Adapted from the Myths/Facts activity in The Practicing Safer Sex Today (PSST!) Education Program, which was developed and implemented by the Department of Health Services Research at the Palo Alto Medical Foundation Research Institute (PAMFRI). Used with permission.

Objective: To dispel myths and reinforce facts about sexually transmitted infections, including HIV.

Minimum Time: 15 minutes

View a detailed guide for this activity on the CD-ROM.

ACTIVITY 2:

Group Activity: The Sexual Transmission Risk Continuum

Adapted from the HIV and STD Risk Continuum activity in The Practicing Safer Sex Today (PSST!) Education Program, which was developed and implemented by the Department of Health Services Research at the Palo Alto Medical Foundation Research Institute (PAMFRI) and the Kaiser Permanente Medical Group. Used with permission.

Objective: To teach participants how to identify high-risk, safe, and safer sexual activities.

Minimum Time: 30 minutes

View a detailed guide for this activity on the CD-ROM.

ACTIVITY 3:

Group Activity: Transmission Case Studies: Scenarios of Risk

Adapted from AIDS 101: How HIV Is Spread, the San Francisco AIDS Foundation. http://www.sfaf.org/aids101/transmission.html

Objective: To teach participants to assess their own risk of acquiring HIV.

Minimum Time: 30 minutes

View a detailed guide for this activity on the CD-ROM.

ACTIVITY 4:

Group Activity: Eliminating Barriers: Identify, Prioritize, Create Solutions

Adapted from the "Safer Sex Efficacy Workshop," in Benner, T. A., Park, M. J., & Peterson, E. C. (1998). PASHA activity sourcebook: Activities for educating teens about pregnancy and STD/HIV/AIDS prevention. *Los Altos, CA: Sociometrics Corporation. Originally developed by Karen Basen-Enquist, PhD, MPH.*

Objective: To help participants understand barriers to using HIV/STI/STD risk-reduction strategies, and to teach participants how to eliminate those barriers.

Minimum Time: 30 minutes

View a detailed guide for this activity on the CD-ROM.

ACTIVITY 5:

Assignment: Tailoring Prevention Strategies

Objective: To understand how different populations require different HIV/AIDS prevention interventions.

Think about the modes of transmission for HIV. In a three- to five-page paper, describe how different groups are affected in different ways by the different modes of infection. Explore the reasons behind these differences, and explain how they affect prevention.

DISCUSSION QUESTIONS

1. What barriers exist that prevent people from using condoms? What can be done to reduce or remove those barriers?
2. What barriers exist to prevent the reduction of IDU-related HIV transmission? What can be done to reduce or remove those barriers?
3. Why have secondary prevention programs become vital to curbing the HIV epidemic?
4. What would be the benefits of an HIV vaccine over current treatments for HIV? What might be the drawbacks of HIV vaccination?

QUIZ

1. List any three behavioral strategies that can reduce or prevent the risk of HIV infection between sexual partners.
2. Which is not a barrier method of HIV prevention?
   a) Male condoms
   b) Dental dams
   c) Microbicides
   d) Female condoms
3. Which of the following is not true of female condoms?
   a) Female condoms can be used with any kind of lubricant.
   b) Female condoms are stronger than male condoms.
   c) Female condoms may offer additional protection against infections than male condoms.

d) Female condoms are less expensive than male condoms.

4. True or False: The use of microbicides eliminates the need for condoms.

5. True or False: Switching from injection to noninjection drugs eliminates HIV transmission risk.

6. List three ways that injection drug users can reduce their risk of HIV transmission.

7. True or False: Antiretroviral therapy should not be used by pregnant women because it does not prevent transmission of HIV to the fetus.

8. List three ways that health care workers can reduce their risk of HIV transmission.

9. Postexposure prophylaxis refers to:
a) Methods for treating HIV exposure
b) Methods for using condoms to prevent HIV transmission
c) Methods for reducing HIV risk during injection drug use

10. Secondary prevention programs refer to:
a) Methods to prevent HIV transmission among HIV− people
b) Methods to prevent HIV transmission among HIV+ people
c) Methods to prevent HIV transmission among health care workers

ANSWERS

1. Abstaining from (not engaging in) sex or having sex with only one, uninfected partner will prevent the sexual transmission of HIV. Engaging in *safer sex*—using condoms, dental dams, or other barriers that prevent or reduce contact with partners' blood, semen, and other body fluids—reduces the likelihood of sexual transmission.

2. C. Barrier methods include male condoms, female condoms, and dental dams.

3. D. Female condoms offer a number of advantages over male condoms; however, they are more expensive and less widely available than male condoms.

4. False. When used correctly, male or female condoms provide better protection against HIV and STIs/STDs than microbicides alone.

5. False. The use of noninjection drugs can still affect the body and mind in ways that put people at risk for HIV and STIs/STDs.

6. Risk of HIV transmission can be reduced by always using new injection equipment, never sharing equipment, and sterilizing equipment between uses with clean water and bleach.

7. False. Antiretroviral therapy can prevent perinatal transmission of HIV.

8. Health care workers should wear gloves, masks, protective eyewear, and gowns; they should wash their hands and skin surfaces after contact with blood or body fluids; and they should take care in handling and disposing of sharp instruments during and after use.

9. A. The CDC has developed postexposure prophylaxis guidelines for treating people who are exposed to bodily fluids that are or may be infected with HIV.

10. B. Secondary prevention programs refer to prevention methods for HIV+ people.

WEB RESOURCES

Overview of Transmission

AIDS 101: How HIV Is Spread (San Francisco AIDS Foundation)

http://www.sfaf.org/aids101/transmission.html

Explains which activities do and do not transmit HIV.

Prevention of Infection Through Sexual Contact

Safer Sex Resources (UCSF HIV InSite)

http://www.hivinsite.com/InSite?page=li-07-11

Provides links to research articles and additional resources about preventing the sexual transmission of HIV.

Instructions for Using a Male Condom

http://www.engenderhealth.org/res/onc/hiv/preventing/miw/hiv6miw3.html

Instructions for Using a Female Condom

http://www.engenderhealth.org/res/onc/hiv/preventing/miw/hiv6miw4.html

Female-Controlled Prevention Technologies: Related Resources (UCSF HIV InSite, 2003)

http://hivinsite.ucsf.edu/InSite.jsp?page=kbr-07-02-04

Lists links to research-based fact sheets, guidelines, FAQs, reports, discussions, interviews, articles, presentations, conference Web sites, conference reports, and additional resources for female-controlled prevention technologies.

Prevention of Infection Through Injection Drug Use

Epidemiology and HIV Transmission in Injection Drug Users: Related Resources (UCSF HIV InSite)

http://www.hivinsite.com/InSite?page=kbr-07-04-01

Provides links to research articles and additional resources relating to injection drug use and HIV/AIDS.

Preventing Parent-to-Child Transmission

Women, Children, and HIV

http://www.womenchildrenhiv.org/

Contains a library of practical, applicable materials on mother and child HIV infection including preventing parent-to-child HIV transmission, safely feeding infants of HIV+ mothers, caring for HIV+ women, children, and orphans, plus up-to-date news on HIV/AIDS.

RECOMMENDED READING

Prevention of Infection Through Sexual Contact

Safer-Sex Methods (Lane & Palacio, 2003)

Lane, T., & Palacio, H. (2003). Safer-sex methods. In L. Pieperl, S. Coffey, O. Bacon, & P. Volberding (Eds.), HIV InSite knowledge base. *San Francisco: Center for HIV Information, University of California, San Francisco.*

This chapter reviews the evidence that has led to the development of safer-sex guidelines, and concludes with specific recommendations for safer-sex practices.

Available online at http://www.hivinsite.com/InSite?page=kb-07-02-02

Preventing Parent-to-Child Transmission

An International Perspective on Preventing Vertical Transmission (Etiebet et al., 2004)

Etiebet, M. A., Fransman, D., Forsyth, B., Coetzee, N., & Hussey, G. (2004). Integrating prevention of mother-to-child HIV transmission into antenatal care: Learning from the experiences of women in South Africa. AIDS Care, 16*(1), 37–46.*

This study showed that routine prenatal HIV testing and interventions to reduce parent-to-child transmission are acceptable to the majority of women in a South African urban township, despite their awareness of discrimination against HIV+ women in the community.

Positive Prevention

Reducing Sexual Transmission of HIV by HIV+ People (Marks, Burris, & Peterman, 1999)

Marks, G., Burris, S., & Peterman, T. A. (1999). Reducing sexual transmission of HIV from those who know they are infected: The need for personal and collective responsibility. AIDS, 13, *297–306.*

This article examines risk-taking of HIV+ people and discusses the roles of personal and collective responsibility in reducing HIV transmission.

Positive Prevention: Reducing HIV Transmission Among People Living With HIV/AIDS (Kalichman, 2004)

Kalichman, S. C. (Ed.). (2004). Positive prevention: Reducing HIV transmission among people living with HIV/AIDS. *New York: Plenum.*

This is a compilation of articles from the top scholars in the field of HIV/AIDS prevention. Topics include unprotected sex among HIV+ gay and bisexual men; whether disclosure leads to safer sex; mental health and HIV among young adults; the impact of HIV diagnosis on sexual risk behaviors; and interventions in community settings. There is also an important chapter on international perspectives on positive prevention.

POWERPOINT SLIDES

(Note: A full-color version of these slides, with graphics, is also available on the CD-ROM.)

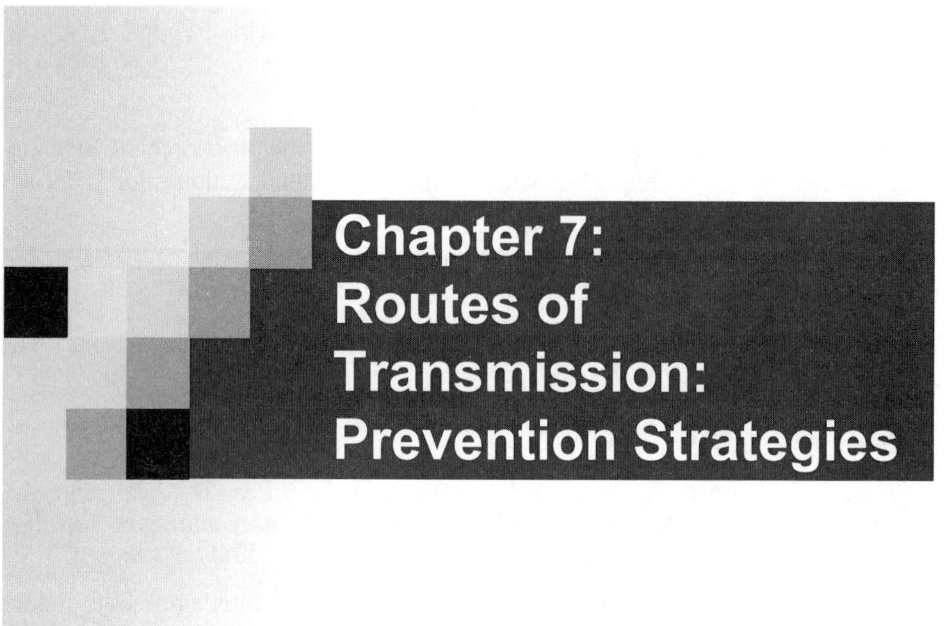

Routes of Transmission: Prevention Strategies

- HIV is not casually transmitted. It is transmitted through a few, very specific practices that bring infected body fluid in close contact with cells.
- In order for HIV to be transmitted:
  - HIV must be present.
  - HIV must be present in sufficient quantity.
  - HIV must get into the bloodstream.

Prevention of Infection Through Sexual Contact

The ABCs of preventing HIV transmission through sexual contact are...

- **A**bstinence
- **B**eing faithful
- **C**ondoms (used correctly/consistently)

Not as Simple as ABC

- The ABCs are sometimes hard to implement.
- Some activists suggest the "DEF" approach:
  - **D**isclosure means telling other people if you are HIV+
  - **E**ducation: Women's vulnerability to infection is linked to their lack of access to education
  - **F**emale-controlled prevention methods (e.g., microbicides and female condoms)

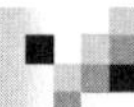

Negotiating Safer Sex

- Safer Sex: Reduces the risk of contracting STIs/STDs, including HIV. Includes using condoms and dental dams.
- Communication: An important part of safer sex.
- Negotiating Safer Sex: This can be extremely challenging, especially for women.

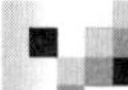

Barrier Methods

- Aside from abstinence or having sex with only one, uninfected partner, using condoms or dental dams is the most effective way of preventing sexual transmission of HIV and other sexually transmitted infections.
- When used consistently and correctly, male condoms are highly effective in preventing transmission of HIV.
- In a study of couples in which one partner had HIV, all 123 couples who used condoms for every sexual act over 4 years prevented HIV transmission. Among the 122 couples who did not use condoms for every sexual act, 12 partners became infected.

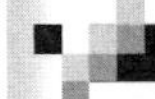

Barrier Methods (continued)

Female Condom
A thin, soft, loose-fitting polyurethane plastic pouch that lines the vagina.

Advantages:
- Female-controlled
- More comfortable to men
- Offers greater protection (covers both internal and external genitalia)
- More convenient (can be inserted before sexual activity begins)
- Stronger (polyurethane is 40% stronger than latex)

Disadvantages:
- Relatively more expensive and less available than the male condom
- The outer ring is visible outside the vagina, which can make some women feel self-conscious
- Some women find it difficult to insert and to remove

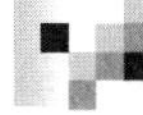

Prevention of Drug Injection-Related Transmission of HIV

- There are several ways to reduce injection drug use-related transmission of HIV. They include, in order of efficacy:
    - Stop injection drug use: Complete abstinence or changing to non-injection drugs (e.g., methadone programs)
    - Always use sterile needles, syringes, and other injection equipment (e.g., needle exchange programs)
    - Never share injecting equipment
    - Sterilize equipment between uses with clean water and bleach

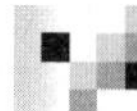

Preventing Parent-To-Child Transmission

- Also known as vertical transmission
- How most children under 10 years of age get HIV
- Infection occurs through:
    - Pregnancy
    - Labor
    - Delivery
    - Breastfeeding
- Has been virtually eliminated in the developed world
- Rates remain high in resource constrained countries
- Breastfeeding increases the risk of mother-to-child HIV transmission by 10–15%

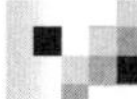

Prevention of HIV Transmission in Health Care Settings

- **HIV Transmission in the Health Care Setting**
    - Workers have been infected with HIV after being stuck with needles containing infected blood or after infected blood gets into open cuts or mucous membranes.
    - Infection due to needle stick injury is rare (about 3 per 1,000 injuries).
- **Universal Precautions**
    - Developed by the CDC to prevent the transmission of blood-borne pathogens (e.g., HIV) in health care settings
    - The CDC recommends that health-care workers consider **all** patients to be potentially infected with HIV.
    - Recommended precautions include using gloves, masks, protective eyewear, and gowns during all procedures that could expose a health care worker to bodily fluids.

HIV Prevention for HIV-Positive People

Treatment is Prevention

- Prevention interventions are increasingly aimed at HIV+ people.
- These efforts strive to:
  - reduce barriers to HIV testing;
  - provide access to quality medical care and treatment; and
  - offer ongoing prevention services to people living with HIV/AIDS.
- Effective treatments reduce the amount of active virus in HIV+ people's body fluids, and therefore decrease the chances of HIV transmission.

Learning Objectives

- Understand the uses and types of HIV counseling, testing, and referral
- Distinguish between confidential and anonymous HIV testing

Key Terms

anonymous testing
confidential testing
CTR
ELISA
individual-level intervention
partner notification programs
rapid serum HIV antibody test
VCT
Western Blot

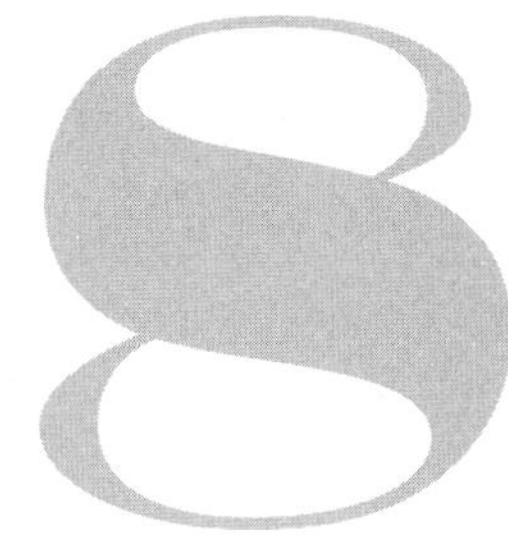

Individual-Level Interventions

Until an effective and safe vaccine is developed, prevention efforts must focus on changing risky behaviors and the factors that lead to those behaviors. Individual-level interventions to prevent HIV are delivered to individuals in one-on-one settings by professionals, peers, and/or media (e.g., videos, DVDs, Web sites). They are commonly based on psychological theories of behavior change (such as the health belief model and stages of change model; see chapter 6) and seek to influence the knowledge, attitudes, skills, intentions, and behaviors that are most closely linked to HIV transmission (CDC, 2006).

Both effective individual- and small group-level interventions may focus on primary and/or secondary prevention, are theory-based, build the behavioral skills needed to reduce risky sexual or drug-using behaviors, and are culturally tailored to their target populations (CDC, 2001a; Wilson & Miller, 2003). This chapter briefly describes several major types of individual-level interventions.

HIV COUNSELING, TESTING, AND REFERRAL

Counseling, Testing, and Referral (CTR), also known as Voluntary Counseling and Testing (VCT), is an important strategy for facilitating behavior change, and is a vital point of entry to other HIV/AIDS care services (CDC, 2001b; FHI, 2003). CTR benefits those who test positive, as well as those who test negative, by informing people of their HIV status; providing high-quality HIV prevention counseling, to reduce likelihood of transmitting or acquiring HIV; and referring people to appropriate medical, preventive, and psychosocial support services.

Counseling

The goal of the counseling component of CTR is to reduce HIV acquisition and transmission by providing information about HIV transmission, prevention, and the meaning of HIV test results (CDC, 2001b). This component includes at least one session of one-on-one prevention counseling that focuses on the client's unique circumstances and risks. It should include an in-depth personalized risk assessment that allows the counselor and the client to identify, acknowledge, and understand the specific behaviors putting the client at risk for acquiring or transmitting HIV.

Confidential and Anonymous HIV Testing

As is discussed in chapter 2, a variety of HIV tests are currently available. Most (including ELISA, the Western Blot test, *rapid serum HIV antibody tests, saliva- and urine-based antibody tests,* and *home HIV antibody testing kits*) test for antibodies that the body develops after it is infected with HIV. HIV RNA tests can detect HIV even earlier, by identifying strands of HIV RNA even before the body has produced antibodies to the virus.

HIV testing may be *anonymous* or *confidential.* In anonymous testing, the person being tested is identified in records by a unique code (e.g., a number, or a fictitious name). The results of the test cannot be associated with the real name, Social Security number, address, or other identifying characteristics of the person being tested, not even by the person administering the test. In this way, anonymous testing can help to allay fears that the findings of the test may be divulged to others without the consent of the person being tested (Constantine, 2001).

In confidential testing, the person being tested is identified in records by his or her real name. Confidential test results become part of the person's medical record, and therefore can legally be divulged to certain parties (e.g., insurance carriers) under particular circumstances. Opting for confidential testing versus anonymous testing is common when official written documentation of test results is required (e.g., for a clinician to begin treatment; for a patient to get Medicaid benefits or worker's compensation) (Constantine, 2001).

Referrals to HIV/AIDS Services

After being counseled and tested, people may be referred to a variety of services. Examples include prevention education or case management, partner counseling, partner notification programs, medical evaluation and treatment, reproductive health services, drug or alcohol abuse treatment, mental health services, legal services, and social services. Referrals for additional testing and/or treatment (e.g., for STIs/STDs) also may be made.

HIV PREVENTION COUNSELING

Counseling interventions conducted separately from HIV testing also can be effective in reducing sex or drug-using risk behaviors among both HIV– and HIV+ persons (Kalichman, 1998; Kalichman et al., 2005; Kamb et al., 1998; Robles et al., 2004). Some of these interventions have been as brief as a single session, demonstrating the promise of these interventions in settings where it is particularly challenging to retain participants in multisession programs. Counseling approaches that are theory-based, interactive, and focused on personal risk reduction seem to be the most promising (Kamb et al., 1998).

PARTNER NOTIFICATION

Partner notification programs locate, counsel, and test the partners of HIV-infected people. Studies have shown that in partner notification programs where *both* partners receive counseling, couples are less likely to break up or acquire new partners and more likely to use condoms (Hoxworth et al., 2003; Kamenga et al., 1991).

HIV/AIDS HOTLINES AND ONLINE FORUMS

Individual-level counseling can also occur without an actual face-to-face encounter with a counselor. The telephone and the computer provide opportunities for individuals to request and receive HIV-related information and advice.

Information Hotlines

AIDS information hotlines are operated by the Centers for Disease Control and Prevention, state health departments, and local community organizations. The main inquiries made to the AIDS hotlines in the United States and abroad focus on HIV transmission and concerns about HIV risk (Benedetti et al., 1989; Polinko, Bradley, Molyneaux, & Lukoff, 1995). A study of over 1,000 U.S. AIDS hotlines found that the most frequently asked questions concerned HIV antibody testing (21%), followed by questions about sexual transmission of HIV (16%), HIV-related symptoms (16%), and situations that do not confer risk of HIV infection (14%) (Kalichman & Belcher, 1997). On the surface, questions that come into HIV hotlines are straightforward, but a deeper level of analysis suggests that individuals are motivated to call hotlines by fears of contracting HIV from actual risk behaviors or to dismiss concerns about contracting HIV through casual modes (Kalichman & Belcher, 1997).

Trained in basic listening and counseling skills, hotline workers are well positioned to offer brief risk-reduction counseling over the phone. Hotline workers may ask questions to identify what motivated the call and to identify additional services to which the person may be referred (Kalichman, 1998).

Online Bulletin Boards and Forums

The Internet is another source for personalized interactive prevention information dissemination. TheBody.com's "Ask the Expert" Question and Answer Forum (http://www.thebody.com/experts.shtml), for example, provides a forum where individuals can write in questions on a variety of issues specific to HIV/AIDS prevention and treatment. An expert in each topical area answers the question and posts the interaction online. Many online bulletin boards and forums are not moderated by experts, however, resulting in the risk that incorrect or misleading information will be disseminated.

REFERENCES

Benedetti, P., Zaccarelli, M., Giuliani, M., Di Fabio, M., Valdarchi, C., Pezzotti, P., et al. (1989). The Italian AIDS "Hot-Line": Providing information to the people. *AIDS Care, 1*(2), 145–152.

Centers for Disease Control and Prevention (CDC). (2001a). *Compendium of HIV prevention interventions with evidence of success*. Atlanta, GA: CDC.

Centers for Disease Control and Prevention (CDC). (2001b). Revised guidelines for HIV counseling, testing, and referral and revised recommendations for HIV screening of pregnant women. *Morbidity and Mortality Weekly Report, 50*(RR19), 1–58.

Centers for Disease Control and Prevention (CDC). (2006). Evolution of HIV/AIDS prevention programs—United States, 1981–2006. *Morbidity and Mortality Weekly Report, 55*(21), 597–603.

Constantine, N. (2001). HIV antibody assays. In L. Pieperl, S. Coffey, O. Bacon, & P. Volberding (Eds.), *HIV InSite knowledge base*. San Francisco: Center for HIV Information, University of California, San Francisco.

Family Health International (FHI). (2003). *Fact sheet: Voluntary counseling and testing for HIV*. Research Triangle Park, NC: FHI.

Hoxworth, T., Spencer, N. E., Peterman, T. A., Craig, T., Johnson, S., & Maher, J. E. (2003). Changes in partnerships and HIV risk behaviors after partner notification. *Sexually Transmitted Diseases, 30*(1), 83–88.

Kalichman, S. C. (1998). *Preventing AIDS: A sourcebook for behavioral interventions*. Mahwah, NJ: Lawrence Erlbaum Associates.

Kalichman, S. C., & Belcher, L. (1997). AIDS information needs: Conceptual and content analyses of questions asked of AIDS information hotlines. *Health Education Research, 12*(3), 279–288.

Kalichman, S. C., Cain, D., Weinhardt, L., Benotsch, E., Presser, K., Zweben, A., et al. (2005). Experimental components analysis of brief theory-based HIV/AIDS risk-reduction counseling for sexually transmitted infection patients. *Health Psychology, 24*(2), 198–208.

Kamb, M. L., Fishbein, M., Douglas, J. M. Jr., Rhodes, F., Rogers, J., Bolan, G., et al. (1998). Efficacy of risk-reduction counseling to prevent human immunodeficiency virus and sexually transmitted diseases: A randomized controlled trial. Project RESPECT Study Group. *Journal of the American Medical Association, 280*(13), 1161–1167.

Kamenga, M., Ryder, R. W., Jingu, M., Mbuyi, N., Mbu, L., Behets, F., et al. (1991). Evidence of marked sexual behavior change associated with low HIV-1 seroconversion in 149 married couples with discordant HIV-1 serostatus: Experience at an HIV counseling center in Zaire. *AIDS, 5*(1), 61–67.

Polinko, P., Bradley, W. F., Molyneaux, B., & Lukoff, C. (1995). HIV in healthcare workers: Managing fear through a telephone information line. *Social Work, 40*, 819–822.

Robles, R. R., Reyes, J. C., Colón, H. M., Sahai, H., Marrero, C. A., Matos, T. D., et al. (2004). Effects of combined counseling and case management to reduce HIV risk behaviors among Hispanic drug injectors in Puerto Rico: A randomized controlled study. *Journal of Substance Abuse Treatment, 27*, 145–152.

Wilson, B. D. M., & Miller, R. L. (2003). Examining strategies for culturally grounded HIV prevention: A review. *AIDS Education and Prevention, 15*(2), 184–202.

Instructor Resources

LEARNING ACTIVITIES

ACTIVITY 1:

Assignment: Local HIV Counseling and Testing Options

Objective: To be aware of the range of local HIV counselling and testing options.

Use the Internet to investigate local HIV counseling and testing options in a community (e.g., city, county, etc.). Make note of the following features of these services:

- Location
- Schedule
- Whether anonymous vs. confidential
- Cost (e.g., free, low-cost, sliding scale, etc.)
- Language in which services are offered
- Type of clients who are specifically targeted by the services
- Related activities or services offered to clients (e.g., STI testing)

Prepare a table showing the features of each local HIV counseling and testing option. Write a short paper that summarizes the range of services available and identifies any groups in the community (e.g., non-English speakers; youth; etc.) for whom there appear to be few or no appropriate services.

ACTIVITY 2: (OPTIONAL)

Assignment: HIV Vaccines

Objective: To describe the development of HIV vaccines.

Vaccines are a powerful and cost-effective disease-prevention tool. An HIV/AIDS vaccine could have advantages over existing HIV prevention interventions because it could reach populations that otherwise have limited access to health care and prevention services.

- Write a two- to three-page summary of the research and development of HIV vaccines.

DISCUSSION QUESTIONS

1. Why might a person opt for anonymous testing over confidential testing, or vice versa?
2. Why might a person opt to use an HIV hotline over other sources of information?

QUIZ

1. Individual interventions are often based on:
   a) Social theories
   b) Psychological theories of behavior change
   c) Community behavioral models
   d) Interpersonal behavioral models
2. Which is not a feature of effective individual interventions?
   a) They focus primarily on primary prevention.
   b) They are culturally targeted to their primary population.
   c) They are based on theory.
   d) They attempt to influence knowledge, attitudes, and behaviors.
3. List three services provided by CTR.
4. In ____ testing, a person's test results cannot be associated with the person being tested.
5. When both partners receive HIV counseling, they are:
   a) More likely to break up
   b) Less likely to break up
   c) Equally likely to break up as without counseling
   d) Neither more or less likely to break up

ANSWERS

1. **B.** Individual-level interventions are commonly based on psychological theories of behavior change such as the health belief model and the stages of change model.
2. **A.** Effective individual interventions may focus on primary and/or secondary intervention.
3. CTR informs people of their HIV status; provides high-quality HIV prevention counseling; and refers people to appropriate medical, preventive, and psychosocial support services.
4. Anonymous.
5. **B.** Studies show that when both partners receive counseling, they are less likely to break up and more likely to use condoms.

WEB RESOURCES

Individual-Level Prevention Strategies

United States AIDS Hotlines

http://www.thebody.com/hotlines/state.html

International HIV/AIDS Service Organizations and Information Resources

http://www.thebody.com/hotlines/internat.html

Medical Level Prevention Strategies

HIV Vaccine Trials Network

http://www.hvtn.org/

Contains links to resources and information about HIV vaccine trials and vaccine advocacy.

Global Campaign for Microbicides

http://www.global-campaign.org/

The Global Campaign for Microbicides is a broad-based, international effort to build support among policy makers, opinion leaders, and the general public for increased investment into microbicides and other user-controlled prevention methods. Through advocacy, policy analysis, and social science research, the campaign works to accelerate product development, facilitate widespread access and use, and protect the needs and interests of users, especially women.

National Institute of Allergy and Infectious Diseases (NIAID) Fact Sheets

http://www.niaid.nih.gov/publications/aidsfact.htm

Includes fact sheets on microbicides, parent-to-child transmission, STI/STD treatment, vaccines, and other medically oriented prevention interventions.

RECOMMENDED READING

Individual-Level Prevention Strategies

Levels of Prevention (Kalichman, 1998)

Kalichman, S. C. (1998). Preventing AIDS: A sourcebook for behavioral interventions. *Mahwah, NJ: Lawrence Erlbaum Associates.*

This highly regarded text summarizes 20 years of research on the behavioral prevention of HIV transmission, reviews HIV risk-reduction theories, and overviews individual-, small group-, and community-level strategies for HIV prevention.

Guidelines for HIV Counseling, Testing, and Referral (CDC, 2001)

Centers for Disease Control and Prevention (CDC). (2001). Revised Guidelines for HIV Counseling, Testing, and Referral: Technical Expert Panel Review of CDC HIV Counseling, Testing, and Referral Guidelines.

These guidelines replace the CDC's 1994 HIV Counseling, Testing, and Referral Standards and Guidelines, and contain recommendations for public- and private-sector policy makers and HIV counseling, testing, and referral (CTR) providers. The new guidelines encourage confidential and anonymous voluntary HIV testing, informed consent, the provision of HIV prevention counseling that focuses on the client's own risk. They also discuss evidence-based recommendations for CTR, acknowledge providers' need for flexibility in implementing the guidelines, recommend that CTR be targeted efficiently through risk screening and other strategies, and address ways to improve the quality and provision of HIV CTR.

Available online at http://www.cdc.gov/mmwr/preview/mmwrhtml/rr5019a1.htm

Medical-Level Prevention Strategies

Preparing for Microbicide Access and Use (Access Working Group of the Microbicide Initiative, 2002)

Access Working Group of the Microbicide Initiative. (2002). Preparing for microbicide access and use. *Silver Spring, MD: International Partnership for Microbicides.*

The Access Working Group seeks to improve reproductive health and reduce HIV transmission by ensuring that women and girls throughout the world have access to safe, effective, affordable, and easy-to-use microbicides. This document reports the group's priorities for action.

Policy Issues in Vaccine Development (UCSF HIV InSite, 2001)

Collins, C. (2001). Policy issues in vaccine development. HIV InSite knowledge base. *San Francisco: Center for HIV Information, University of California, San Francisco.*

This article overviews the history and application of HIV vaccine research.

Available online at http://hivinsite.ucsf.edu/InSite.jsp?page=kb-08-01-11

POWERPOINT SLIDES

(Note: A full-color version of these slides, with graphics, is also available on the CD-ROM.)

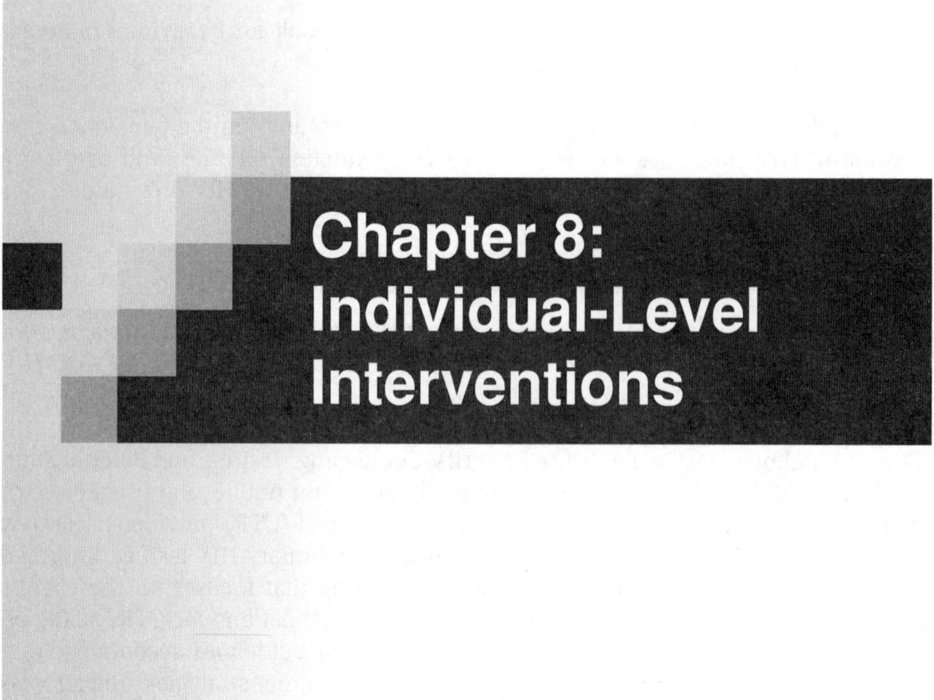

Individual-Level Interventions

HIV Counseling, Testing, and Referral (CTR)

- A cost-effective strategy for facilitating behavior change
- Benefits those who test positive, as well as those who test negative, by:
  - □ informing people of their HIV status;
  - □ providing HIV prevention counseling; and
  - □ referring people to appropriate support

Individual-Level Interventions (continued)

- Best practices in HIV CTR include:
  - □ providing information and education to support HIV risk reduction;
  - □ assessing individuals' risk levels;
  - □ ensuring that test results are given in person;
  - □ providing information and referrals to other services; and
  - □ facilitating partner notification.

HIV Counseling

- The goal of HIV counseling is to reduce HIV acquisition and transmission by providing:
  - **INFORMATION** about HIV transmission, prevention, and the meaning of HIV test results;
  - **PREVENTION COUNSELING** that focuses on the client's unique circumstances and risks; and
  - **PERSONALIZED RISK ASSESSMENT** that allows the counselor and the client to identify, acknowledge, and understand the specific behaviors putting the client at risk for acquiring or transmitting HIV.

HIV Testing

Anonymous testing:

- The person being tested is identified in records by a code.
- The test results cannot be associated with the person, not even by the person administering the test.
- Helps to allay fears of violated confidentiality.
- May attract people at high risk who are not yet willing to be tested in a confidential setting.

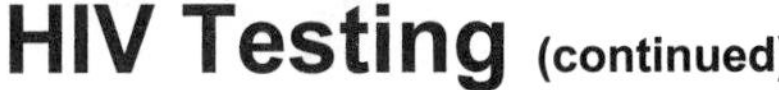

HIV Testing (continued)

Confidential testing:

- The person being tested is identified in records by his or her real name.
- Confidential test results become part of the person's medical record.
- While efforts to maintain confidentiality in HIV testing should be taken seriously, confidentiality cannot be guaranteed.
- Opting for confidential testing is common when official written documentation of test results is required (e.g., for a clinician to begin treatment; to get Medicaid benefits or worker's compensation).

Couples Counseling and Partner Notification

Because HIV is often transmitted between people in relationships, couples are an important target for HIV prevention interventions.

- **Couples Counseling:** After testing positive for HIV, people often reduce or discontinue behaviors that might transmit HIV. Safer-sex counseling sessions can lead to more frequent condom use.
- **Partner Notification:** Partner notification programs locate, counsel, and test the partners of HIV-infected people.

HIV/AIDS Hotlines

- Operated by the CDC, state health departments, and local community organizations
- Most hotline callers in the United States and abroad ask about HIV transmission and their own risks of getting and giving HIV.
- Callers are often motivated by their fears of contracting HIV.

HIV/AIDS Online Forums

Online Bulletin Boards and Forums

- The Internet is another source of personalized interactive HIV/AIDS prevention information.
- The Body.com's "Ask the Expert" question-and-answer forum (http://www.thebody.com/experts.html) allows people to send questions about a wide variety of HIV/AIDS concerns.

STI Prevention, Diagnosis, and Treatment

STIs/STDs Increase HIV's Impact

- People with another STI/STD have up to 10 times the risk of getting and giving HIV than people without STIs/STDs.
- This is true for both infections that cause sores on the genitalia, such as syphilis and herpes, and for infections that do not cause sores, such as gonorrhea and chlamydia.
- The presence of other STIs/STDs can speed up the development of AIDS.

STI Prevention, Diagnosis, and Treatment (continued)

Early Detection and Treatment

- An effective strategy for preventing sexually transmitted HIV infection
- STI diagnosis and prevention includes:
  - counseling to ensure follow-up treatment, and
  - strategies to notify partners for treatment.

Microbicides

Benefits of Microbicides:

- Currently under development, microbicides are creams, gels, and foams that can be inserted into the vagina or rectum
- They work by killing or inactivating viruses and bacteria.
- Microbicides may be another way that women and men can protect themselves from HIV and STIs/STDs.
- When inserted in the body during childbirth, microbicides may also reduce the transmission of HIV and STIs/STDs from mothers to infants during childbirth.
- However, microbicides do not eliminate the need for condoms and they do not necessarily protect against all STIs/STDs.

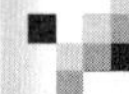

Microbicides (continued)

Possible Barriers to Microbicide Use:

- Non-supportive cultural practices, like dry sex
- Lack of discretion in packaging and application
- Lack of availability
- Difficulty in use or application
- Unacceptable odor or taste
- Contraceptive properties (or lack thereof)

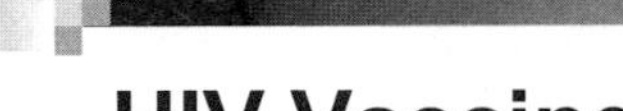

HIV Vaccines

The Promise of HIV Vaccines

- Vaccines are medicines made of dead or weakened pathogens (viruses, bacteria) that strengthen the body's immune system against a particular disease.
- Vaccines are among the most powerful and cost-effective disease prevention tools available.

The Reality of HIV Vaccines

- In anticipation of the potential increased risk behaviors in response to future HIV vaccine availability, prevention messages and interventions should:
  - educate people about vaccines' partial efficacy.
  - combat people's belief in an HIV vaccine as a "magic bullet" that can cure HIV/AIDS.

Learning Objectives

- Understand the strengths and drawbacks of small group interventions as compared to other methods
- Define the characteristics of effective small group interventions

Key Terms

serodiscordant

small group intervention

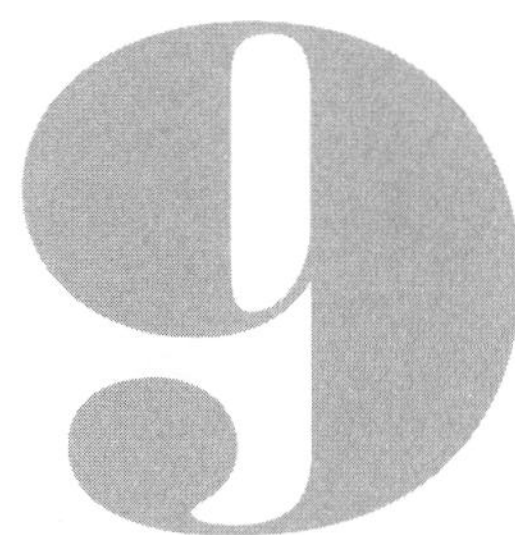

Small Group-Level Interventions

Small group-level interventions are delivered to couples, small groups, or families by professionals, peers, and/or media (e.g., videos, DVDs, Web sites). They seek to influence the knowledge, attitudes, skills, intentions, and behaviors that are most closely linked to HIV transmission (CDC, 2006). Effective small group-level interventions may focus on primary and/or secondary prevention, and they may last one or many sessions. They based on a variety of psychological and social theories about behavior and behavior change (see chapter 6). They build the skills needed to reduce risky sexual or drug-using behaviors, and are culturally tailored to their target populations (CDC, 2001; Wilson & Miller, 2003).

A relatively large number of small group interventions have been rigorously evaluated and shown to be effective in reducing HIV risk behaviors (see Figure 9-1). Research shows that small group interventions can decrease HIV risk behaviors in many populations, including men who have sex with men, heterosexual women, heterosexual men, adolescents, injection drug users (IDUs), and HIV-positive persons (Card, Benner, Shields, & Feinstein, 2001; CDC, 2001; Copenhaver et al., 2006).

However, small group interventions also have some limitations. In particular, not everyone likes participating in groups, and it can be difficult to get several people together at the same time on a consistent basis. Additionally, the strong leaders with good interpersonal skills who are necessary for small group interventions are not always available (Kalichman, 1998). The remainder of this chapter briefly describes two types of small group interventions, couples counseling and group educational and skills-building interventions.

COUPLES COUNSELING

After testing positive for HIV, people often reduce or discontinue behaviors that might transmit HIV (Colfax et al., 2002). However, risk behavior may not be eliminated entirely, leaving HIV– partners vulnerable to initial infection and HIV+ partners vulnerable to infection with a different strain of HIV. Couples counseling can lead to the diagnosis of sex and needle-sharing partners with previously undiagnosed infections (CDC, 2003). In addition, even brief safer-sex counseling sessions (addressing such issues as condom use, safer-sex negotiation, and disclosure of HIV

For more information about effective small group-level interventions see:

- The CDC's "Replicating Effective Programs" project Web site at http://www.cdc.gov/hiv/projects/rep
- The CDC's "Diffusion of Effective Behavioral Interventions" project Web site at http://www.effectiveinterventions.org
- Sociometrics Corporation's "HIV/AIDS Prevention Program Archive (HAPPA)" Web site at http://www.socio.com/happa.htm
- Sociometrics Corporation's "Program Archive on Sexuality, Health & Adolescence (PASHA)" Web site at http://www.socio.com/pasha.htm

Figure 9-1

serostatus) can lead to more frequent condom use and sexual abstinence among *serodiscordant* couples (in which one partner is HIV+ and the other is HIV–) (Padian, O'Brien, Chang, Glass, & Francis, 1993).

EDUCATIONAL AND SKILLS-BUILDING GROUP INTERVENTIONS

Most small-group HIV prevention interventions focus on: (1) communicating information about HIV (what it is, how it spreads); (2) building skills to avoid risky behaviors that promote HIV transmission; or (3) building skills to practice safer behaviors that protect against HIV transmission (e.g., using a condom at every intercourse). These interventions are typically delivered by a health educator to small groups of relatively homogeneous participants.

Intervention Content

Single- and multi-session group interventions may be conducted in a variety of settings, including community-based organizations, clinics, schools, faith-based organizations, prisons, and other settings. The content of most effective group HIV prevention interventions includes (Kalichman, 1998):

- Basic education about HIV transmission, local prevalence of HIV and AIDS, AIDS myths, and HIV antibody tests.
- Examination of participants' own behavior to assess personal risk and to motivate behavior change.
- Behavioral skills training, including techniques for examining personal risk behaviors and for reducing personal risk.
- Sexual communication and relationship-building skills, often presented through role-playing activities, including techniques for putting condoms on, for persuading partners to use condoms, for asserting sexual preferences, and for refusing sex.

Interventions that target IDUs generally provide training in how to properly sterilize needles and other equipment ("works") used to inject drugs. Many also address sexual risk reduction among this population. Examples of effective educational and skills-building small group-level HIV prevention programs are given in Table 9-1. Replication kits for all these programs, containing all the materials needed to deliver the program, can be obtained from the HIV/AIDS Prevention Program Archives (HAPPA) at http://www.socio.com/happa.htm and the Program Archive on Sexuality, Health, and Adolescence (PASHA) at http://www.socio.com/pasha.htm. Both HAPPA and

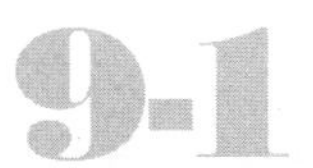

Examples of Effective STI/HIV Prevention Programs

PROGRAM NAME (DEVELOPERS)	REFERENCE(S)
STI/HIV Prevention Programs for Youth (see http://www.socio.com/pasha.htm for program descriptions)	
A Clinic-Based AIDS Education Program for Female Adolescents (Rickert, Gottlieb, & Jay)	Rickert et al., 1990 Rickert et al., 1992
Adolescents Living Safely: AIDS Awareness, Attitudes, and Actions (Rotheram-Borus et al.)	Rotheram-Borus et al., 1991 Rotheram-Borus et al., 1994a
Adolescents Living Safely: AIDS Awareness, Attitudes, and Actions for Gay, Lesbian and Bisexual Teens (Miller, Hunter, & Rotheram-Borus)	Rotheram-Borus et al., 1994b
AIDS Prevention and Health Promotion among Women (Hobfoll et al.)	Hobfoll et al., 1994 Levine et al., 1993
AIDS Prevention for Adolescents in School (Walter & Vaughan)	Walter & Vaughan, 1993
AIDS Risk Reduction Education and Skills Training Program (ARREST) (Kipke)	Kipke et al., 1993
AIDS Risk Reduction for College Students (Kimble et al.)	Fisher et al., 1996
ASSESS for Adolescent Risk Reduction (Boekeloo et al.)	Boekeloo, Schamus, & O'Connor, 1998 Boekeloo, et al., 1996a Boekeloo, et al., 1996b Boekeloo, et al., 1998 Boekeloo, et al., 1999
Draw the Line/Respect the Line: Middle School Intervention to Reduce Sexual Risk Behavior (University of California, San Francisco, The Center for AIDS Prevention Studies, & ETR Associates)	Coyle et al., 2004
FOCUS: Preventing Sexually Transmitted Infections and Unwanted Pregnancies Among Young Women (Boyer et al.)	Boyer et al., 2005
Focus on Kids: An Adolescent HIV Risk Prevention Program (Stanton et al.)	Stanton et al., 1996 Stanton et al., 1997
Get Real About AIDS® (Comprehensive Health Education Foundation)	Main et al., 1994
Information-Motivation-Behavioral Skills (IMB) HIV Prevention Program (Fisher et al.)	Fisher et al., 2002 Fisher & Fisher, 1992 Misovich, 2002
Poder Latino: A Community AIDS Prevention Program for Inner-City Latino Youth (New England Research Institutes & Hispanic Office of Planning & Evaluation)	Sellers et al., 1994
Rikers Health Advocacy Project (RHAP) (Magura, Shapiro, & Sung-Yeon)	Magura et al., 1994
Safer Choices: A High-School Based Program to Prevent STDs, HIV, and Pregnancy (ETR Associates & Center for Health Promotion Research and Development, University of Texas)	Basin-Enquist et al., 1997 Coyle et al., 1996 Coyle et al., 1999 Coyle et al., 2001 Kirby et al., 2004
Safer Sex Efficacy Workshop (Basen-Enquist)	Basen-Enquist, 1994
SiHLE: Health Workshops for Young Black Women (DiClemente et al.)	DiClemente et al., 2004
What Could You Do? Interactive Video Intervention fo Reduce Adolescent Females' STD Risk (Downs et al.)	Downs et al., 2004
Youth AIDS Prevention Project (YAPP) (Levy et al.)	Levy et al., 1995a Levy et al., 1995b
Youth and AIDS Project's HIV Prevention Program (Remafedi)	Remafedi, 1994
STI/HIV Prevention Programs for Adults (see http://www.socio.com/happa.htm for program descriptions)	
Brother to Brother—Hot, Healthy, and Safe (Peterson et al.)	Peterson et al., 1996
Doing Something Different (Cohen)	Cohen, Dent, & MacKinnon, 1991 Cohen et al., 1992a Cohen et al., 1992b
Hot, Healthy, and Keeping It Up! (Choi et al.)	Choi et al., 1995 Choi et al., 1996
Let's Chat (Kalichman)	Kalichman et al., 1995
Point For Point (San Francisco AIDS Foundation HIV Prevention & The Prevention Point Research Group)	Watters, 1996 Watters et al, 1994

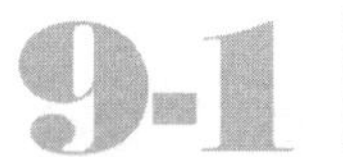 (*continued*)

PROGRAM NAME (DEVELOPERS)	REFERENCE(S)
Project S.A.F.E.: Sexual Awareness for Everyone (Shain et al.)	Shain et al., 1999 Shain et al., 2002
Project Smart (Lewis)	McCusker et al., 1992 McCusker et al., 1993 McCusker et al., 1995
Safety Point (Rhodes)	Rhodes & Wood, 1999
Sniffer (Des Jarlais et al.)	Casriel et al., 1990 Des Jarlais et al., 1992
The SISTA Project (DiClemente & Wingood)	DiClemente & Wingood, 1995
Turning Point (Falck, Carlson, & Siegal)	Siegal et al., 1995
WILLOW: HIV Transmission Reduction Among Women Living with HIV (Wingood et al.)	Wingood et al., 2004

PASHA are operated by Sociometrics Corporation with funding from the National Institutes of Health.

Intervention Processes

In small group HIV/AIDS prevention interventions, the way in which an intervention unfolds is as important as the activities conducted in the intervention. Group facilitators can build group cohesiveness by creating a sense of shared interests and trust. Examples of strategies to build group cohesiveness include involving all participants in group projects, encouraging all participants to share their experiences, valuing all contributions equally, teaching participants how to disagree respectfully, and protecting participants' reputations and feelings by enforcing confidentiality (Kalichman, 1998).

Youth Group Interventions

Implementing effective HIV prevention interventions in school settings can be particularly challenging. In many schools and school districts, parents and school boards insist on abstinence-only sex education programs that teach that abstinence from all sexual activity is the only appropriate option for unmarried people. These programs do not provide much, if any, discussion about contraception, condom use, or other safer-sex practices (Collins, Alagiri, & Summers, 2002). To date, there is very little evidence that abstinence-only programs significantly delay the onset of intercourse or reduce the frequency of sexual activity (Kirby, 2001, 2002; Manlove, Romano-Papillo, & Ikramullah, 2004; Santelli et al., 2006).

At the same time, there is strong research-based evidence that sexuality and HIV/AIDS education programs that include a discussion of condoms and contraception (including those conducted with young adolescents) do not promote sexual intercourse, do not hasten the onset of sexual intercourse, do not increase the frequency of sexual intercourse, and do not increase the number of sexual partners (Kirby, 2001). Indeed, research on these more comprehensive sexuality and HIV education programs has demonstrated that they can increase condom use and reduce frequency of intercourse among students (Card, Niego, Mallari, & Farrell, 1996; Kirby, 2001, 2002). Characteristics that have been shown to be common to effective sex and HIV education curricula for youth are shown in Figure 9-2.

Characteristics describing the development of the curriculum:

1. Included multiple individuals (and sometimes groups) with expertise in different areas in the design of the curriculum.

2. Assessed the relevant needs and assets of the young people that they were targeting.

3. Used a logic model approach to develop the curriculum.

4. Designed activities consistent with community values and available resources (staff time, staff skills, facility space and supplies).

5. Pilot-tested the program.

Characteristics describing the contents of the curriculum itself:

6. Focused on at least one of three health goals: the prevention of HIV, other STDs, and/or unintended pregnancy.

7. Focused narrowly on specific behaviors leading to these health goals, gave clear messages about these behaviors, and addressed situations that might lead to them and how to avoid them.

8. Focused on specific sexual psychosocial factors that affect the specified behaviors, and changed some of those factors.

9. Attempted to create a safe environment for youth to participate.

10. Included multiple instructionally sound activities designed to change each of the targeted risk and protective factors.

11. Employed instructionally sound teaching methods that actively involved the participants, that helped participants personalize the information, and that were designed to change each group of risk and protective factors.

12. Employed activities, instructional methods, and behavioral messages that were appropriate to the youths' culture, developmental age, and sexual experience.

13. Covered topics in a logical sequence.

Characteristics describing the implementation of the curriculum:

14. Secured at least minimal support from appropriate authorities.

15. Selected educators with desired characteristics (whenever possible), trained them, and provided monitoring, supervision, and support.

16. Implemented needed activities to recruit and retain youth.

17. Implemented curricula with reasonable fidelity.

Figure 9-2 Characteristics common to effective youth sex and HIV education curricula (Kirby, Laris, & Rolleri, 2006).

REFERENCES

Academy for Education Development (AED). (2006). *Voices/Voces fact sheet.* Washington, DC: AED.

Basen-Enquist, K. (1994). Evaluation of a theory-based HIV prevention intervention for college students. *AIDS Education and Prevention, 6,* 412–424.

Basen-Enquist, K., Parcel, G., Harrist, R., Kirby, D., Coyle, K., Banspach, S., et al. (1997). The Safer Choices project: Methodological issues in school-based health promotion intervention research. *Journal of School Health, 67,* 365–371.

Boekeloo, B. O., Schamus, L. A., Cheng, T. L., & Simmens, S. J. (1996a). Young adolescents' comfort with discussion about sexual problems with their physician. *Archive of Pediatric and Adolescent Medicine, 150,* 1146–1152.

Boekeloo, B. O., Schamus, L. A., & O'Connor, K. (1998). The effect of patient-education tools on physicians' discussions with young adolescents about sex. *Academic Medicine, 73,* s84–s87.

Boekeloo, B. O., Schamus, L. A., Simmens, S. J., & Cheng, T. L. (1996b). Tailoring STD/HIV prevention messages for young adolescents. *Academic Medicine, 71,* s97–s99.

Boekeloo, B. O., Schamus, L. A., Simmens, S. J., & Cheng, T. L. (1998). Ability to measure sensitive adolescent behaviors via telephone. *American Journal of Preventive Medicine, 14,* 209–216.

Boekeloo, B. O., Schamus, L. A., Simmens, S. J., Cheng, T. L., O'Connor, K., & D'Angelo, L. J. (1999). A STD/HIV prevention trial among adolescents in managed care. *Pediatrics, 103*, 107–115.

Boyer, C. B., Shafer, M. A., Shaffer, R. A., Brodine, S. K., Pollack, L. M., Betsinger, K., et al. (2005). Evaluation of a cognitive-behavioral, group, randomized controlled intervention trial to prevent seuxally transmitted infections and unintended pregnancies in young women. *Preventive Medicine, 40*, 420–431.

Card, J. J., Benner, T., Shields, J. P., & Feinstein, N. (2001). The HIV/AIDS Prevention Program Archive (HAPPA): A collection of promising prevention programs in a box. *AIDS Education and Prevention, 13*(1), 1–28.

Card, J. J., Niego, S., Mallari, A., & Farrell, W. S. (1996). The Program Archive on Sexuality, Health and Adolescence: Promising "prevention programs in a box." *Family Planning Perspectives, 28*(5), 210–220.

Casriel, C., Des Jarlais, D. C., Rodriguez, R., Friedman, S. R., Stepherson, B., & Khuri, E. (1990). Working with heroin sniffers: Clinical issues in preventing drug injection. *Journal of Substance Abuse Treatment, 7*, 1–10.

Centers for Disease Control and Prevention (CDC). (2001). *Compendium of HIV prevention interventions with evidence of success.* Atlanta, GA: CDC.

Centers for Disease Control and Prevention (CDC). (2003). Partner counseling and referral services to identify persons with undiagnosed HIV—North Carolina, 2001. *Morbidity and Mortality Weekly Report, 52*(48), 1181–1184.

Centers for Disease Control and Prevention (CDC). (2006). Evolution of HIV/AIDS prevention programs—United States, 1981–2006. *Morbidity and Mortality Weekly Report, 55*(21), 597–603.

Choi, K.-H., Coates, T. J., Catania, J. A., Lew, S., & Chow, P. (1995). High HIV risk among gay Asian and Pacific Islander men in San Francisco [letter]. *AIDS, 9*, 306–308.

Choi, K.-H., Lew, S., Vittinghoff, E., Catania, J., Barrett, D. C., & Coates, T. J. (1996). The efficacy of brief group counseling in HIV risk reduction among homosexual Asian and Pacific Islander men. *AIDS, 10*, 81–87.

Cohen, D., Dent, C., & MacKinnon, D. (1991). Condom skills education and sexually transmitted disease reinfection. *The Journal of Sex Research, 28*(1), 139–144.

Cohen, D., Dent, C., MacKinnon, D., & Hahn, C. (1992a). Condoms for men, not women: Results of brief promotion programs. *Sexually Transmitted Diseases, 19*(5), 245–251.

Cohen, D., MacKinnon, D., Dent, C., Mason, H., & Sullivan, E. (1992b). Group counseling at STD clinics to promote use of condoms. *Public Health Reports, 107*(6), 727–731.

Colfax, G. N., Buchbinder, S. P., Cornelisse, P. G., Vittinghoff, E., Mayer, K., & Celum, C. (2002). Sexual risk behaviors and implications for secondary HIV transmission during and after HIV seroconversion. *AIDS, 16*(11), 1529–1535.

Collins, C., Alagiri, P., & Summers, T. (2002, March). *Abstinence only vs. comprehensive sex education. Policy Monograph Series, March 2002.* San Francisco: AIDS Research Institute, University of California, San Francisco.

Copenhaver, M. M., Johnson, B. T., Lee, I. C., Harman, J. J., Carey, M. P., & the SHARP Research Team. (2006). Behavioral HIV risk reduction among people who inject drugs: Meta-analytic evidence of efficacy. *Journal of Substance Abuse Treatment, 31*(2), 163–71.

Coyle, K., Basen-Enquist, K., Kirby, D., Parcel, G., Banspach, S., Collins, J., et al. (2001). Safer Choices: Reducing teen pregnancy, HIV, and STDs. *Public Health Reports, 116*(Suppl), 82–93.

Coyle, K., Basen-Enquist, K., Kirby, D., Parcel, G., Banspach, S., Harrist, R., et al. (1999). Short-term impact of Safer Choices: A mulitcomponent, school-based HIV, other STD, and pregnancy prevention program. *Journal of School Health, 69*, 181–188.

Coyle, K., Kirby, D., Marín, B., Gómez, C., & Gregorich, S. (2004). Draw the Line/Respect the Line: A randomized trial of a middle school intervention to reduce sexual risks. *American Journal of Public Health, 94*, 843–851.

Coyle, K., Kirby, D., Parcel, G., Basen-Enquist, K., Banspach, S., Rugg, D., et al. (1996). Safer Choices: A multicomponent school-based HIV/STD and pregnancy prevention program for adolescents. *Journal of School Health, 66*, 89–94.

Des Jarlais, D. C., Casriel, C., Friedman, S. R., & Rosenblum, A. (1992). AIDS and the transition to illicit drug injection—results of a randomized trial prevention program. *British Journal of Addiction, 87*, 493–498.

DiClemente, R. J., & Wingood, G. M. (1995). A randomized controlled trial of an HIV sexual risk-reduction intervention for young African-American women. *Journal of the American Medical Association, 274*(16), 1271–1276.

DiClemente, R. J., Wingood, G. M., Harrington, K. F., Lang, D. L., Davies, S. L., Hook, E. W., et al. (2004). Efficacy of an HIV prevention intervention for African American adolescent girls: A randomized controlled trial. *Journal of the American Medical Association, 292,* 171–179.

Downs, J. S., Murray, P. J., Bruin de Bruine, W., Penrose, J., Palmgren, C., & Fischholf, B. (2004). Interactive video behavioral intervention to reduce adolescent females STD risk: A randomized controlled trial. *Social Science & Medicine, 59,* 1561–1572.

Fisher, J. D., & Fisher, W. A. (1992). Changing AIDS risk behavior. *Psychological Bulletin, 111,* 455–474.

Fisher, J. D., Fisher, W. A., Bryan, A. D., & Misovich, S. J. (2002). Information-motivation-behavioral skills model-based HIV risk behavior change intervention for inner-city high school youth. *Health Psychology, 21*(2), 177–186.

Fisher, J. D., Fisher, W. A., Misovich, S. J., Kimble, D. L., & Malloy, T. E. (1996). Changing AIDS risk behavior: Effects of an intervention emphasizing AIDS risk reduction information, motivation, and behavioral skills in a college student population. *Health Psychology, 15*(2), 114–123.

Hobfoll, S. E., Jackson, A. P., Lavin, J., Britton, P. J., & Shepherd, J. B. (1994). Reducing inner-city women's AIDS risk activities: A study of single, pregnant women. *Health Psychology, 13*(5), 397–403.

Kalichman, S. C. (1998). *Preventing AIDS: A sourcebook for behavioral interventions.* Mahwah, NJ: Lawrence Erlbaum Associates.

Kalichman, S. C., Sikkema, J., Kelly, J. A., & Bulto, M. (1995). Use of a brief behavioral skills intervention to prevent HIV infection among chronic mentally ill adults. *Psychiatric Services, 46*(3), 275–280.

Kipke, M. D., Boyer, C., & Hein, K. (1993). An evaluation of an AIDS Risk Reduction Education and Skills Training (ARREST) program. *Journal of Adolescent Health, 14*(7), 533–539.

Kirby, D. (2001). *Emerging answers: Research findings on programs to reduce teen pregnancy.* Washington, DC: National Campaign to Prevent Teen Pregnancy.

Kirby, D. (2002). *Do abstinence-only programs delay the initiation of sex among young people and reduce teen pregnancy?* Washington, DC: National Campaign to Prevent Teen Pregnancy.

Kirby, D., Baumler, E., Coyle, K., Basen-Enquist, K., Parcel, G., Harrist, R., et al. (2004). The Safer Choices intervention: Its impact on the sexual behaviors of different subgroups of high school students. *Journal of Adolescent Health, 35,* 442–452.

Kirby, D., Laris, B. A., & Rolleri, L. (2006). *Sex and HIV prevention programs for youth: Their impact and important characteristics.* Scotts Valley, CA: ETR Associates.

Levine, O. H., Britton, P. J., James, T. C., Jackson, A. P., Hobfoll, S. E., & Lavin, J. P. (1993). The empowerment of women: A key to HIV prevention. *Journal of Community Psychology, 21,* 320–334.

Levy, S. R., Perhats, C., Weeks, K., Handler, A., Zhu, C., & Flay, B. R. (1995b). Impact of a school-based AIDS prevention program on risk and protective behaviors for newly sexually active students. *Journal of School Health, 65*(4), 145–151.

Levy, S. R., Weeks, K., Handler, A., Perhats, C., Franck, J. A., Hedeker, D., et al. (1995a). A longitudinal comparison of the AIDS-related attitudes and knowledge of parents and their children. *Family Planning Perspectives, 27*(1), 4–10, 17.

Magura, S., Kang, S. Y., & Shapiro, J. L. (1994). Outcomes of intensive AIDS education for male adolescent drug users in jail. *Journal of Adolescent Health, 15*(6), 457–463.

Main, D. S., Iverson, D. C., McGloin, J., Banspach, S., Collins, J. L., Rugg, D. L., et al. (1994). Preventing HIV infection among adolescents: Evaluation of a school-based education program. *Preventive Medicine, 23*(4), 409–417.

Manlove, J., Romano-Papillo, A., & Ikramullah, E. (2004). *Not yet: Programs to delay first sex among teens.* Washington, DC: National Campaign to Prevent Teen Pregnancy.

McCusker, J., Bigelow, C., Luippold, R., Zorn, M., & Lewis, B. F. (1995). Outcomes of a 21-day drug detoxification program: Retention, transfer to further treatment, and HIV risk reduction. *American Journal of Drug and Alcohol Abuse, 21*(1), 1–16.

McCusker, J., Stoddard, A. M., Zapka, J. G., & Lewis, B. F. (1993). Behavioral outcomes of AIDS educational intervention for drug users in shot-term treatment. *American Journal of Public Health, 83*(10), 1463–1466.

McCusker, J., Stoddard, A. M., Zapka, J. G., Morrison, C. S., Zorn, M., & Lewis, B. F. (1992). AIDS education for drug abusers: Evaluation of short-term effectiveness. *American Journal of Public Health, 82*(4), 533–540.

Misovich, S. J. (2002). *Information-motivation-behavioral skills HIV prevention program. Program overview.* Manual produced as part of an overall program of research by J. D. Fisher, W. A. Fisher, S. J. Misovich, & A. D. Bryan. Storrs, CT: University of Connecticut Center for HIV Intervention and Prevention.

Padian, N. S., O'Brien, T. R., Chang, Y., Glass, S., & Francis, D. P. (1993). Prevention of heterosexual transmission of human immunodeficiency virus through couple counseling. *Journal of Acquired Immune Deficiency Syndromes*, *6*(9), 1043–1048.

Peterson, J. L., Coates, T. J., Catania, J., Hauck, W. W., Acree, M., Daigle, D., et al. (1996). Evaluation of an HIV risk reduction intervention among African-American homosexual and bisexual men. *AIDS*, *10*(3), 319–325.

Remafedi, G. (1994). Cognitive and behavioral adaptations to HIV/AIDS among gay and bisexual adolescents. *Journal of Adolescent Health*, *15*, 142–148.

Rhodes, F., & Wood, M. M. (1999). *A cognitive-behavioral intervention to reduce HIV risks among active drug users*. Paper presented at the 127th Annual Meeting of the American Public Health Association, Chicago, IL.

Rickert, V. I., Gottlieb, A., & Jay, M. S. (1990). A comparison of three clinic-based AIDS education programs on female adolescents' knowledge, attitudes and behavior. *Journal of Adolescent Health Care*, *11*(4), 298–303.

Rickert, V. I., Gottlieb, A., & Jay, M. S. (1992). Is AIDS education related to condom acquisition? *Clinical Pediatrics*, *31*(4), 205–210.

Rotheram-Borus, M. J., Feldman, J., Rosario, M., & Dunne, E. (1994b). Preventing HIV among runaways: Victims and victimization. In R. J. DiClemente & J. L. Peterson (Eds.), *Preventing AIDS: Theories and methods of behavioral intervention* (pp. 175–188). New York: Plenum.

Rotheram-Borus, M. J., Koopman, C., Haignere, C., & Davies, M. (1991). Reducing HIV sexual risk behaviors among runaway adolescents. *Journal of the American Medical Association*, *266*, 1237–1241.

Rotheram-Borus, M. J., Reid, H., & Rosario, M. (1994a). Factors mediating changes in sexual HIV risk behaviors among gay and bisexual male adolescents. *American Journal of Public Health*, *84*, 1938–1946.

Santelli, J., Ott, M. A., Lyon, M., Rogers, J., Summers, D., & Schleifer, R. (2006). Abstinence and abstinence-only education: A review of U.S. policies and programs. *Journal of Adolescent Health*, *38*(1), 72–81.

Sellers, D. E., McGraw, S. A., & McKinlay, J. B. (1994). Does the promotion and distribution of condoms increase teen sexual activity? Evidence from an HIV prevention program for Latino youth. *American Journal of Public Health*, *84*, 1952–1959.

Shain, R. N., Perdue, S. T., Piper, J. M., Holden, A. E., Champion, J. D., Newton, E. R., et al. (2002). Behaviors changed by intervention are associated with reduced STD recurrence: The importance of context in measurement. *Sexually Transmitted Diseases*, *29*(9), 520–529.

Shain, R. N., Piper, J. M., Newton, E. R., Perdue, S. T., Ramos, R., Champion, J. D., et al. (1999). A randomized, controlled trial of a behavioral intervention to prevent sexually transmitted disease among minority women. *The New England Journal of Medicine*, *340*(2), 93–100.

Siegal, H. A., Falck, R. S., Carlson, R. G., & Wang, J. (1995). Reducing HIV needle risk behaviors among injection-drug users in the midwest: An evaluation of the efficacy of standard and enhanced interventions. *AIDS Education and Prevention*, *7*(4), 308–319.

Stanton, B. F., Fang, X., Li, X., Feigelman, S., Galbraith, J., & Ricardo, I. (1997). Evolution of risk behaviors over 2 years among a cohort of urban African-American Adolescents. *Archives of Pediatrics and Adolescent Medicine*, *151*(4), 398–406.

Stanton, B. F., Li, X., Ricardo, I., Galbraith, J., Feigelman, S., & Kaljee, L. (1996). A randomized, controlled effectiveness trial of an AIDS prevention program for low-income African-American youths. *Archives of Pediatrics and Adolescent Medicine*, *150*(4), 363–372.

Walter, H. J., & Vaughan, R. D. (1993). AIDS risk reduction among a multiethnic sample of urban high school students. *Journal of the American Medical Association*, *270*, 725–730.

Watters, J. K. (1996). Impact of HIV risk and infection and the role of prevention services. *Journal of Substance Abuse Treatment*, *13*(5), 375–385.

Watters, J. K., Estilo, M. J., Clark, G. L., & Lorvick, J. (1994). Syringe and needle exchange as HIV/AIDS prevention for injection drug users. *Journal of the American Medical Association*, *271*(2), 115–120.

Wilson, B. D. M., & Miller, R. L. (2003). Examining strategies for culturally grounded HIV prevention: A review. *AIDS Education and Prevention*, *15*(2), 184–202.

Wingood, G. M., DiClemente, R. J., Mikhail, I., Lang, D. L., Hubbard McCree, D., Davies, S. L., et al. (2004). A randomized controlled trial to reduce HIV transmission risk behaviors and sexually transmitted diseases among women living with HIV: The WiLLOW program. *Journal of Acquired Immune Deficiency Syndromes*, *82*(Suppl 2), s58–s67.

Instructor Resources

LEARNING ACTIVITIES

ACTIVITY 1:

Assignment: Designing a Prevention Intervention

Objective: To create an HIV/AIDS prevention for a particular community.

Minimum Time: 45 minutes

View a handout for this activity on the CD-ROM.

DISCUSSION QUESTIONS

1. What are some advantages of small group interventions over individual interventions? What are some disadvantages?
2. Why do you think some parents and schools insist on abstinence-only education programs? Do you think these programs work?

QUIZ

1. Where would small group interventions not be conducted?
   a) Schools
   b) Health clinics
   c) Prisons
   d) Religious institutions
   e) None of the above
   f) All of the above
2. Which is not true of small group interventions?
   a) They do not require skilled leadership.
   b) They may last one or more sessions.
   c) They focus on primary and/or secondary transmission.
   d) They can decrease risk behaviors in many populations.
3. Which has shown to be more effective in reducing the frequency of intercourse among students?
   a) Abstinence-only programs
   b) Comprehensive sexuality and HIV/AIDS education programs
   c) Neither; both are equally effective

ANSWERS

1. **E.** Small group interventions could be conducted in any of the settings listed.
2. **A.** Small group interventions must be led by facilitators with strong interpersonal skills.
3. **B.** Research suggests that comprehensive sexuality and HIV education programs can increase condom use and decrease frequency of intercourse among students. There is little evidence that abstinence-only programs significantly delay the onset of intercourse or reduce the frequency of sexual activity.

WEB RESOURCES

Small Group Prevention Strategies

The Centers for Disease Control: Replicating Effective Programs Plus

http://www.cdc.gov/hiv/projects/rep/default.htm

Identifies HIV/AIDS prevention programs that have been shown to work.

Diffusion of Effective Behavioral Interventions for HIV

http://www.effectiveinterventions.org/

Provides high quality training and ongoing technical assistance for selected evidence-based HIV/STD prevention interventions to state and community program staff.

Sociometrics Corporation: Program Archives

http://www.socio.com/program.htm

Effective HIV/AIDS prevention programs can be found in the "HIV/AIDS Prevention Program Archive" (HAPPA) and the "Program Archive on Sexuality, Health, and Adolescence" (PASHA).

Center for AIDS Prevention Services (CAPS) Model Prevention Programs

http://www.caps.ucsf.edu/projects/

Describes HIV prevention programs that have been designed by CAPS researchers and have either been evaluated or are in the process of being evaluated.

AIDS Videos

http://psychology.ucdavis.edu/rainbow/html/vid_aids.html

Links to lists and descriptions of videos made for several different audiences (African American audiences, Latino/Latina audiences, gay/bisexual men, or women) to use in HIV/AIDS prevention education settings. In addition to a brief description, each entry includes information about the target audience, format, length, distributor, and language.

RECOMMENDED READING

Activities

Activity Manual: Program Archive on Sexuality, Health and Adolescence Activity (PASHA) Sourcebook (Sociometrics, 1998)

Benner, T. A., Park, M. J., & Peterson, E. C. (Eds.). (1998). PASHA activity sourcebook. Los Altos, CA: Sociometrics Corporation.

The PASHA Activity Sourcebook contains a diverse array of group-based activities that reinforce sexual health education among young people. Activities include role-plays, group discussions, homework assignments, and group activities. To purchase the PASHA Activity Sourcebook, go to http://www.socio.com/srch/summary/pasha/paspubl3.htm.

Small Group-Level Prevention Strategies

Levels of Prevention (Kalichman, 1998)

Kalichman, S. C. (1998). Preventing AIDS: A sourcebook for behavioral interventions. *Mahwah, NJ: Lawrence Erlbaum Associates.*

This highly regarded text summarizes 20 years of research on behavioral prevention of HIV, reviews HIV risk-reduction theories, and overviews of individual-, small group-, and community-level strategies for HIV prevention.

POWERPOINT SLIDES

(Note: A full-color version of these slides, with graphics, is also available on the CD-ROM.)

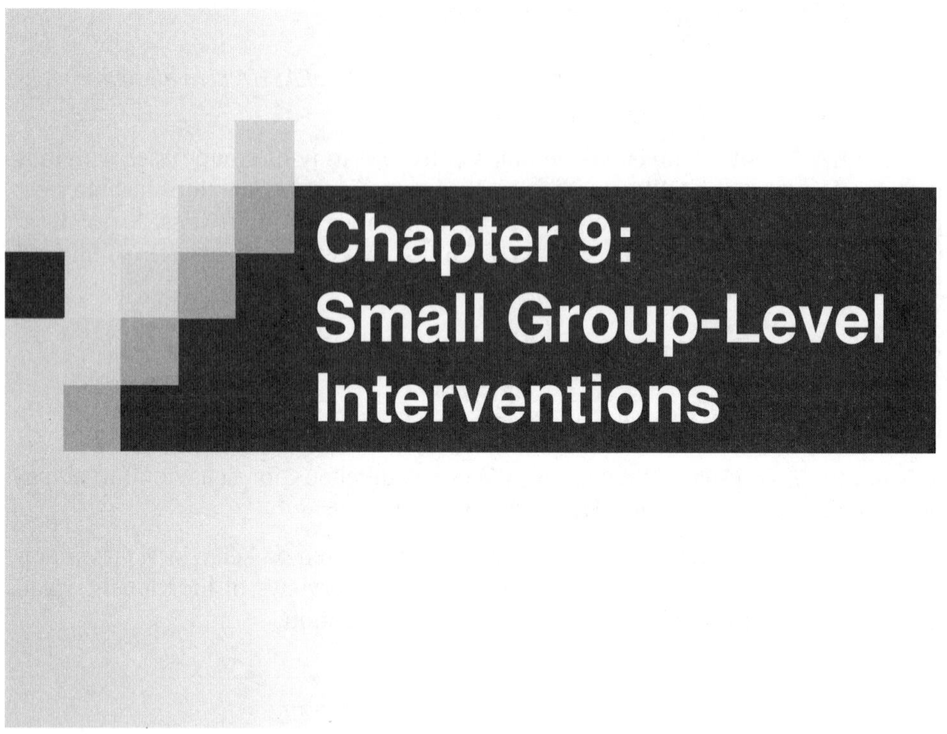

Small Group-Level Interventions

- Most small group HIV/AIDS prevention interventions include:
  - basic education about HIV transmission, local prevalence of HIV and AIDS, AIDS myths, and HIV antibody tests;
  - examination of participants' own behavior to assess personal risk and to motivate behavior change;
  - behavioral skills training; and
  - sexual communication and relationship-building skills.

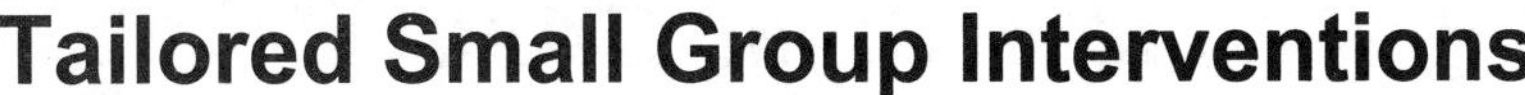

Tailored Small Group Interventions

- Small group HIV/AIDS prevention interventions are tailored to the contexts in which they take place.
- Strategies for tailoring intervention components to be culturally and personally relevant include:
  - □ interviewing key community contacts to learn the values, concerns, and practices of the target population;
  - □ conducting focus groups with members of the target population;
  - □ using examples, language, and images that resonate with participants; and
  - □ selecting group facilitators who are of the same age, ethnic background, gender, and sexual orientation as participants.

Group Process

The way in which an intervention unfolds is as important as the activities conducted in the intervention. Group facilitators can build group cohesiveness by creating a sense of shared interests and trust.

Examples of strategies to build group cohesiveness include:

- involving all participants in group projects;
- encouraging all participants to share experiences;
- valuing all contributions equally;
- teaching participants how to disagree respectfully; and
- protecting participants' reputations and feelings by enforcing confidentiality.

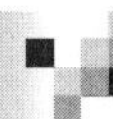

Best Practices in Small Group Interventions

- Small group interventions decrease HIV risk behaviors in many populations.
- They increase knowledge, motivation for behavior change, and sexual communication skills.
- They use multiple-hour formats, from many group sessions to single-session workshops.

Limitations of Small Group Interventions

- Not everyone likes participating in groups.
- It is difficult to get people together on a consistent basis.
- Only a few people can be targeted at a time.
- Strong facilitators are not always available.

Learning Objectives

- Describe the process of social influence interventions
- Understand the benefits and components of outreach interventions
- Explain the uses and techniques of social marketing and media interventions

Key Terms

behavior change agent
community
community-level intervention
opinion leader
outreach intervention
public service announcement
social influence intervention
social marketing
social norm

10

Community-Level Interventions

A *community* is a group of people who share something. What they share may be a geographic area, a cultural background, a religious affiliation, or a common set of interests, beliefs, or practices. Community-level interventions seek to influence the knowledge, attitudes, skills, and behaviors of an entire community both directly and indirectly, often through a focus on changing social norms (CDC, 2006). This chapter briefly summarizes the major types of HIV prevention interventions that operate at the community level. For further information on effective community-level interventions, see the sources shown in Figure 10-1.

SOCIAL INFLUENCE INTERVENTIONS

Many community-level interventions seek out people who are capable of influencing others and of disseminating an intervention throughout their social networks. These are referred to as *social influence interventions*. Social influence interventions generally follow these steps (Kalichman, 1998):

1. Identification and recruitment of popular opinion leaders
2. Training of opinion leaders to become risk-reduction behavior change agents
3. Dissemination of risk-reduction messages by opinion leaders to friends and other members of their social networks

Social influence interventions are commonly based on theories about behavior and behavior change that focus on the importance of social norms, such as the theory of reasoned action, social cognitive theory, and the diffusion of innovations theory. See Figure 10-2 for an example of an effective social influence intervention.

Social influence interventions target and train key members of a social group to act as behavior agents.

OUTREACH INTERVENTIONS

Outreach interventions are relatively low-cost interventions that target large numbers of people in their natural environments, where they may not otherwise be exposed to HIV-prevention messages. Outreach activities are most closely identified

For more information about effective community-level interventions see:

- The CDC's "Replicating Effective Programs" project Web site at http://www.cdc.gov/hiv/projects/rep
- The CDC's "Diffusion of Effective Behavioral Interventions" project Web site at http://www.effectiveinterventions.org
- Sociometrics Corporation's "HIV/AIDS Prevention Program Archive (HAPPA)" Web site at http://www.socio.com/happa.htm
- Sociometrics Corporation's "Program Archive on Sexuality, Health & Adolescence (PASHA)" Web site at http://www.socio.com/pasha.htm

Figure 10-1

with efforts to reach injection drug users, the sex partners of injection drug users, and commercial sex workers. Outreach interventions also may involve crack cocaine abusers, men who have sex with men (MSM), and people living in high HIV-prevalence areas.

Intervention activities include providing both prevention information and prevention materials (e.g., condoms, clean needles, bleach for sterilizing drug injection equipment) where they are needed. Often, outreach activities also serve as a means of alerting the community to the existence of other prevention (or treatment) programs and services and recruiting new program participants.

Main Components of Outreach Interventions

The main components of outreach interventions include:

- Dissemination and distribution of prevention information and materials (e.g., informational brochures, condoms, bleach) to people in mass transit stations, bath houses, brothels, parks, crack houses, shooting galleries (injection drug using sites), and other places where at-risk people are accessible.
- Behavior change counseling targeted at specific risk behaviors.

POL is a social influence intervention that was designed to reduce unprotected sex among male patrons of gay bars. POL uses popular "opinion leaders" (i.e., bar patrons whom other patrons seem to look up to) to deliver safer-sex messages, while creating the impression that safer sex is the norm among people who are respected and admired.

The opinion leaders are identified by bartenders, based on their observations of who comes to the bar frequently and is greeted by many other patrons. When a person is identified as an opinion leader by more than one bartender, the person is asked if he would be interested in using this influence to save others' lives by delivering safer-sex messages to peers. The leaders are also each asked to invite another influential friend to participate. Each opinion leader is trained in a series of four sessions to communicate HIV prevention messages to his peers. Training methods include didactic presentations, group discussions, modeling of appropriate messages, and role-playing exercises. Opinion leaders then sign a contract to have a minimum number of sexual risk reduction conversations with peers at the bar. Posters hung in the bars and matching lapel buttons for opinion leaders also help stimulate safer-sex conversations.

In the original evaluation of the program, which was conducted in three U.S. cities, in each city, following intervention implementation, unprotected anal intercourse among bar patrons decreased significantly. In comparison sites (i.e., sites that had not yet received the intervention), there was little or no change in behavior during the same period.

Figure 10-2 The popular opinion leaders programs (POL) (Kelly et al., 1991; Kelly et al., 1992).

- Recruitment of clients for HIV risk-reduction programs and drug treatment programs.

Outreach Staffing and Processes

Effective outreach workers are able to blend into the community in which they are working, or even be part of the community. For example, it is common for recovering injection drug addicts to serve as outreach workers in IDU communities. Effective outreach workers also know how to earn the trust and confidence of community members. In addition, they know how to keep themselves safe in the challenging environments in which they work.

Once entering a community, outreach workers commonly establish initial contact with the target population through a brief and usually nonverbal exchange. They build trust with community members and maintain contact until individuals become motivated and use services being offered by the outreach agency. They also follow up with clients to reassess needs, revisit strategies, and deliver ongoing services (Kalichman, 1998; Leviton & Schuh, 1991; Valentine & Wright-DeAgüero, 1996; Wiebel, 1993).

SOCIAL MARKETING AND MEDIA INTERVENTIONS

Outreach interventions can leverage the reach of commercial marketing methods—including advertisements and public service announcements in newspapers, billboards, radio, and television—to expand their effectiveness in reaching their target populations.

Social Marketing Interventions

Social marketing of HIV prevention uses commercial marketing methods to promote HIV antibody testing and safer sex (Kalichman, 1998; Ling, Franklin, Lindsteadt, & Gearon, 1992; Winett et al., 1995). To be effective, HIV prevention social marketing campaigns should (Maibach, Kreps, & Bonaguro, 1993):

- Target campaigns to particular audiences and involve those target audiences in planning the campaign
- Reflect the needs, concerns, and cultures of target audiences in the messages and delivery channels
- Incorporate theories of human behavior and behavior change
- Take into account social structures and institutions that influence behavior, such as policies, practices, economies, and corporate systems
- Focus on realistic health behavior objectives
- Demonstrate that benefits of behavior change far outweigh the costs
- Employ a wide range of communication strategies and channels
- Empower people to get involved in campaign-related programs

Media Interventions

A variety of mass media can be used to deliver HIV prevention messages. For example, public service announcements (PSAs) in the form of newspaper and bus advertisements, billboards, informational brochures, and radio and television spots can help raise awareness of HIV/AIDS and how it is transmitted, reduce stigma against people who are infected with HIV, promote HIV testing, and keep HIV/AIDS in the public eye (Kalichman, 1998). Culturally tailored AIDS information and motivational videotapes can provide information about HIV and AIDS disease processes, HIV antibody testing, behaviors that produce risk for HIV transmission, and self-protective behaviors (Kalichman, 1998). Public awareness of HIV/AIDS is furthered by television, radio, and Internet coverage of newsworthy HIV/AIDS-related events, such as basketball star Earvin "Magic" Johnson's 1991 announcement of his HIV+ serostatus (Kalichman, 1998). Art, including theater, film, and visual art, also can directly and indirectly promote awareness for HIV/AIDS (Green, 2003).

Messages delivered through the mass media can stimulate interpersonal discussions about a health issue. A public service announcement about prevention of HIV and other sexually transmitted infections might prompt sex partners to discuss condom use (Freimuth, Linnan, & Potter, 2000). For example, a Tanzanian program that used radio and newspapers ads to promote the female condom showed that exposure to the mass media campaign significantly increased the chances that people would discuss using female condoms with their partner. This discussion strengthened people's intentions to use the female condom in the future (Agha & Van Rossem, 2002).

REFERENCES

Agha, S., & Van Rossem, R. (2002). Impact of mass media campaigns on intentions to use the female condom in Tanzania. *International Family Planning Perspectives, 28*(3), 151–158.

Centers for Disease Control and Prevention (CDC). (2006). Evolution of HIV/AIDS prevention programs—United States, 1981–2006. *Morbidity and Mortality Weekly Report, 55*(21), 597–603.

Freimuth, V., Linnan, H. W., & Potter, P. (2000). Communicating the threat of emerging infections to the public. *Emerging Infectious Diseases, 6*(4), 337–347.

Green, J. (2003, December 7). When political art mattered. *New York Times Magazine.*

Kalichman, S. C. (1998). *Preventing AIDS: A sourcebook for behavioral interventions.* Mahwah, NJ: Lawrence Erlbaum Associates.

Kelly, J. A., St. Lawrence, J. S., Diaz, Y. E., Stevenson, L. Y., Hauth, A. C., Kalichman, S. C., et al. (1991). HIV risk behavior reduction following intervention with key opinion leaders of population: An experimental analysis. *American Journal of Public Health, 81*(2), 168–171.

Kelly, J. A., St. Lawrence, J. S., Stevenson, L. Y., Hauth, A. C., Kalichman, S. C., Diaz, Y. E., et al. (1992). Community AIDS/HIV risk reduction: The effects of endorsements by popular people in three cities. *American Journal of Public Health, 82*(11), 1483–1489.

Leviton, L. C., & Schuh, R. G. (1991). Evaluation of outreach as a project element. *Evaluation Review, 15,* 420–440.

Ling, J. C., Franklin, B., Lindsteadt, J., & Gearon, S. (1992). Social marketing: Its place in public health. In G. S. Omenn, J. E. Fielding, & L. B. Lave (Eds.), *Annual Review of Public Health, 13,* 341–362. Palo Alto, CA: Annual Review.

Maibach, E. W., Kreps, G. L., & Bonaguro, E. W. (1993). Developing strategic communication campaigns for HIV/AIDS prevention. In S. C. Ratzan (Ed.), *AIDS: Effective health communication for the 90s* (pp. 15–35). Washington, DC: Taylor & Francis.

Valentine, J., & Wright-DeAgüero, L. K. (1996). Defining the components of street outreach for HIV prevention: The contact and the encounter. *Public Health Reports, 111*(Suppl), 69–74.

Wiebel, W. (1993). *The indigenous leader outreach model: Intervention manual.* Rockville, MD: National Institute of Drug Abuse.

Winett, R. A., Anderson, E., Desiderato, L., Solomon, L., Perry, M., Kelly, J., et al. (1995). Enhancing social diffusion theory as a basis for prevention intervention: A conceptual and strategic framework. *Applied and Preventive Psychology, 4,* 233–245.

Instructor Resources

LEARNING ACTIVITIES

ACTIVITY 1:

Assignment: Designing a Prevention Intervention

Objective: To create an HIV/AIDS prevention for a particular community.

Minimum Time: 45 minutes

View a handout for this activity on the CD-ROM.

DISCUSSION QUESTIONS

1. Why is recruitment of opinion leaders an important factor in social influence interventions?
2. How are outreach interventions different from individual or small group interventions?
3. Have you personally encountered any HIV prevention media interventions (such as PSAs, advertisements, or television or radio spots)? Did you think they were effective? Why or why not?

QUIZ

1. Which is *not* commonly a feature of outreach interventions?
   a) They alert the community to other programs and services.
   b) They target relatively small numbers of people.
   c) They are relatively low cost
   d) They attempt to reach people in their natural environments
2. Describe any two characteristics of an effective outreach worker.
3. Describe any two characteristics of an effective HIV prevention social marketing campaign.

ANSWERS

1. **B.** Outreach interventions are relatively low-cost interventions that target large numbers of people in their natural environments and alert them to other programs and services.

2. Effective outreach workers are able to blend into the community in which they are working, or even be part of the community. Effective outreach workers also know how to earn the trust and confidence of community members. In addition, they know how to keep themselves safe in the challenging environments in which they work.
3. To be effective, HIV prevention social marketing campaigns should target campaigns to particular audiences; reflect the needs, concerns, and cultures of target audiences in the messages and delivery channels; incorporate theories of human behavior and behavior change; take into account social structures and institutions that influence behavior; focus on realistic health behavior objectives; demonstrate that benefits of behavior change far outweigh the costs; employ a wide range of communication strategies and channels; and empower people to get involved in campaign-related programs.

WEB RESOURCES

Community-Level Prevention Strategies

The Centers for Disease Control: Replicating Effective Programs Plus

http://www.cdc.gov/hiv/projects/rep/default.htm

Identifies HIV/AIDS prevention programs that have been shown to work.

Diffusion of Effective Behavioral Interventions for HIV

http://www.effectiveinterventions.org/

Provides high-quality training and ongoing technical assistance for selected evidence-based HIV/STD prevention interventions to state and community HIV/STI program staff.

Sociometrics Corporation: Program Archives

http://www.socio.com/program.htm

Effective HIV/AIDS prevention programs can be found in the "HIV/AIDS Prevention Program Archive" (HAPPA) and the "Program Archive on Sexuality, Health, and Adolescence" (PASHA).

Center for AIDS Prevention Services (CAPS) Model Prevention Programs

http://www.caps.ucsf.edu/projects/

Describes HIV prevention programs that have been designed by CAPS researchers and have either been evaluated or are in the process of being evaluated.

AIDS Activist Central

http://www.thebody.com/govt/activist.html

Offers activist guides and links to governmental and nongovernmental advocacy and activist organizations, information, and resources.

RECOMMENDED READING

Community-Level Prevention Strategies

Levels of Prevention (Kalichman, 1998)

Kalichman, S. C. (1998). Preventing AIDS: A sourcebook for behavioral interventions. *Mahwah, NJ: Lawrence Erlbaum Associates.*

This highly regarded text summarizes 20 years of research on behavioral prevention of HIV, reviews HIV risk-reduction theories, and overviews individual-, small group-, and community-level strategies for HIV prevention.

POWERPOINT SLIDES

(Note: A full-color version of these slides, with graphics, is also available on the CD-ROM.)

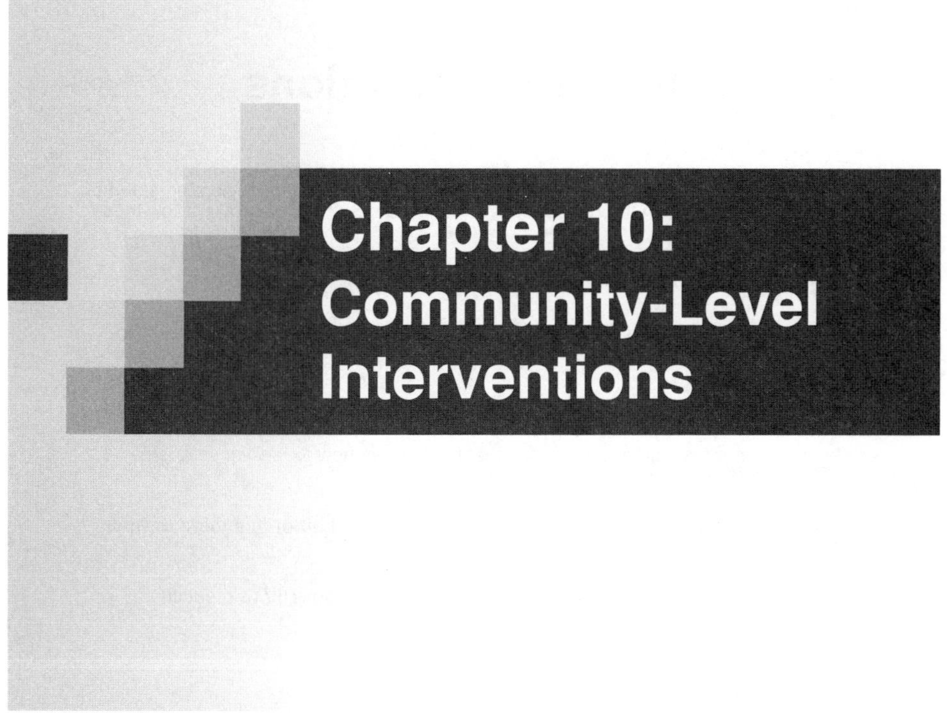

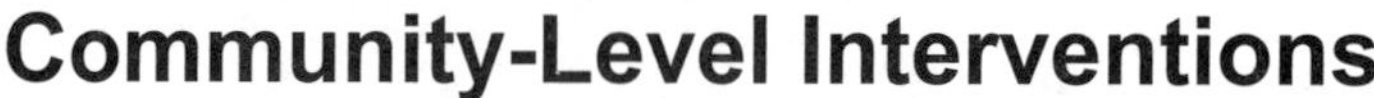

Community-Level Interventions

Community-level interventions seek to influence the knowledge, attitudes, skills, and behaviors of an entire community.

- Social Influence Interventions
- Outreach Interventions
- Social Marketing and Media Interventions

Social Influence Interventions

Social influence interventions seek out people who are capable of influencing others and of disseminating an intervention throughout their social networks. They generally follow these steps:

1. Identification and recruitment of popular opinion leaders

Example: bartenders in gay bars who are well-liked, respected, and trusted by gay men become opinion leaders for the bars' patrons

2. Training of opinion leaders to become risk-reduction behavior change experts

Example: bartenders may attend workshops that teach them how to deliver safer-sex messages and establish safer-sex norms

3. Dissemination of risk-reduction messages to friends and other members of their social networks

Example: trained bartenders may converse with bar patrons about HIV risk reduction

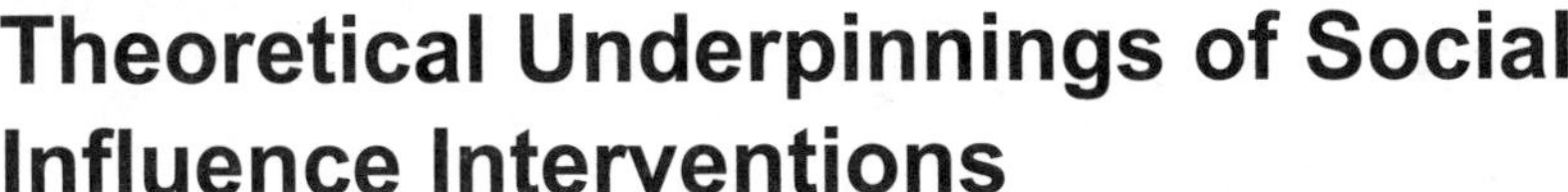

Theoretical Underpinnings of Social Influence Interventions

Social Cognitive Theory:
Trusted and credible role models who support behavior change are critical to learning new behaviors. Role models can endorse safer sex, reinforce safer-sex practices, and make condoms available.

Theory of Reasoned Action/Planned Behavior:
Social norms (other people's expectations) influence behavior. Norms generated by influential members of the community often powerfully shape individual actions.

Diffusion of Innovations Theory:
Innovations (new products, technologies, and behaviors) spread among people through several different channels. Group leaders and early adopters are critical to this spread.

Theoretical Underpinnings of Social Influence Interventions (continued)

School-based HIV interventions are offered in multiple formats and seek to accomplish multiple goals:

Large group sessions that present basic HIV/AIDS information, guest speakers, and panel discussions

Small group sessions that teach communication and negotiation exercises, ways to assess risk levels, and ways to access resources

School-wide activities that are intended to alter sex and drug-use norms; methods include placing AIDS awareness ads and stories in the school newspaper, putting up an AIDS bulletin board, declaring an AIDS awareness week, etc.

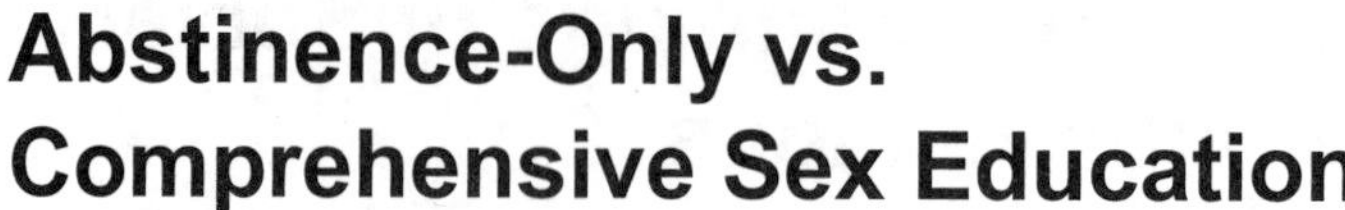

Abstinence-Only vs. Comprehensive Sex Education

- HIV/AIDS education can be embedded in a comprehensive sex education program.
- The most controversial question is how much to emphasize condom use versus abstinence.
- Abstinence-only sex education programs teach that abstinence from all sexual activity is the only appropriate option for unmarried people.
- Research on abstinence-only programs has **not** shown that these programs reduce rates of intercourse or delay the onset of intercourse among youth.
- However, studies show that abstinence-plus programs may delay the onset of sexual intercourse.

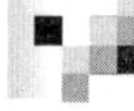

Outreach Interventions

Features of Outreach Interventions

Main Prevention Components:
- Distribution of prevention information and materials in places where at-risk people are accessible
- Recruitment of clients for treatment programs
- Behavior change counseling targeted at specific risk behaviors

Objectives:
- Serve as primary prevention for "at-risk" populations
- Provide secondary prevention for people who are already infected
- Alert the community to the presence of a prevention program
- Maintain low-cost, high-volume HIV prevention services

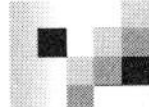

Outreach Interventions (continued)

Features of Outreach Interventions

Characteristics of Outreach Workers:

- Able to blend into the community in which they are working, or even be part of the community (e.g., recovering injection drug addicts)
- Know how to be safe and effective in the community

Elements of an Outreach Encounter:

- Establish initial contact with target population
- Maintain contact until clients become motivated and use services
- Follow up to reassess needs, revisit strategies, and deliver services

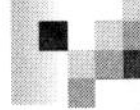

Social Marketing and Media Interventions

Even the best-crafted message is useless if it fails to reach the intended audience.

A message delivered through the mass media can stimulate discussions about a health issue. For example, a public service announcement about prevention of HIV might prompt sex partners to discuss condom use.

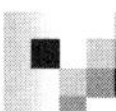

Social Marketing and Media Interventions (continued)

Principles for Implementing Social Marketing Campaigns

- Employ a wide range of communication strategies
- Reflect the concerns and cultures of target audiences
- Involve target audiences in planning the campaign
- Target campaigns to particular audiences
- Focus on realistic health behavior objectives
- Use many communication channels

Social Marketing and Media Interventions (continued)

Principles for Implementing Social Marketing Campaigns

- Demonstrate that benefits of behavior change far outweigh costs
- Incorporate theories of human behavior at the individual, group, and population levels
- Take into account social structures and institutions that influence behavior
- Address audience needs
- Empower people to get involved in campaign-related programs
- Be evaluated throughout the planning and implementation phases

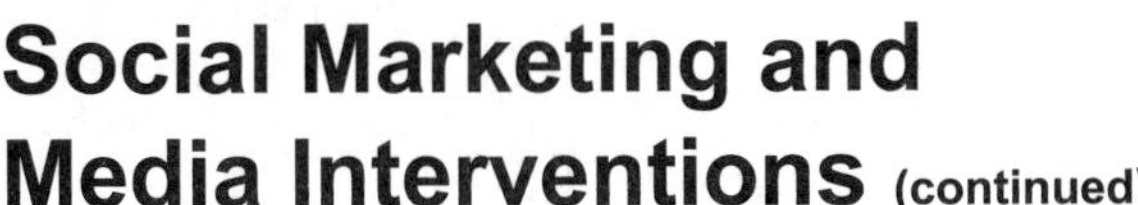

Social Marketing and Media Interventions (continued)

Media Interventions include:

- public service announcements (PSAs);
- AIDS informational and motivational videotapes;
- mass-media coverage of HIV/AIDS related material; and
- art that directly or indirectly promotes awareness of HIV/AIDS.

Learning Objectives

- Understand how laws, policies, structures, and institutional practices may help or hinder HIV prevention efforts
- Give examples of specific structural interventions that can benefit high-risk populations
- Define HIV/AIDS strategies such as containment-and-control, cooperation-and-inclusion, and harm-reduction
- Describe the impact of condom distribution and needle exchange programs

Key Terms

containment-and-control strategy
cooperation-and-inclusion strategy
harm-elimination approach
harm-reduction approach
law
policy
structural barrier
structural intervention

11

Structural Interventions

Many laws, policies, structures, and institutional practices are counterproductive to fighting HIV/AIDS, such as the prohibition of condoms in prisons, lack of funding for drug and alcohol treatment, and mandated abstinence-only education programs in schools. In addition, the absence of certain laws, policies, structures, or institutional practices—or the failure to fund and enforce those that exist—also can contribute to HIV risk. Structural interventions indirectly influence risk behavior by effecting changes to policies, laws, organizational practices, or other structures that are related either to risk behaviors or to access to behavioral prevention information, tools, or services (CDC, 2006). For example, by increasing the number of condoms in a person's environment, a Louisiana condom distribution effort reduced a barrier to safer sex (Cohen et al., 1999). Alternatively, by criminalizing unprotected sex with sex workers, Nevada's criminal justice system increased barriers to this risky behavior (Albert, Warner, Hatcher, Trussell & Bennett, 1995).

Evidence suggests that not only can structural interventions complement behavioral programs, but they may also surpass them in effectiveness. Most structural interventions reach more people than individual- or small group-level interventions and they can effect long-term environmental modifications that support sustained behavior change (Des Jarlais, 2000; Hovell et al., 1994). Indeed, a recent analysis showed several structural interventions (e.g., higher alcohol taxes, mass media campaigns, condom distribution) to be more cost-effective than many behavioral interventions at reducing HIV risk behaviors (Cohen, Wu, & Farley, 2004). This chapter briefly describes several structural approaches in HIV prevention.

STRUCTURAL INTERVENTIONS FOR HIGH-RISK POPULATIONS: AN OVERVIEW

Many populations face structural barriers to reducing risk behaviors and increasing protective behaviors for HIV. These barriers can be reduced through advocacy efforts that mobilize community members, lawmakers, policy makers, and other stakeholders to effect changes to relevant laws, policies, structures, and institutional practices. An overview of the types of structural interventions that can benefit specific high-risk populations are provided in the following sections.

Injection Drug Users (IDUs)

Structural interventions that target IDUs focus on provision of sterile injecting equipment and improving access to drug treatment programs, condoms, health care, and HIV/AIDS prevention and treatment services (FHI, 2003).

Sex Workers

Preventing the transmission of HIV through sex workers is difficult, in part, because sex work continues to be illegal in many countries. Structural interventions that benefit sex workers include policies that require condom use education and distribution of condoms in brothels, as well as the provision of free medical services (Hamand, 2001).

Children and Young People

Many young people are put at risk of HIV infection because they are denied access to HIV education, information, health care, and means of prevention (Gruskin & Tarantola, 2002). Ensuring that schools provide comprehensive sex and HIV education is crucial to stemming the increasing infection rate among this age group. Legal and policy efforts that reduce sexual exploitation and abuse are also crucial structural interventions for this population.

Migrants and Refugees

Migrants and refugees often have little or no access to HIV information, health services, and prevention materials (Brummer, 2002; McGinn, Purdin, Krause, & Jones, 2001). Legal, policy, and other institutional changes can reduce logistical and perceived barriers to accessing services (Hamand, 2001).

Armed Forces Personnel

Military personnel have higher rates of sexually transmitted infections – 2 to 5 times higher than in civilian populations during peace time and 50 times higher during conflict (UNAIDS, 2003). Structural interventions that work with senior military and defense ministry personnel to institutionalize prevention education and condom distribution can reduce HIV infection risk (Hamand, 2001).

Prisoners

Overcrowding, sharing drug injection equipment, unprotected anal sex, and male rape are significant factors in the transmission of HIV in prison environments (Kantor, 2003). Advocacy seeks to change prison policies so that clean syringes, sterilizing bleach, and lubricated condoms are made available to prisoners (Hamand, 2001).

HIV/AIDS-RELATED POLICIES AND LAWS

Policies can be created by governments and by non-governmental bodies; *laws* begin as legislation, and are subsequently interpreted by courts. Many policies are clarified through the legal system, and many laws are implemented through administrative policies (Smith, 2001). Changes to laws and policies at the national, regional, and local levels can have a profound, positive impact on HIV risk behaviors and use of prevention services, particularly when those laws and policies are data-driven, appropriately funded, and fully implemented. For example, laws that criminalize unprotected commercial sex, deregulate syringe sales and possession, and provide

Taiwan established a nationwide surveillance system for HIV infection in 1989 and adopted a policy to provide all HIV-infected citizens with free access to HAART beginning in 1997. After free access to HAART was established, the estimated HIV transmission rate decreased by 53%. There was no statistically significant change in the incidence of syphilis, in the general population or among HIV+ patients, during the same period, suggesting that the drop in transmission could not be accounted for by changes in sexual behavior. Researchers have concluded that providing free HAART to all HIV-infected citizens contributed to the control of the HIV epidemic in Taiwan.

Figure 11-1 Making free HAART available to HIV-positives in Taiwan (Fang et al., 2004).

free access to HAART to all HIV-positives have shown positive effects on sexual risk-taking behavior and/or HIV infection rates (Albert et al., 1995; Fang et al., 2004; Groseclose et al., 1995) (see Figure 11-1).

There are several different approaches to HIV/AIDS-related policy and law. These approaches sometimes come into conflict with each other, complicating efforts to develop and implement laws and policies that will stem the tide of HIV infection (Smith, 2001).

For example, the *containment-and-control* strategy focuses on the coercive power of the state to force compliance with laws. It emphasizes the protection of HIV– people from exposure to the virus by regulating individual behavior. Containment and control objectives are enforced by legal and monetary penalties for violation.

The *cooperation-and-inclusion* strategy, by contrast, relies on the participation of all heavily impacted communities. It emphasizes the voluntary participation of HIV+ people in reducing HIV transmission. Cooperation and inclusion goals are met through persuasion and material incentives (Schubert & Peterson, 2002). The tension between these two approaches is apparent for sex workers. Sex work is illegal in most places, which makes it difficult for sex workers to access health care services. Indeed, in some places, a woman may be arrested and fined for carrying a large number of condoms, making it problematic for condom distribution programs to conduct outreach to sex workers. Thus, laws against sex work, whose original intention was partly to reduce the spread of STIs/STDs, often heighten the risk of HIV infection for sex workers and their clients (Feinstein & Prentice, 2001). Several studies have found that sanctioning *unprotected sex* among sex workers has been an effective way to reduce HIV (Albert et al., 1995; Celentano et al., 1998; Hanenberg, Rojanapithayakorn, Kunasol, & Sokal, 1994).

Another example is provided by the harm-elimination and hard-reduction approaches. A *harm-elimination* approach seeks to strengthen people's ability to abstain from all risk behaviors, whereas a *harm-reduction* approach tries to make risk behaviors less dangerous. The tension between these two approaches is apparent for injection drug users. In the United States, not only is it illegal to possess narcotics, but it is also illegal to possess drug-using paraphernalia. Although abiding by these laws would eliminate the risk of HIV transmission through injection drug use, clearly not everyone abides by these laws.

One harm-reduction strategy of reducing the risk of injection drug use is to decriminalize the possession of injection equipment. When it is legal to possess injection equipment, people perceive less of a need to share needles (Gostin, Lazzarini, Jones, & Flaherty, 1997), and therefore may be less likely to transmit HIV through shared needles. Harm-elimination laws may therefore deter physicians, pharmacists, and public health professionals from reducing the risk of getting and giving HIV among injection drug users. Evidence for the benefit of decriminalizing possession of injection equipment comes from Connecticut. There, officials partially deregulated the sale and possession of syringes. Pharmacy sales of sterile syringes to IDUs increased, and the use of contaminated syringes fell (Groseclose et al., 1995).

A number of other (often hotly debated) policy and law issues affect HIV prevention efforts. Health care reform, insurance coverage, confidentiality and partner notification in the context of HIV testing, immigration and travel restrictions for HIV+ people, educational policy (concerning sex and HIV education in primary and secondary schools), and funding for prevention efforts all have an impact on risk behaviors and access to prevention and treatment services.

CONDOM DISTRIBUTION AND NEEDLE EXCHANGE PROGRAMS

Other environmental interventions, beyond policies and laws, can lead to reductions in HIV risk behavior. Two prime examples are condom distribution programs and syringe exchange and access programs.

Condom Distribution Programs

The promotion of male and female condoms for protection against HIV and other STIs/STDs and unwanted pregnancy can have spectacular results. For example, Thailand's 100% condom campaign has averted 2 million infections, saving an estimated U.S. $6 billion (Hamand, 2001). In addition, a program in Louisiana distributed 33 million free condoms through public health clinics, community mental health centers, substance abuse treatment sites, and businesses in neighborhoods with high rates of STIs/STDs. Surveys among 275,000 African Americans showed that condom use increased by 30%, and that number of sexual partners did not increase. The program was estimated to have averted over $33 million in medical care costs (Bedimo, Pinkerton, Cohen, Gray, & Farley, 2002; Cohen et al., 1999).

Needle Exchange and Access Programs

The aim of syringe and needle exchange programs is to increase the availability of sterile injecting equipment and to remove contaminated syringes from circulation. Some programs also refer injection drug users (IDUs) to appropriate services. They also may provide information and advice on safer sex, and may distribute condoms for use by IDUs and their sexual partners. IDUs who use needle exchange programs reduce the likelihood of HIV transmission by decreasing their use of needles and syringes that are contaminated. IDUs who do not participate in the exchange also benefit from the decreased proportion of contaminated needles in circulation.

A number of studies both in the United States and abroad have found that needle exchange programs are associated with reduced high-risk injection behavior (Bedimo et al., 2002). In San Francisco, a 47% decline in needle sharing was reported after introduction of a needle exchange program (Hagan, Des Jarlais, Friedman, Purchase, & Alter, 1995). A decline in needle sharing from 12% to 4% of IDUs was associated with a needle exchange program in New York City (Heimer, Khoshnood, Bigg, Guydish, & Junge, 1998).

There is clear evidence from the United States and Western Europe that needle exchange schemes do not increase either drug use, the frequency of injection, or the number of new injection drug users (Hagan et al., 1995; Heimer et al., 1998; Pouget et al., 2005).

REFERENCES

Albert, A. E., Warner, D. L., Hatcher, R. A., Trussell, J., & Bennett, C. (1995). Condom use among female commercial sex workers in Nevada's legal brothels. *American Journal of Public Health, 85*(11), 1514–1520.

Bedimo, A. L., Pinkerton, S. D., Cohen, D. A., Gray, B., & Farley, T. A. (2002). Condom distribution: A cost-utility analysis. *International Journal of STD and AIDS, 13*(6), 384–392.

Brummer, D. (2002). *Labour migration and HIV/AIDS in Southern Africa*. International Organization for Migration, Regional Office For Southern Africa.

Celentano, D. D., Nelson, K. E., Lyles, C. M., Beyrer, C., Eiumtrakul, S., Go, V. F., et al. (1998). Decreasing incidence of HIV and sexually transmitted diseases in young Thai men: Evidence for success of the HIV/AIDS control and prevention program. *AIDS, 12*(5), F29–F36.

Centers for Disease Control and Prevention (CDC). (2006). Evolution of HIV/AIDS prevention programs—United States, 1981-2006. *Morbidity and Mortality Weekly Report, 55*(21), 597–603.

Cohen, D. A., Farley, T. A., Bedimo-Etame, J. R., Scribner, R., Ward, W., Kendall, C., et al. (1999). Implementation of condom social marketing in Louisiana, 1993 to 1996. *American Journal of Public Health, 89*(2), 204–208.

Cohen, D. A., Wu, S. Y., & Farley, T. A. (2004). Comparing the cost-effectiveness of HIV prevention interventions. *Journal of Acquired Immune Deficiency Syndromes, 37*(3), 1404–1414.

Des Jarlais, D. C. (2000). Structural interventions to reduce HIV transmission among injecting drug users. *AIDS, 14*(Suppl 1), S41–S46.

Family Health International (FHI). (2003). *Fact sheet: Reducing HIV in injecting drug users (IDU)*. Arlington, VA: FHI.

Fang, C. T., Hsu, H. M., Twu, S. J., Chen, M. Y., Chang, Y. Y., Hwang, J. S., et al. (2004). Decreased HIV transmission after a policy of providing free access to highly active antiretroviral therapy in Taiwan. *The Journal of Infectious Diseases, 190*(5), 879–885.

Feinstein, N., & Prentice, B. (2001). *The UNAIDS gender and AIDS almanac*. Los Altos, CA: Sociometrics Corporation.

Gostin, L. O., Lazzarini, Z., Jones, T. S., & Flaherty, K. (1997). Prevention of HIV/AIDS and other blood-borne diseases among injection drug users. A national survey on the regulation of syringes and needles. *Journal of the American Medical Association, 277*(1), 53–62.

Groseclose, S. L., Weinstein, B., Jones, T. S., Valleroy, L. A., Fehrs, L. J., & Kassler, W. J. (1995). Impact of increased legal access to needles and syringes on practices of injecting-drug users and police officers—Connecticut, 1992–1993. *Journal of Acquired Immune Deficiency Syndromes and Human Retrovirology, 10*(1), 82–89.

Gruskin, S., & Tarantola, D. (2002). Human rights and HIV/AIDS. In L. Pieperl, S. Coffey, O. Bacon, & P. Volberding (Eds.), *HIV InSite knowledge base*. San Francisco: Center for HIV Information, University of California, San Francisco.

Hagan, H., Des Jarlais, D. C., Friedman, S. R., Purchase, D., & Alter, M. J. (1995). Reduced risk of hepatitis B and hepatitis C among injection drug users in the Tacoma syringe exchange program. *American Journal of Public Health, 85*(11), 1531–1537.

Hamand, J. (2001). *Advocacy guide for HIV/AIDS*. London: International Planned Parenthood Federation.

Hanenberg, R. S., Rojanapithayakorn, W., Kunasol, P., & Sokal, D. C. (1994). Impact of Thailand's HIV-control programme as indicated by the decline of sexually transmitted diseases. *Lancet, 344*(8917), 243–245.

Heimer, R., Khoshnood, K., Bigg, D., Guydish, J., & Junge, B. (1998). Syringe use and reuse: Effects of syringe exchange programs in four cities. *Journal of Acquired Immune Deficiency Syndromes and Human Retrovirology, 18*(Suppl 1), S37–S44.

Hovell, M. F., Hillman, E. R., Blumberg, E., Sipan, C., Atkins, C., Hofstetter, C. R., et al. (1994). A behavioral-ecological model of adolescent sexual development: A template for AIDS prevention. *Journal of Sex Research, 31*(4), 267–281.

Kantor, E. (2003). HIV transmission and prevention in prisons. In L. Pieperl, S. Coffey, O. Bacon, & P. Volberding (Eds.), *HIV InSite knowledge base*. San Francisco: Center for HIV Information, University of California, San Francisco.

McGinn, T., Purdin, S. J., Krause, S., & Jones, R. K. (2001). Forced migration and transmission of HIV and other sexually transmitted infections: Policy and programmatic responses. In L. Pieperl, S. Coffey, O. Bacon, & P. Volberding (Eds.), *HIV InSite knowledge base*. San Francisco: Center for HIV Information, University of California, San Francisco.

Pouget, E. R., Deren, S., Fuller, C. M., Blaney, S., McMahon, J. M., Kang, S. Y., et al. (2005). Receptive syringe sharing among injection drug users in Harlem and the Bronx during the New York State Expanded Syringe Access Demonstration Project. *Journal of Acquired Immune Deficiency Syndromes, 39*(4), 471–477.

Schubert, J. N., & Peterson, S. A. (2002). Measuring substantive AIDS policies in the American states. *State and Local Government Review, 34*(1), 45–50.

Smith, R. (Ed.). (2001). *Encyclopedia of AIDS: A social, political, cultural, and scientific record of the HIV epidemic*. New York: Penguin Putnam.

United Nations Program on HIV/AIDS (UNAIDS). (2003). *Fact sheet: HIV/AIDS and uniformed services*. Geneva, Switzerland: UNAIDS.

Instructor Resources

LEARNING ACTIVITIES

ACTIVITY:

Assignment: Public Health and Human Rights

Objective: To understand how HIV policies and laws attempt to preserve public liberties while also protecting public health.

Liberals have generally emphasized the need to insulate people with HIV/AIDS from discrimination, whereas conservatives often have framed the epidemic as a danger to the general population resulting from social decay and personal immorality. Partner notification has emerged as an important strategy in the fight against AIDS, and some state and national governments have adopted laws that encourage or mandate notification, often without the patient's consent.

Write a five- to seven-page paper exploring:

1. the implications of mandatory notification laws from a public health perspective, and
2. the implications of mandatory notification laws from a human rights perspective.

DISCUSSION QUESTIONS

1. Are you aware of any laws or policies in your school or state that impact HIV/AIDS transmission or treatment? What are they?
2. Why do you think harm-reduction models are so controversial? What can be done to make them less controversial?

QUIZ

1. Which of the following is *not* an example of a structural intervention?
   a) Free medical services for sex workers
   b) Condom distribution on military bases
   c) Offering clean syringes to prison populations
   d) Couples counseling for serodiscordant partners
2. Laws against sex work could be an example of which strategy?
   a) Containment-and-control
   b) Cooperation-and-inclusion
   c) Harm-elimination
   d) Harm-reduction

3. Decriminalizing the possession of injection equipment can be an example of which strategy?
a) Containment-and-control
b) Cooperation-and-inclusion
c) Harm-elimination
d) Harm-reduction

4. Studies in Louisiana show that the distribution of condoms did all of the following except:
a) Increased condom use
b) Decreased infection rates
c) Increased numbers of sexual partners
d) Saved money in health care costs

5. Studies in San Francisco show that needle exchange program caused a decline of nearly ___ in needle sharing.
a) 20%
b) 40%
c) 50%
d) 70%

ANSWERS

1. D. Couples counseling is an example of a small group intervention, not a structural intervention.

2. A. The *containment-and-control* strategy focuses on the coercive power of the state to force compliance with laws. It emphasizes the protection of HIV-negative people from exposure to the virus by regulating individual behavior. Containment and control objectives are enforced by legal and monetary penalties for violation.

3. D. When it is legal to possess injection equipment, people perceive less of a need to share needles, and therefore may be less likely to transmit HIV through shared needles.

4. C. Surveys show that the numbers of sexual partners did not increase.

5. C. In San Francisco, a 47% decline in needle sharing was reported after the introduction of a needle exchange program.

WEB RESOURCES

Sexual Orientation: Science, Education, and Policy

http://psychology.ucdavis.edu/rainbow/index.html

http://www.AIDSstigma.net

Features work by Dr. Gregory M. Herek, an internationally recognized authority on sexual prejudice, hate crimes, and AIDS stigma; promotes the use of scientific knowledge for education and enlightened public policy related to sexual orientation and HIV/AIDS.

HIV/AIDS and Human Rights Related Resources (UCSF HIV Insite)

http://hivinsite.ucsf.edu/InSite?page=kbr-08–01–07#S1X

Lists links to organizations and projects on HIV/AIDS and human rights.

Human Rights Watch: HIV/AIDS and Human Rights

http://hrw.org/doc/?t=hivaids&document_limit=0,2

Describes research and provides information on the relationship between human rights abuses and HIV/AIDS in the United States and around the world.

United Nations Population Fund Interactive Population Center (UNFPA) Interactive Population Center: Working to Empower Women

http://www.unfpa.org/intercenter/beijing/index.htm

Discusses women and poverty, education and training of women, women and health, violence against women, women and armed conflict, women and the economy, women in power and decision making, institutional mechanisms for the advancement of women, human rights of women, women and the media, women and the environment, and the girl-child.

United Nations Population Fund Interactive Population Center (UNFPA) Interactive Population Center: Women's Empowerment and Reproductive Health

http://www.unfpa.org/intercenter/cycle/

Describes the international consensus reached at the Fourth World Conference on Women (FWCW) in Beijing in 1995 about empowering women and ending gender inequality, defines key human rights concepts, and examines issues of reproductive health and rights that affect women throughout their lives.

Activity Manual: Gender, HIV and Human Rights: A Training Manual (UNIFEM, 2000)

http://www.unifem.org/resources/item_detail.php?ProductID=5

United Nations Development Fund for Women (UNIFEM). (2000). Gender, HIV and human rights: A training manual. *New York: UNIFEM.*

This guide contains information and activities for educators and practitioners to address gender inequality, legal, and ethical concerns in the context of HIV.

Advocacy Guide for HIV/AIDS (Hamand, 2001)

http://www.ippfwhr.org/publications/download/monographs/HIV_Guide_e.pdf

Hamand, J. (2001). Advocacy guide for HIV/AIDS. *London: International Planned Parenthood Federation.*

Describes what advocacy can do, often at little cost, to prevent HIV/AIDS.

RECOMMENDED READING

HIV/AIDS and Human Rights: International Guidelines (UNAIDS, 1998)

Office of the United Nations High Commissioner for Human Rights and the Joint United Programme on HIV/AIDS. (1998). HIV/AIDS and human rights: International guidelines. *UN Doc HR/PUB/98/1.*

Resolutions of the U.N. Commission on Human Rights and the 1998 International Guidelines on HIV/AIDS and Human Rights provide advocates and policy makers with useful tools for helping to ensure increased attention to both HIV/AIDS and human rights.

Global Crisis—Global Action (UNAIDS, 2001)

Joint United Nations Programme on HIV/AIDS (UNAIDS). (2001). Declaration of Commitment on HIV/AIDS: Global Crisis—Global Action. United Nations General Assembly Special Session on HIV/AIDS, New York, NY, 2001.

Informative document for advocacy and accountability in relation to HIV/AIDS and human rights.

POWERPOINT SLIDES

(Note: A full-color version of these slides, with graphics, is also available on the CD-ROM.)

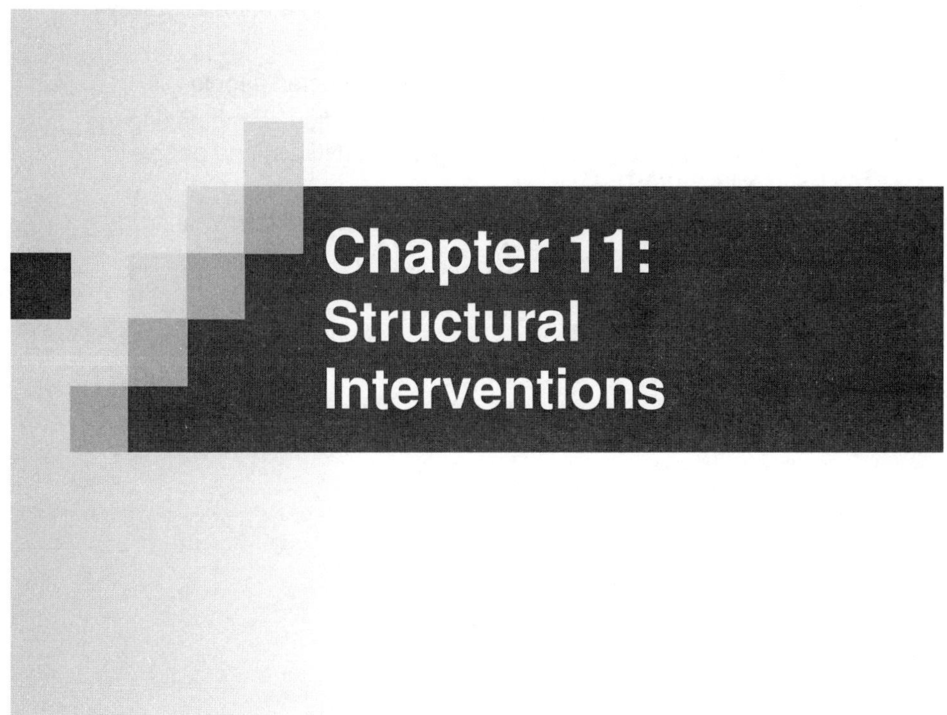

Structural Interventions

HIV/AIDS advocacy has produced cultural changes that reduce HIV transmission.

What Is Advocacy?

▪ Advocacy promotes good policies and practices and upholds the rights of HIV+ people. The goals of advocacy include:

- □ creating awareness of the magnitude of HIV/AIDS;
- □ redressing discriminatory practices; and
- □ removing barriers to prevention and care activities.

Social Action

▪ Social action targets policies that are counterproductive to fighting HIV/AIDS, such as:

- □ prohibiting condoms in prisons;
- □ reducing funding for drug and alcohol treatment; and
- □ mandating abstinence-based education programs.

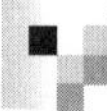

The Application of Advocacy in HIV/AIDS Prevention

- Advocacy supports HIV/AIDS prevention efforts in a number of ways:
  - □ Educates people about how HIV is spread
  - □ Reduces the stigmatization of HIV/AIDS-affected people
  - □ Mobilizes HIV/AIDS prevention programs, often strengthening the ties between non-governmental agencies (NGOs) and people living with HIV/AIDS
  - □ Initiates and supports campaigns for making antiretroviral drugs widely available and affordable

Major Areas of Advocacy for HIV/AIDS

Human Rights:
When human rights are protected, fewer people get HIV/AIDS, and people affected by HIV/AIDS can better cope with the disease.

HIV and Gender:
Advocacy that improves women's access to educational and economic resources can increase women's power in sexual relationships.

Involving People with HIV/AIDS:
Involving people with HIV/AIDS in policy design, planning, and implementation ensures that the needs of HIV+ people are better recognized, reduces discrimination, helps destigmatize HIV/AIDS, and increases understanding of the impact of HIV/AIDS.

Major Areas of Advocacy for HIV/AIDS (continued)

HIV Testing:
Advocacy for HIV testing addresses the need for high-quality, voluntary, confidential, and easily accessible HIV testing and counseling, and discourages mandatory testing.

Microbicides and Vaccines:
Advocacy is directed at governments to support research and development of microbicides and effective vaccines against HIV.

Parent-to-Child Transmission of HIV:
A short antiretroviral course offered to pregnant, HIV+ women reduces transmission to their infants by at least 50%. Advocating for governments to integrate such prevention interventions into reproductive health services can help reduce HIV infection in children.

Major Areas of Advocacy for HIV/AIDS (continued)

Promotion of Condoms:
The promotion of male and female condoms for protection against STIs/HIV/AIDS and unwanted pregnancy can have spectacular results.

Children and Young People:
Advocacy issues concerning young people include efforts to stop sexual exploitation and abuse and to involve young people in the design, implementation, and evaluation of HIV/AIDS advocacy campaigns.

Sex Workers:
Prevention strategies for this particularly vulnerable group include encouraging protection of sex workers and their clients through 100% condom use.

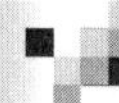

Major Areas of Advocacy for HIV/AIDS (continued)

Injection Drug Users (IDUs):

- Providing sterile injecting equipment
- Providing education about HIV risks and safe practices
- Making available drug treatment programs
- Providing access to counseling and support for HIV-infected injectors
- Providing access to health care services
- Providing condoms

Men who have Sex with Men (MSM):

- Peer education
- Distribution of high-quality condoms and water-based lubricants
- Safer sex campaigns and skills training
- Strengthening of other organizations for self-identified gay men
- Education among health care providers to overcome prejudice

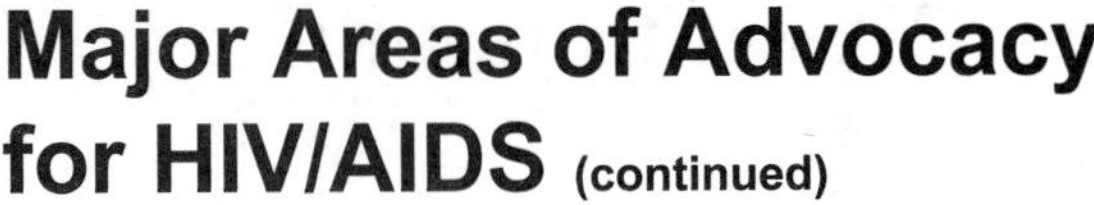

Major Areas of Advocacy for HIV/AIDS (continued)

Armed Forces:
Advocacy promotes providing effective HIV prevention information and ultimately reducing the infection rate in the armed forces. Advocacy directed at senior military and defense ministry personnel has the highest impact.

Prisoners:
Advocacy issues to be brought to the attention of senior prison officials include providing clean, free syringes and sterilizing bleach for drug users, and providing lubricated condoms for everyone.

Migrants and Refugees:
Reducing discrimination against migrants and refugees and providing services for them can help reduce HIV infection.

Approaches to HIV/AIDS Policy and Law

Containment-and-Control versus Cooperation-and-Inclusion:

Containment-and-Control:

- Emphasizes the protection of HIV- people from exposure to the virus by regulating individual behavior.
- Enforced by legal and monetary penalties for violation.

Cooperation-and-Inclusion:

- Emphasizes voluntary participation of HIV+ people in reducing HIV transmission.
- Goals are met through persuasion and material incentives.

Harm-Elimination versus Harm-Reduction:

- Harm-elimination attempts to stop all risk behaviors.
- Harm-reduction attempts to make risk behaviors less dangerous.

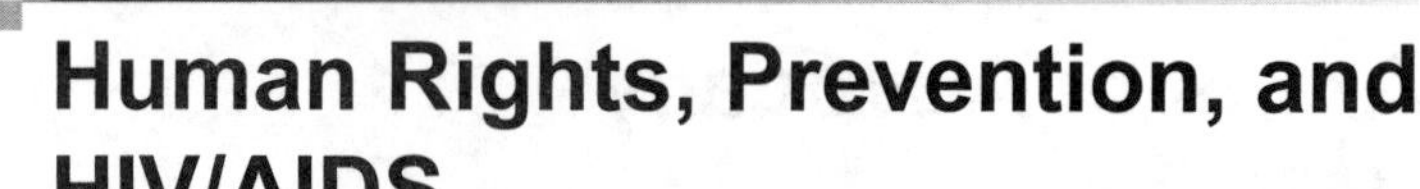

Human Rights, Prevention, and HIV/AIDS

Human Rights Abuses Increase Vulnerability to HIV Infection
Human rights violations further stigmatize those at highest risk of infection, blocking access to information, preventive services, and treatment. Such violations come in a variety of forms, including:

- sexual violence and coercion against women and girls;
- discrimination and violence against men having sex with men;
- discrimination and violence against sex workers and injection drug users;
- violations of the right of young people to information on HIV transmission; and
- confiscation of property from women whose husbands have died of AIDS.

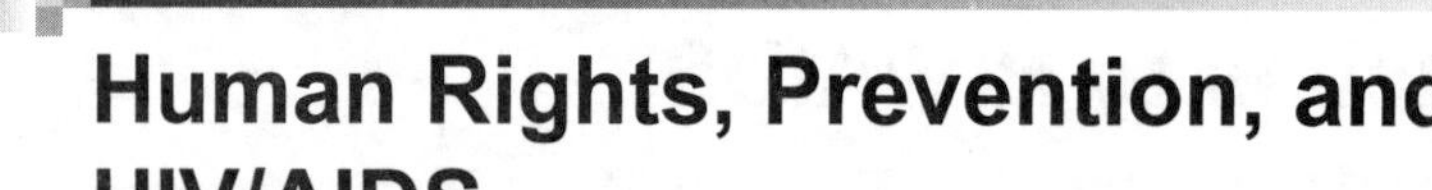

Human Rights, Prevention, and HIV/AIDS (continued)

Human Rights Abuses Increase Vulnerability to HIV Infection
Human rights violations further stigmatize those at highest risk of infection, blocking access to information, preventive services, and treatment. Such violations come in a variety of forms, including:

- Human rights violations against children who have lost parents to AIDS or whose parents are living with the disease, including losing inheritance rights, having to take on hazardous labor including prostitution, and being forced to live on the streets where they are subject to police violence and other abuses.
- Discrimination against people with HIV and AIDS including the many issues raised by names reporting, partner notification, and confidentiality that may deter people from getting tested and/or from disclosing their status to their partners.

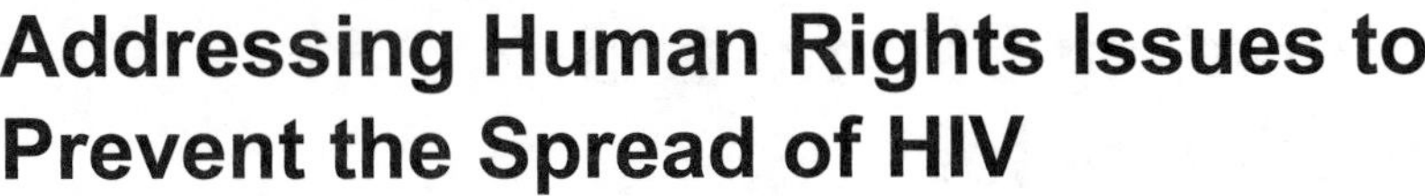

Addressing Human Rights Issues to Prevent the Spread of HIV

Governmental Obligations in the Context of HIV/AIDS

Respect:
Governments should respect the rights of people living with HIV/AIDS, affected by HIV/AIDS, and vulnerable to HIV/AIDS.

Protect:
Governments should prevent rights violations against people living with HIV/AIDS and provide some legal means for redressing rights violations.

Fulfill:
Governments should take administrative, judicial, and other measures toward realization of the rights of people living with HIV/AIDS and affected by HIV/AIDS; should also work to minimize people's vulnerability to HIV/AIDS.

Addressing Gender Norms and Inequalities

Strategies to Address Gender Inequality

1) Promote awareness of gender issues in HIV/AIDS.
2) Provide women with HIV prevention technologies that they can control.
3) Promote women's economic empowerment and access to education, information, and skills.
4) Ensure women's access to medical and social support.
5) Focus on strategies to include men and boys.

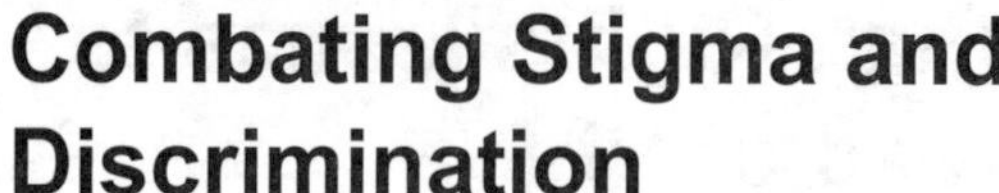

Combating Stigma and Discrimination

- HIV-related stigma refers to all unfavorable attitudes, beliefs, and policies directed toward people perceived to be infected with HIV.
- HIV-related stigma reinforces existing social inequalities, especially those related to gender, sexuality, and race.
- Fear of discrimination prevents people from getting tested and treated for HIV.

Combating Stigma and Discrimination (continued)

The Stigma of Being a Woman

- Women are often blamed for the spread of HIV to their families because they are often the first ones in their families to be tested.
- In many parts of the world, HIV is misperceived as a ‘woman's disease’or a “prostitute's disease.”

Homophobia

- Homophobia is the fear of or aversion to men who have sex with men and women who have sex with women.
- Because of homophobia, men who have sex with men often keep their sexual behavior secret and deny their sexual risk. This increases their own risk of getting and giving HIV.

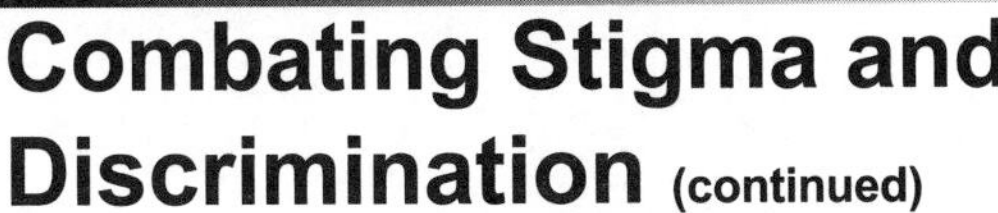

Combating Stigma and Discrimination (continued)

The Stigma of Illicit Drug Use

- The stigma associated with addiction and illicit drug use hinders HIV prevention efforts.
- Illicit drug users are often very hard to reach for prevention interventions.
- In addition, discrimination against drug users can be seen in the lack of funding for health promotion programs directed at this population.

PART III

Living with HIV/AIDS

HIV+ people are living longer, healthier lives, in large part because of advances in anti-HIV drug therapies. Part 3 describes these therapies, as well as the medical issues that people living with HIV/AIDS face. It then addresses the psychological and social challenges of living with HIV/AIDS. Part 3 closes with a discussion of HIV prevention efforts that are aimed at HIV+ people.

Learning Objectives

- Describe how antiretroviral therapies work to treat HIV/AIDS
- Compare and contrast the four classes of antiretroviral medications
- Understand the critical factors in successful HIV/AIDS treatment
- Describe the measures used to handle complications in HIV/AIDS treatment

Key Terms

antiretroviral therapy
AZT
fusion inhibitors
HAART
HIV coreceptor blockers
integrase inhibitors
non-nucleoside reverse transcriptase inhibitors
nucleoside reverse transcriptase inhibitors
opportunistic infections
protease inhibitors
resistance

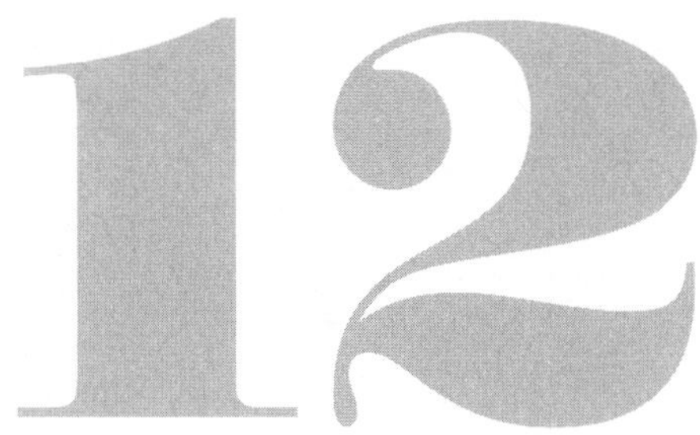

The Medical Side of Living With HIV/AIDS

The advent of antiretroviral therapies has changed the face of the HIV/AIDS epidemic. This chapter describes the development of antiretroviral therapies, how they work, and why they sometimes do not work. This chapter also discusses HIV/AIDS-related complications and their treatment.

ADVANCES IN THE MEDICAL TREATMENT OF HIV/AIDS

Where antiretroviral therapy has been available, HIV morbidity and mortality have decreased.

In the early years of the epidemic, an AIDS diagnosis meant a rapid decline in health and imminent death. Then in 1987, the first antiretroviral drug, AZT (*azidothymidine*; generic name *zidovudine*), was approved by the U.S. Food and Drug Administration to slow the progression of HIV disease (Kanabus & Fredricksson, n.d.). This was followed by the approval of other antiretroviral drugs.

In 1996, the use of three antiretroviral medications in combination (referred to as Highly Active Antiretroviral Therapy [HAART], or simply antiretroviral therapy) became the new treatment standard. HAART revolutionized the treatment of HIV/AIDS and improved the outlook for many HIV+ people (Omobosola & Henry, 2003; Palella et al., 1998). Combinations of drugs are more effective than individual drugs against HIV/AIDS because HIV's genetic material mutates very quickly and becomes resistant to individual drugs. Combinations of drugs overwhelm HIV, keeping it from multiplying and mutating as quickly.

In 1996, scientists also developed tests that measure the level of HIV-1 RNA (that is, viral load) in the plasma of HIV+ people. These tests help clinicians to better monitor how an individual's disease is advancing, and how he or she is responding to antiretroviral medications (Mellors et al., 1997; Riddler & Mellors, 1998).

Many people treating AIDS in the late 1990s adopted the dogma of "hit early, hit hard," and prescribed HAART right after HIV was diagnosed. Since that time, health care providers have learned to wait to prescribe HAART until people enter the more advanced stages of HIV disease, as HAART is often accompanied by many negative side effects (Dybul, Fauci, Bartlett, Kaplan, & Pau, 2002; Hare, 2004; Office of AIDS Research Advisory Council [OARAC], 2006). These side effects range from fatigue and nausea to diabetes and permanent liver damage. Researchers also have developed ways to treat the opportunistic infections that often accompany HIV/AIDS, such as yeast infections and herpes (Omobosola & Henry, 2003). The Department

The U.S. Department of Health and Human Services (DHHS) provides guidelines for the medical management of HIV infection and other issues surrounding HIV infection. These guidelines contain information that is useful not only to health care providers but also to patients, their friends, and their family members, who are encouraged to review the guidelines with their health care providers.

For the most up-to-date treatment guidelines for adults and adolescents, children, and pregnant women, see the Health and Human Services AIDS info Web site at http://aidsinfo.nih.gov/Guidelines/.

Figure 12-1 HIV/AIDS treatment standards for adults, adolescents, and children.

of Health and Human Services makes available regularly updated guidelines that represent the official U.S. treatment standards for the management of HIV infection in adults, adolescents, and children (see Figure 12-1).

SLOWING DOWN HIV

Although there is no cure for HIV to date, there are treatment options that can slow the effects of HIV on the body.

Antiretroviral drugs work by keeping HIV from multiplying. There are four kinds of antiretroviral drugs approved by the U.S. Food and Drug Administration (FDA), which attack three different phases of the HIV reproductive cycle (Department of Health and Human Services [DHHS], 2005).

Current Antiretroviral Medications

Current antiretroviral medications fall into four classes:

- nucleoside reverse transcriptase inhibitors (NRTIs)
- non-nucleoside reverse transcriptase inhibitors (NNRTIs)
- protease inhibitors
- fusion inhibitors

Here is how each class of antiretroviral drug works:

1. Nucleoside Reverse Transcriptase Inhibitors (NRTIs). To make copies of itself, HIV uses an enzyme called reverse transcriptase to convert its RNA into DNA after the virus enters the host cell. The viral DNA then enters the host cell's nucleus and hijacks it for its own reproduction (refer to Part 1). NRTIs are faulty versions of reverse transcriptase. When the HIV attempts to turn its RNA into DNA, NRTIs take the place of real reverse transcriptase, which results in incomplete DNA that cannot create new copies of the virus.

2. Non-Nucleoside Reverse Transcriptase Inhibitors (NNRTIs). Like NRTIs, NNRTIs also interfere with reverse transcriptase. Instead of replacing reverse transcriptase with a faulty fake, NNRTIs chemically bind to reverse transcriptase and make it unable to do its job.

3. Protease Inhibitors (PIs). After HIV hijacks a cell's nucleus to make copies of itself, it needs an enzyme called protease to chop its long chains of proteins into infectious bits. Protease inhibitors chemically bind to protease, so that protease cannot cleave the HIV proteins into mature viral particles.

4. Fusion Inhibitors. To make copies of itself, HIV first uses its spikes to fuse with the host cell's membrane, and then thrusts its contents inside. Fusion inhibitors work by attaching themselves to one of the proteins on HIV's spikes (i.e., glycoprotein 41), which makes the HIV spike unable to fuse with the host cell.

Future Antiretroviral Medications

New antiretroviral medications that are currently being developed could include drugs that are easier for the body to absorb and circulate, drugs that last longer in the body, drugs with fewer negative side effects, and drugs that interfere with different stages of the HIV reproduction cycle. This last group includes *integrase inhibitors*, which would keep HIV's newly formed DNA from being spliced into the host cell's DNA, and *HIV coreceptor blockers*, which would keep HIV from binding with the host cell membrane (Hare, 2004).

SUCCESSFUL ANTIRETROVIRAL THERAPY

Front and center of the battle against HIV are antiretroviral therapies that keep the virus from multiplying, thereby extending the life and improving the quality of life of HIV+ patients.

Goals of Antiretroviral Therapy

Antiretroviral therapy (sometimes called Highly Active Antiretroviral Therapy, or HAART) typically combines three or more antiretroviral drugs that work together to keep HIV from multiplying. Although antiretroviral drugs improve health and delay death, they do not cure HIV/AIDS. Eventually, HIV overwhelms the drugs and the body's defenses, and fatal infections set in.

Once the decision is made to initiate antiretroviral therapy, the goals of that treatment (OARAC, 2006) are to:

- reduce HIV-related morbidity and mortality,
- improve quality of life,
- restore and preserve immunologic function, and
- maximally and durably suppress viral load.

Initiating Antiretroviral Therapy

The decision to initiate therapy should be made by both the patient and the physician, taking into account the patient's willingness and readiness to begin therapy, risk of progression to AIDS (as measured by the patient's viral load and CD4+ cell count), level of immunodeficiency (as measured by the patient's CD4+ cell count), and likelihood of adhering to the medication regimen. The decision also should be informed by an assessment of the risks versus benefits of initiating therapy at that point in time.

The Pros and Cons of Initiating Therapy Early or Later

Some people choose to put off therapy for as long as it is safely possible. Others decide to begin therapy earlier in the course of their disease. Both strategies have merit, and both are supported by research. The decision to initiate therapy should weigh the benefits and risks of starting treatment early versus later in the progression of HIV disease (see Table 12-1).

Critical Factors for Successful HIV/AIDS Treatment

Provider's Level of Experience

An HIV specialist should supervise treatment. Patients who have an experienced provider to manage their care live longer and are healthier than those who do not have an experienced provider (Paterson et al., 2000).

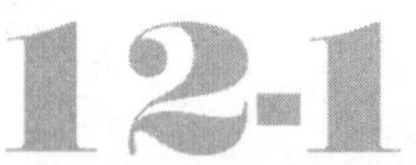

Benefits and Risks of Early and Deferred Antiretroviral Therapy (OARAC, 2006)

	BENEFITS	RISKS
EARLY THERAPY	■ More likely to achieve and maintain control of HIV reproduction ■ Delays or prevents immune system compromise ■ Lowers risk of drug resistance if HIV reproduction is completely suppressed ■ Decreased risk of HIV transmission	■ Drug-related reduction in quality of life because of antiretroviral therapy side effects ■ More drug-related side effects and health problems ■ Earlier development of drug resistance if complete HIV suppression is not achieved ■ Fewer drugs to use in future, if HIV develops resistance to drugs that are used early on
DEFERRED THERAPY	■ Avoids negative effects of therapy on quality of life ■ Avoids drug-related adverse events ■ Delays development of drug resistance ■ Preserves maximum number of future drug options for when HIV disease risk is highest	■ Irreversible immune system depletion ■ Greater difficulty in suppressing viral replication ■ Increased risk of HIV transmission

Patient's Level of Adherence

It is critically important that patients take all of the right pills at the right times (Kalichman & Rompa, 2003). When people do not take the correct medicines in the correct doses, at the correct times, the levels of the drugs in their bodies drop, allowing HIV to multiply (OARAC, 2006). The more HIV multiplies, the more likely it is to mutate into a form that the drugs are not designed to combat. When this happens, HIV is said to be *resistant* to a drug. Because there is a limited number of anti-HIV drugs—some of which many people cannot take because of their side effects—people quickly run out of drugs that work against their HIV disease.

Why Adherence to Antiretroviral Therapy May Be Difficult

Although antiretroviral therapy may prolong HIV+ people's lives, many people have difficulty taking the right doses of the right medicines at the right times, for several reasons. First, antiretroviral therapy is expensive, so many people cannot afford it. In addition, antiretroviral therapy requires taking at least three drugs. Remembering to take the right drugs in the right doses at the right times is difficult for many people—especially for people suffering from AIDS-related dementia, for people with drug or alcohol problems, or for people with mental illness. Antiretroviral therapy is time-consuming. Having the time and the place to take the drugs is difficult for some people. Finally, HAART has many negative side effects, which make taking the drugs unpleasant. These side effects include fatigue, nausea, vomiting, abdominal pain, diarrhea, muscle pain, wasting (loss of strength and weight), liver problems, diabetes, abnormal fat distribution, high cholesterol, skin rashes, inflammation of the pancreas, nerve problems, and increased bleeding (in patients with hemophilia).

HIV+ people first develop mild symptoms of opportunistic infections 7–8 years (on average) after exposure to HIV.

TREATING HIV DISEASE-RELATED COMPLICATIONS

Almost inevitably, with the passage of time, HIV+ individuals will develop the symptoms of full-blown AIDS.

Opportunistic Infections

As HIV damages the immune system, many different bacteria, viruses, fungi, and protozoa take this opportunity to invade and infect the body. People may be HIV+ for many years before they develop such opportunistic infections. There are some opportunistic infections, such as herpes and yeast infections, which people without HIV commonly get, and some opportunistic infections, such as Kaposi's sarcoma, that people rarely get unless they have HIV or another immune-suppressing condition. There are 26 HIV-related opportunistic infections that are considered AIDS-defining opportunistic infections. If a person has HIV antibodies in his or her blood, a CD4+ cell count of fewer than 200 per cubic millimeter of blood, and one of these 26 AIDS-defining opportunistic infections, he or she is said to have AIDS (Bartlett, 2004; NIAID, 2005).

Initial Symptoms of Opportunistic Infections

HIV+ people first develop mild symptoms of opportunistic infections 7–8 years (on average) after exposure to HIV. Their symptoms include:

- Swollen lymph nodes that persist for more than 3 months
- Fatigue
- Weight loss
- Frequent fevers and sweats
- Persistent or frequent yeast infections (oral, esophageal, or vaginal)
- Persistent skin rashes and flaky skin
- Pelvic inflammatory disease (PID) that does not respond to treatment
- Short-term memory loss
- Frequent or severe herpes infections with oral, genital, or anal sores
- Shingles (a painful flare-up of the chickenpox virus in the nervous system)

AIDS-Defining Opportunistic Infections

The following opportunistic infections, when accompanied by a positive HIV test and a low CD4+ cell count, indicate AIDS (refer to Part 1):

- Pneumocystis carinii pneumonia (PCP) (a kind of pneumonia)
- Kaposi's sarcoma (KS) (a kind of cancer)
- HIV wasting syndrome (extreme weight loss)
- Non-Hodgkin's lymphoma (a kind of cancer)
- HIV encephalopathy (AIDS dementia)
- Candidiasis (yeast infection) of the esophagus, trachea, bronchi, or lungs
- Cryptosporidiosis, chronic intestinal (a bacterial infection of the intestines)
- Cytomegalovirus disease (CMV)
- Tuberculosis (outside of the lungs)
- Herpes simplex virus infection
- Progressive multifocal leukoencephalopathy (PML) (a nervous system disorder)
- Primary lymphoma of the brain (a kind of cancer)
- Toxoplasmosis of the brain (a parasitic infection of the brain)
- Coccidioidomycosis (a fungal infection)
- Salmonella septicemia (a bacterial infection)
- Bacterial infections, recurrent
- Pulmonary tuberculosis
- Recurrent bacterial pneumonia (two or more episodes in 1 year)
- Invasive cervical cancer

The current definition of AIDS was created in 1993. It includes a list of opportunistic infections and cancers, known as diagnostic indicators. The definition also emphasizes the importance of the level of CD4+ cells in the blood (Bartlett, 2004).

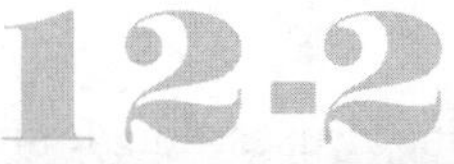

Some HIV-Related Symptoms and Opportunistic Infections and Treatments

SYMPTOM OR INFECTION	TREATMENTS
Weight Loss	- Eat more calories - Eat a balanced diet - Exercise moderately - Take appetite stimulants - Take nutritional supplements, like Ensure - Treat diarrhea and opportunistic infections of the stomach and intestines
Yeast Infections	- Use antifungal creams, suppositories, and lozenges - Use antifungal pills - For serious cases, administer Amphotericin B by IV
Herpes	- Shorten (but not cure) outbreaks with acyclovir or valacyclovir
Shingles	- Take anti-herpes drugs, as shingles is caused by a virus similar to the one that causes herpes - Use pain-relief therapies, including nerve-blockers and skin treatments
Pulmonary Tuberculosis	- If the disease is not active, take isoniazid for 6 months - If the disease is active, take a combination of antibiotics for 6 months

Treating HIV-Related Symptoms and Opportunistic Infections

Antiretroviral drugs delay the onset or weaken the symptoms of opportunistic infections because they preserve some immune system functioning. Some HIV-related symptoms and opportunistic infections, like those shown in Table 12-2, can be diagnosed and treated in medical settings with minimal resources, and sometimes even at home. Others require more advanced medical technology for diagnosis and treatment, and therefore are rarely diagnosed or treated in resource-poor countries. These include such infections as toxoplasmosis, Mycobacterium avium complex disease (MAC), and Cytomegalovirus infection (CMV).

It is important for HIV+ people to keep their immune systems as strong as possible by eating nutritionally sound foods, making sure that food and water are clean and safe, getting vaccines for common opportunistic infections, and having acute illnesses diagnosed and treated as soon as possible.

REFERENCES

Bartlett, J. G. (2004). Acquired immunodeficiency syndrome. *Microsoft Encarta online encyclopedia*. Retrieved February 6, 2004, from http://encarta.msn.com/Acquired_Immunodeficiency_Syndrome.html

Department of Health and Human Services (DHHS). (2005, May). *Approved medications to treat HIV infection*. Washington, DC: DHHS.

Dybul, M., Fauci, A. S., Bartlett, J. G., Kaplan, J. E., & Pau, A. K. (2002). Guidelines for using antiretroviral agents among HIV-infected adults and adolescents. *Annals of Internal Medicine, 137*(5 Pt 2), 381–433.

Hare, C. B. (2004). Clinical overview of HIV disease. In L. Pieperl, S. Coffey, O. Bacon, & P. Volberding (Eds.), *HIV InSite knowledge base*. San Francisco: Center for HIV Information, University of California, San Francisco.

Kalichman, S. C., & Rompa, D. (2003). HIV treatment adherence and unprotected sex practices in people receiving antiretroviral therapy. *Sexually Transmitted Infections, 79*, 59–61.

Kanabus, A., & Fredricksson, J. (n.d.). *The history of AIDS 1987–1992*. Horsham,West Sussex, UK: AVERT.org. Retrieved February 4, 2004, from http://www.avert.org/his87_92.htm

Mellors, J. W., Munoz, A., Giorgi, J. V., Margolick, J. B., Tassoni, C. J., Gupta, P., et al. (1997). Plasma viral load and CD4+ lymphocytes as prognostic markers of HIV-1 infection. *Annals of Internal Medicine, 126*(12), 946–954.

National Institute of Allergy and Infectious Diseases (NIAID). (2005, March). *HIV infection and AIDS: An overview*. Bethesda, MD: NIAID.

Office of AIDS Research Advisory Council (OARAC). (2006, May 6). *Guidelines for the use of antiretroviral agents in HIV-1-infected adults and adolescents*. Department of Health and Human Services (DHHS) Panel on Antiretroviral Guidelines for Adults and Adolescents. Washington, DC: DHHS.

Omobosola, A., & Henry, K. (2003). Current trends in the treatment of HIV infection, 2003. *Minnesota Medicine, 86*(6), 39–44.

Palella, F. J. Jr., Delaney, K. M., Moorman, A. C., Loveless, M. O., Fuhrer, J., Satten, G. A., et al. (1998). Declining morbidity and mortality among patients with advanced human immunodeficiency virus infection. HIV Outpatient Study Investigators. *New England Journal of Medicine, 338*(13), 853–860.

Paterson, D. L., Swindells, S., Mohr, J., Brester, J., Vergis, E. M., Squier, C., et al. (2000). Adherence to protease inhibitor therapy and outcomes in patients with HIV infection. *Annals of Internal Medicine, 133*, 21–30.

Riddler, S. A., & Mellors, J. W. (1998). Clinical applications of viral load testing. In L. Pieperl, S. Coffey, O. Bacon, & P. Volberding (Eds.), *HIV InSite knowledge base*. San Francisco: Center for HIV Information, University of California, San Francisco.

Instructor Resources

LEARNING ACTIVITIES

ACTIVITY 1:

Assignment and Group Activity: Increasing Adherence to Antiretroviral Therapy

Objective: To understand the issues with antiretroviral therapy adherence.

Although adherence to antiretroviral therapy can prolong the lives of HIV+ people, many people have difficulty taking the right combinations of medications, in the right doses, and at the right times. A number of strategies have been developed to help increase adherence to prescribed therapy regimens, including:

- Special pill organizers
- Brief provider-delivered psychosocial and educational interventions that address patient knowledge, attitudes, skills, and behaviors related to adherence
- *Directly observed therapy (DOT)*, in which providers, outreach workers, or peers deliver every medication dose and watch the patient ingest it
- Electronic dosing reminder systems, such as pagers

Pick a particular HIV+ population (such as HIV+ middle-class men-who-have-sex-with-men, migrant workers, or injection drug users in inner city settings), and write a two- to three-page summary of the potential pros and cons of using each of these strategies to increase antiretroviral adherence among that group.

Option: Once the summaries have been prepared, have a 20-minute group discussion about the pros and cons of the various strategies among diverse populations.

ACTIVITY 2:

Assignment: Approval of an Antiretroviral Drug

Objective: To understand the process behind drug testing and approval.

Pick an antiretroviral drug that has been approved for use in the United States (see http://www.fda.gov/oashi/aids/virals.html for a current list). Investigate the history and current uses of that drug, including:

- The development, testing, and approval process for the drug
- The drug's benefits and drawbacks, including side effects and costs

- How the drug is currently being used in the United States and abroad
- Prepare a visual drug history timeline and a one- to two-page written summary of your findings.

ACTIVITY 3:

Assignment: Opportunistic Infections

Objective: To understand the incidence and impact of opportunistic infections.

Pick an HIV+ group in a specific country or region of the world. Examples:

- Injection drug users in Eastern Europe
- Women in South Africa
- Men who have sex with men in the United States

Investigate the three most common opportunistic infections among that population. What are the key challenges in preventing and treating those infections? What strategies can best address those challenges? Prepare a three- to five-page summary of your findings.

DISCUSSION QUESTIONS

1. The development of antiretroviral therapies has transformed HIV/AIDS from a disease which led to imminent death to one that can be lived with for many years. How has this transformation changed the entire face of HIV? What are the implications of living with HIV from a biological, sexual, psychological, and social standpoint?

QUIZ

1. Match the antiretroviral drug class with a brief description of how it works.

a) NRTIs	1) Prevents protease from cleaving HIV proteins into mature viral particles.
b) NNRTIs	2) Disables reverse transcriptase.
c) PIs	3) Makes HIV spike unable to fuse with the host cell.
d) Fusion inhibitors	4) Results in incomplete DNA that cannot create new copies of the virus.
e) Integrase inhibitors	5) Keeps HIV from binding with the host cell membrane.
f) HIV coreceptor blockers	6) Keeps HIV's DNA from being spliced into the host cell DNA.

2. True or False: There is no danger in occasionally missing a dosage of HIV medication.
3. True or False: There is a danger in taking drugs to which a strain of HIV is already resistant.
4. List any three reasons why adherence to antiretroviral therapy may be difficult.

5. HIV+ people first develop mild symptoms of opportunistic infections ___ years on average after exposure to HIV.
   a) 2–3
   b) 5–6
   c) 7–8
   d) 10 or more

6. List any three ways, in addition to taking HIV medications, that HIV+ people can keep their immune systems strong.

ANSWERS

1. **A–4; B–2; C–1; D–3; E–6; F–5.** Nucleoside Reverse Transcriptase Inhibitors (NRTIs) are faulty versions of reverse transcriptase. When HIV attempts to turn its RNA into DNA, NRTIs take the place of real reverse transcriptase, which results in incomplete DNA that cannot create new copies of the virus. Non-Nucleoside Reverse Transcriptase Inhibitors (NNRTIs) also interfere with reverse transcriptase. Instead of replacing reverse transcriptase with a faulty fake, NNRTIs chemically bind to reverse transcriptase and make it unable to do its job. Protease inhibitors (PIs) chemically bind to protease, so that it cannot cleave the HIV proteins into mature viral particles. Fusion inhibitors work by attaching themselves to one of the proteins on HIV's spikes, which makes the HIV spike unable to fuse with the host cell. Integrase inhibitors keep HIV's newly formed DNA from being spliced into the host cell's DNA. HIV coreceptor blockers keep HIV from binding with the host cell membrane.

2. **False.** When people do not take the correct medicines in the correct doses, at the correct times, the levels of the drugs in their bodies drop, allowing HIV to multiply. The more HIV multiplies, the more likely it is to mutate into a form that the drugs are not designed to combat. When this happens, HIV is said to be *resistant* to a drug. Because there is a limited number of anti-HIV drugs—some of which many people cannot take because of their side effects—people quickly run out of drugs that work against their HIV disease.

3. **True.** Continuing to take drugs to which a strain of HIV is already resistant actually increases the speed with which the drug-resistant strain multiplies.

4. Antiretroviral therapy is expensive; it is difficult to remember to take the right doses at the right times; it is time-consuming; and it has many negative side effects.

5. **C.** HIV+ people first develop mild symptoms of opportunistic infections 7–8 years (on average) after exposure to HIV.

6. HIV+ individuals can keep their immune systems as strong as possible by eating nutritionally sound foods, making sure that food and water are clean and safe, getting vaccines for common opportunistic infections, and having acute illnesses diagnosed and treated as soon as possible.

WEB RESOURCES

Antiretroviral Therapy

Avert: Introduction to HIV/AIDS Treatment

http://www.avert.org/introtrt.htm

Provides an overview of antiretroviral treatments and links to more detailed information.

U.S. Food and Drug Administration (FDA): Drugs Used in the Treatment of HIV Infection

http://www.fda.gov/oashi/aids/virals.html

Presents an up-to-date listing of FDA-approved drugs for treating HIV/AIDS.

HIV InSite: Fact Sheets: Antiretrovirals and Immune-Based Therapies

http://hivinsite.ucsf.edu/InSite?page=md-rr-20

Provides links to patient-oriented clinical fact sheets on HIV/AIDS therapies (in English, French, and Spanish, targeting various reading levels) that are produced by numerous agencies.

HIV InSite: Adherence to HIV Antiretroviral Therapy: Related Resources

http://hivinsite.ucsf.edu/InSite?page=kbr-03–02–09

Provides links to HIV InSite Web pages on various antiretroviral therapy topics, as well as links to relevant journal articles, reports, guidelines, newsletters, clinical support tools, and patient and community education materials.

HIV InSite: U.S. Treatment Guidelines

http://hivinsite.ucsf.edu/InSite?page=md-01–01

Offers links to treatment guidelines for various HIV-infected populations, including:

- DHHS Panel on Antiretroviral Guidelines for Adults and Adolescents: Guidelines for the Use of Antiretroviral Agents in HIV-1-Infected Adults and Adolescents (October 10, 2006)
- http://www.aidsinfo.nih.gov/ContentFiles/AdultandAdolescentGL.pdf
- Public Health Service Task Force: Recommendations for Use of Antiretroviral Drugs in Pregnant HIV-1-Infected Women for Maternal Health and Interventions to Reduce Perinatal HIV-1 Transmission in the United States (October 12, 2006)
- http://www.aidsinfo.nih.gov/ContentFiles/PerinatalGL.pdf
- National Pediatric and Family HIV Resource Center, Health Resources and Services Administration, and National Institutes of Health: Guidelines for the Use of Antiretroviral Agents in Pediatric HIV Infection (October 26, 2006)
- http://www.aidsinfo.nih.gov/contentfiles/PediatricGuidelines.pdf

Opportunistic Infections

Avert: HIV-Related Opportunistic Infection: Prevention and Treatment

http://www.avert.org/aidscare.htm

Discusses the prevention and treatment of opportunistic inf0ctions.

The Body: Opportunistic Infections

http://www.thebody.com/nmai/oi.html

Discusses the identification, prevention, and treatment of opportunistic infections.

AIDSInfo: Treatment of Opportunistic Infections Guidelines

http://www.aidsinfo.nih.gov/Guidelines/GuidelineDetail.aspx?MenuItem=Guidelines&Search=Off&GuidelineID=14&ClassID=4

Offers links to opportunistic infections treatment guidelines, including:

- Recommendations from CDC, the National Institutes of Health, and the HIV Medicine Association/Infectious Diseases Society of America: Treating Opportunistic Infections Among HIV-Infected Adults and Adolescents (December 17, 2004)
  http://www.aidsinfo.nih.gov/ContentFiles/TreatmentofOI_AA.pdf
- Recommendations from CDC, the National Institutes of Health, and Infectious Diseases Society of America: Treating Opportunistic Infections Among HIV-Exposed and Infected Children (December 3, 2004)
  http://www.aidsinfo.nih.gov/ContentFiles/TreatmentofOI_Children.pdf

HIV InSite: Fact Sheets: Complications (Opportunistic Infections and Malignancies, Symptoms, and Side Effects)

http://hivinsite.ucsf.edu/InSite?page=md-rr-21

Provides links to patient-oriented clinical fact sheets on HIV/AIDS complications (in English, French, and Spanish, targeting various reading levels) that are produced by numerous agencies.

RECOMMENDED READING

Overview of Medication Adherence Issues and Strategies

Medication Adherence in HIV/AIDS (Laurence, 2004)

Laurence, J. (Ed.). (2004). Medication adherence in HIV/AIDS. *Larchmont, NY: Mary Ann Liebert.*

Addresses the barriers to medication adherence among diverse populations (including adolescents, ethnic and racial minorities, pregnant women, and drug users), as well as proposed strategies for addressing these challenges. The book is written for clinicians as well as other health and social service professionals.

Techniques for Improving Antiretroviral Therapy Adherence

Antiretroviral Adherence Interventions: A Review of Current Literature and Ongoing Studies (Simoni et al., 2003)

Simoni, J. M., Frick, P. A., Pantalone, D. W., & Turner, B. J. (2003). Antiretroviral adherence interventions: A review of current literature and ongoing studies. Topics in HIV Medicine, 11*(6), 185–198.*

Provides a review and meta-analysis of antiretroviral therapy intervention adherence studies.

Efficacy of Interventions in Improving Highly Active Antiretroviral Therapy Adherence and HIV-1 RNA Viral Load (Simoni et al., 2006)

Simoni, J. M., Pearson, C. R., Pantalone, D. W., Marks, G., & Crepaz, N. (2006). Efficacy of interventions in improving highly active antiretroviral therapy adherence and HIV-1 RNA viral load. Journal of Acquired Immune Deficiency Syndromes, 43*(Suppl 1), S23–S35.*

Provides an updated review and meta-analysis of antiretroviral therapy intervention adherence studies.

Antiretroviral Therapy in the Developing World

Scaling Up Treatment for the Global AIDS Pandemic (Curran et al., 2004)

Curran, H. D., Arya, M., Kelley, P., Knobler, S., & Pray, L. (Eds.). (2004). Scaling up treatment for the global AIDS pandemic. *Washington, DC: National Academies Press.*

Reviews and assesses rapid scale-up antiretroviral therapy programs worldwide, identifies the components of effective antiretroviral implementation programs, and offers recommendations concerning implementation of antiretroviral programs in resource-poor settings.

Management of HIV

Management of the HIV-Infected Patient (Crowe, Hoy, & Mills, 2002)

Crowe, S., Hoy, J., & Mills, J. (2002). Management of the HIV-infected patient *(2nd ed.). London: Martin Dunitz.*

Addresses the clinical presentation, diagnosis, and management of the various manifestations of HIV infection, including medical, psychological, and social dimensions.

POWERPOINT SLIDES

(Note: A full-color version of these slides, with graphics, is also available on the CD-ROM.)

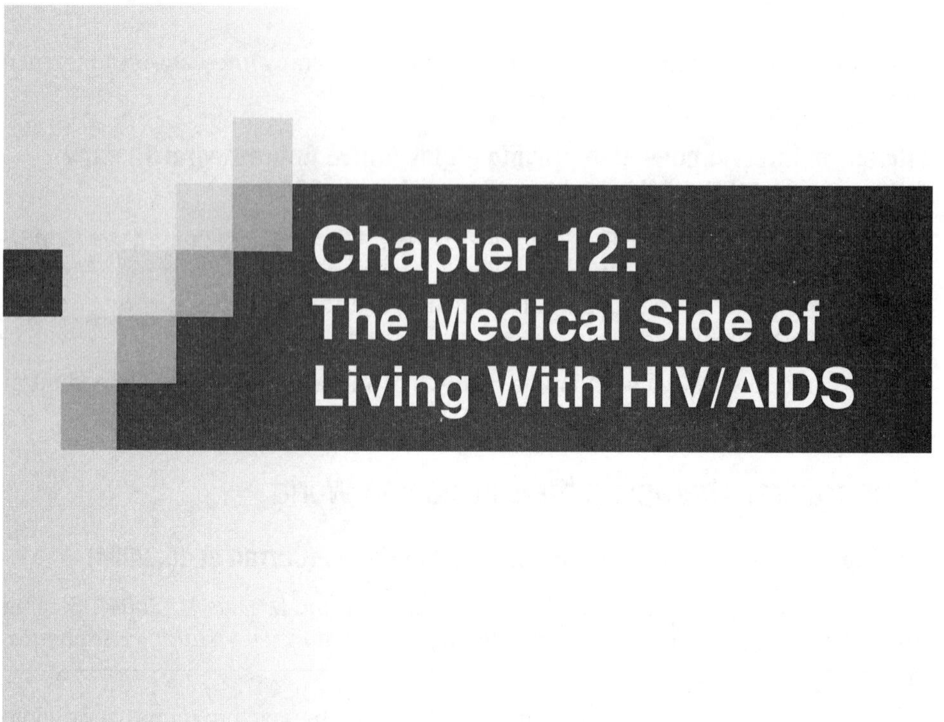

The Medical Side of Living With HIV/AIDS

- HIV+ people are living longer, healthier lives, in large part because of advances in anti-HIV drug therapies.
- Despite these therapies, people living with HIV/AIDS face many medical, psychological, and social challenges.

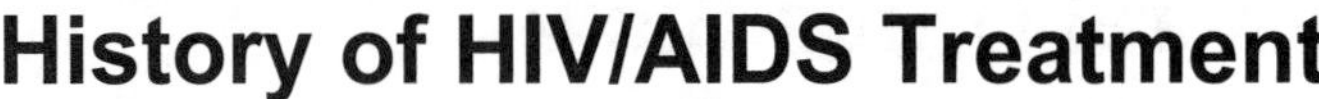

History of HIV/AIDS Treatment

- In the early years of the epidemic, an AIDS diagnosis meant a rapid decline in health and imminent death.
- In 1987, the first antiretroviral drug, AZT, slowed the progress of HIV.
- In 1996, scientists created tests that measured viral load in plasma of HIV+ people, enabling measurement of disease progression.
- In the late 1990s it was believed that high doses of HAART right after HIV was diagnosed would be most effective at slowing disease progression.

History of HIV/AIDS Treatment (continued)

- Now physicians wait until the more advanced stages of HIV disease to prescribe HAART as HAART is accompanied by many negative side effects.
- Many ways to treat the opportunistic infections that often accompany HIV/AIDS have been developed.
- The federal Department of Health and Human Services and the Henry J. Kaiser Family Foundation developed and regularly update guidelines for the management of HIV infection in adults and adolescents.

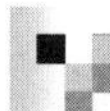

Antiretroviral Drugs Slow HIV Replication

- Antiretroviral drugs work by keeping HIV from multiplying.
- There are **four** kinds of antiretroviral drugs:

Nucleoside Reverse Transcriptase Inhibitors (NRTIs)

- HIV uses a reverse transcriptase to convert RNA to DNA in order to reproduce itself.
- NRTIs are *faulty* versions of reverse transcriptase that prevent DNA from creating new viruses.

Non-Nucleoside Reverse Transcriptase Inhibitors (NNRTIs)

- NNRTIs also interfere with reverse transcriptase.
- NNRTIs chemically bind to reverse transcriptase and make it unable to do its job.

Antiretroviral Drugs Slow HIV Replication (continued)

Protease Inhibitors (PIs)

- After HIV hijacks a cell's nucleus to make copies of itself, it needs an enzyme called protease to chop its long chains of proteins into infectious bits.
- Protease inhibitors chemically bind to protease so that it cannot cleave the HIV proteins into mature viral particles.

Fusion Inhibitors

- To make copies of itself, HIV first uses its spikes to fuse with the host cell's membrane, and then thrusts its contents inside.
- Fusion inhibitors work by attaching themselves to one of the proteins on HIV spikes, which makes the HIV spike unable to fuse with the host cell.

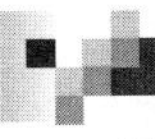

New Antiretroviral Medications

New antiretroviral medications that are currently being developed could include the following improvements:

- Drugs that are easier for the body to absorb and circulate
- Drugs that last longer in the body
- Drugs with fewer negative side effects
- Drugs that interfere with different stages of HIV replication, such as
    - integrase inhibitors (which would keep HIV's newly formed DNA from incorporating itself in the host cell's DNA), and
    - HIV coreceptor blockers (which would keep HIV from binding with the host cell membrane).

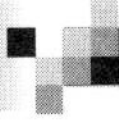

Goals of Antiretroviral Therapy

- Antiretroviral therapy (sometimes called Highly Active Antiretroviral Therapy, or HAART) typically combines three or more antiretroviral drugs that work together to keep HIV from multiplying.

- The goals of antiretroviral therapy are:
    - Reduce a person's viral load as much as possible, for as long as possible
    - Restore the number of CD4+ cells to within the normal range
    - Strengthen the immune system so that it responds to pathogens
    - Halt disease progression
    - Prevent or reduce resistant variants of HIV
    - Conserve the number of non-HIV-resistant drugs available to the patient in the future
    - Minimize side effects
    - Maximize patient adherence (that is, make sure the patient takes all the right drugs in the right amounts at the right times)

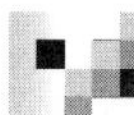

Initiating Antiretroviral Therapy

- Some people choose to put off therapy for as long as safely possible.
- Others decide to begin therapy earlier.
- Both strategies have merit, and both are supported by research.
- The decision to initiate therapy should be made by patient and physician, taking into account the patient's
  - willingness and readiness to begin therapy;
  - risk of progression to AIDS (as measured by the patient's viral load and CD4+ cell count);
  - level of immunodeficiency (as measured by the patient's CD4+ cell count);
  - assessment risks versus benefits of initiating therapy; and
  - likelihood of adhering to the medication regimen.

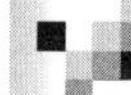

Critical Factors for Successful HIV/AIDS Treatment

- ***Provider's level of experience***
  - An HIV specialist should supervise treatment.
  - Patients with an experienced provider live longer and are healthier than those who do not.

- ***Patient's level of adherence***
  - Patients must take all of the right pills at the right times, or levels of the drugs in their bodies drops, allowing the HIV to multiply.
  - The more the HIV multiply, the more likely they are to mutate into a drug-resistant form of the disease.
  - Since there are only about 20 anti-HIV drugs—some of which many people cannot take because of their side effects—people quickly run out of drugs that work against their HIV disease.

Adherence to Antiretroviral Treatment May Be Difficult

- Many people have difficulty taking the medications, because:
  - they cannot afford it;
  - remembering to take the right drugs in the right doses at the right times is difficult; and
  - having the time and the place to take the drugs is difficult for some people.
- HAART has many negative side effects, including:
  - Fatigue
  - Diabetes
  - Nausea
  - High cholesterol
  - Wasting
  - Abdominal pain
  - Diarrhea
  - Skin rashes
  - Vomiting

Opportunistic Infections

- As HIV damages the immune system, many different bacteria, viruses, fungi, and protozoa invade and infect the body.
- HIV+ people first develop mild symptoms of opportunistic infections 7-8 years (on average) after exposure to HIV. Symptoms include:
  - Swollen lymph nodes that persist for more than 3 months
  - Fatigue
  - Weight loss
  - Frequent fevers and sweats
  - Persistent or frequent yeast infections
  - Persistent skin rashes and flaky skin
  - Pelvic inflammatory disease that does not respond to treatment
  - Short-term memory loss
  - Frequent or severe herpes infections
  - Shingles

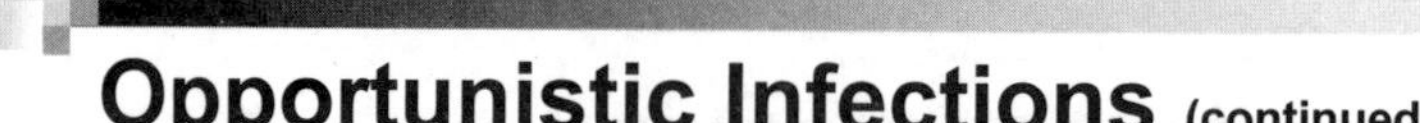

Opportunistic Infections (continued)

The opportunistic infections that, accompanied by a positive HIV test, indicate AIDS include the following:

- Pneumocystis Carinii Pneumonia (PCP) (a kind of pneumonia)
- Kaposi's sarcoma (KS) (a kind of cancer)
- HIV wasting syndrome (extreme weight loss)
- Non-Hodgkin's lymphoma (a kind of cancer)
- HIV encephalopathy (AIDS dementia)
- Candidiasis (yeast infection) of the esophagus, trachea, bronchi, or lungs
- Cryptosporidiosis, chronic intestinal (a bacterial infection of the intestines)
- Cytomegalovirus disease (CMV) (a kind of eye infection)
- Tuberculosis (outside of the lungs)

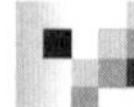

Opportunistic Infections (continued)

The opportunistic infections that, accompanied by a positive HIV test, indicate AIDS include the following:

- Herpes simplex virus infection
- Progressive Multifocal Leukoencephalopathy (PML) (a nervous system disorder)
- Primary lymphoma of the brain (a kind of cancer)
- Toxoplasmosis (a parasitic infection of the brain)
- Coccidioidomycosis (a fungal infection)
- Salmonella septicemia (a bacterial infection)
- Bacterial infections, recurrent
- Pulmonary tuberculosis
- Recurrent bacterial pneumonia (two or more episodes in 1 year)
- Invasive cervical cancer

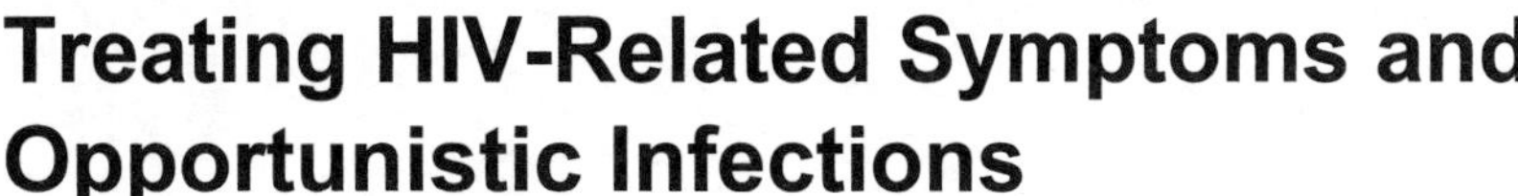

Treating HIV-Related Symptoms and Opportunistic Infections

Symptom or Infection	Treatments
Weight loss	■ eat more calories (take appetite stimulants) ■ eat a balanced diet and/or nutritional supplements ■ exercise moderately ■ treat diarrhea and opportunistic infections of the stomach and intestines
Yeast infections	■ use antifungal creams, suppositories, and lozenges ■ use antifungal pills
Herpes	■ shorten outbreaks with antiviral medications
Shingles	■ take anti-herpes drugs ■ use pain-relief therapies, including nerve-blockers and skin treatments
Pulmonary Tuberculosis	■ if the disease is not active, take isoniazid for 6 months ■ if the disease is active, then take a combination of antibiotics for 6 months

Learning Objectives

- Define and describe the psychological challenges of living with HIV/AIDS
- Define and describe the social supports that can help people living with HIV/AIDS
- Understand the medical, personal, and social uncertainties that can arise while living with HIV/AIDS
- Discuss the sources HIV/AIDS-related grief, stigma, and discrimination

Key Terms

chronic somatic preoccupation
HIV-associated dementia
minor cognitive-motor disorder
prognosis
stigma

13

Psychological and Social Challenges of Living With HIV/AIDS

People living with HIV/AIDS face unique psychological and social challenges. Chapter 13 first describes the psychological difficulties that arise from HIV disease itself, from anti-HIV treatment, from HIV/AIDS-related stress and uncertainty, and from grieving the loss of HIV+ loved ones. Chapter 13 then discusses the stigma and discrimination faced by people living with HIV/AIDS.

PSYCHOLOGICAL ISSUES IN HIV/AIDS

HIV/AIDS does not just affect the body. It also affects a person's psychological and emotional well-being.

HIV/AIDS-Related Psychological Disorders

HIV and opportunistic diseases of the brain and nervous system can alter people's brain and nervous system, causing psychological disorders (Horwath, 2003). Psychological disorders associated with HIV include *HIV-associated dementia* (HAD), which includes symptoms such as forgetfulness, apathy, difficulty concentrating, speech problems, tremors, and delusions; *minor cognitive-motor disorder* (MCMD), which includes mild impairments in memory, movement, and concentration; mood disorders, such as depression; anxiety disorders; and brain tumors.

Psychological Side Effects of Anti-HIV Drugs

Some HIV treatments also have psychological side effects. These can range from moodiness and aggressive behavior to severe depression, suicidal thoughts, paranoia, delusions, and hallucinations.

HIV/AIDS-Related Psychological Distress

Additionally, people living with HIV/AIDS may suffer psychological distress as a result of the many physical, social, and economic effects of the disease on their lives. Among the various stressors are chronic physical pain, physical disfigurement, the possibility of infecting other people, and discrimination, abuse, and loss of fundamental human rights. Other challenges include changes in lifestyle to accommodate the illness itself and the financial burdens that treatment brings for oneself and one's family. HIV+ persons often also face loss of independence; physical, social, and emotional isolation; uncertainty concerning the timing and nature of treatment and disease progression; and uncertainty in their personal and social lives. Additionally, many HIV positives are simultaneously coping with grief from already having lost loved ones to AIDS (Cline, 1990; De Gagne, 1994). As a result of these many stressors, people diagnosed with HIV infection often suffer from a number of psychological symptoms, including anger, frustration, anxiety, depression, and *chronic somatic preoccupation* (i.e., a fixation on physical symptoms) (Kelly et al., 1993b).

Psychological Benefits and Challenges of HIV/AIDS Therapy

The advent of highly active antiretroviral therapies (HAART) for treating HIV infection was a major breakthrough in managing the HIV/AIDS crisis. These combinations of drugs target different stages of the HIV replication cycle, slow HIV disease progression, and prolong life. Using HAART, many HIV+ people who have been diagnosed with AIDS become healthy enough to return to work or school. Returning to work or school is often considered the benchmark of successful HIV treatment (Brooks & Klosinski, 1999).

HAART also may give hope and optimism to HIV+ people. Researchers have found that having hope and an optimistic outlook, in turn, improves people's physical health, decreases their levels of depression, and even extends their life spans (Low-Beer et al., 2000; Taylor, Kemeny, Reed, Bower, & Gruenewald, 2000). Despite these benefits, however, antiretroviral therapy can present significant psychological challenges to both those who respond well to the treatment and those who do not (Brashers et al., 1999).

Challenges for People Who Respond Well to Treatment

Those who experience renewed health after being diagnosed with AIDS and treated with HAART must often recalibrate and renegotiate a number of aspects of their lives. These include:

- Feelings of hope and future orientation (e.g., "Will recovery last?")
- Social roles and identities (e.g., "How do I live as a person with a chronic illness?")
- Interpersonal relations (e.g., "Will people accept me if I try to reenter the workforce?")
- Quality of life (e.g., "What activities do I have to give up to stay healthy?")

Challenges for People Who Do Not Respond Well to Treatment

Although antiretroviral therapy makes many HIV+ people healthier, between 15% and 35% of research participants in antiviral therapy studies do not improve with antiretroviral therapy, and even more people who are not research participants do not respond well to the treatment (Kelly & Kalichman, 2002). In addition, some people's health may initially improve with therapy, but then quickly deteriorate (Stone & Smith, 2004).

People whose treatments fail may feel a sense of personal injustice, like they were cheated, betrayed, or misled about the effects of antiretroviral therapy. They also may engage in self-blame for not having been able to tolerate a potentially effective treatment, especially when they had to discontinue therapy because of severe side effects. A sense of hopelessness and an unwillingness to try new therapies are also common (Rabkin & Ferrando, 1997).

Meeting HIV+ People's Needs Helps Everyone

There is a clear need for services that will improve the psychological health of people with HIV/AIDS (Demmer, 2001). Improved psychological services for HIV+ people not only help them but also may help the general public (Kelly et al., 1993a). High levels of depression and maladaptive coping with HIV infection have been associated with substance use and risky sexual activities, which put others at risk for acquiring HIV (Kelly et al., 1993b).

Support Groups

The stress of HIV/AIDS can be buffered by the social support provided by support groups (Green & Smith, 2004; Kalichman, Sikkema, & Somlai, 1996). For example, in a study of HIV+ men who were experiencing moderate depression, 86% of participants who attended a social-support group showed improved mental health, whereas about 67% of the participants who did not attend the social-support group showed worsened mental health (Kelly et al., 1993a). Support groups that target specific sources of emotional distress, improve the number and quality of friendships, and give health information are especially beneficial (Kalichman et al., 1996).

Coping and Stress Management Programs

Coping and stress management programs that are based on cognitive and behavioral theories and delivered to small groups can positively affect the mental health of people living with HIV/AIDS (Kelly & Kalichman, 2002). These interventions first teach people how to tell the difference between stressors that they can control or change and stressors that they cannot control or change. In response to the controllable stressors, these interventions then teach people how to address their problems in constructive and efficient ways. In response to the uncontrollable stressors, these programs teach people how to view their situations more positively and to deal with their negative emotions (Chesney, Chambers, Taylor, Johnson, & Folkman, 2003). Some of these interventions also teach people how to relax and avoid anxiety (Eller, 1999).

LIVING WITH THE UNCERTAINTY OF HIV/AIDS

Because of the success of antiretroviral therapies in the United States, HIV/AIDS is increasingly treated as a long-term, chronic illness. People who live with chronic illnesses such as HIV/AIDS often face uncertainty in the medical, personal, and social aspects of their lives (Brashers, Neidig, Reynolds, & Haas, 1998). Such uncertainty is stressful and can impair HIV+ people's quality of life (Brashers et al., 1998; McCain & Cella, 1995; Regan-Kubinski & Sharts-Hopko, 1995; Weitz, 1989). To maintain a good quality of life, people living with HIV/AIDS must learn to cope with this unpredictability and uncertainty (Murdaugh, 1998).

Medical Uncertainties

Medical uncertainties include uncertainties about diagnosis, symptom patterns, treatments and care, and disease progression and *prognosis* (i.e., the probable future course and outcome of a person's disease) (Brashers et al., 2003).

Changing or Unclear Diagnoses

CD4+ counts rise and fall, so that people diagnosed with AIDS in the past, based on their low CD4+ counts, can recover and have CD4+ counts that do not meet the CDC's diagnostic criteria for AIDS. This can be confusing for HIV+ people, both psychologically ("Do I still have AIDS?") and financially ("Do I still qualify for disability benefits?"). In addition, the various numbers used to monitor HIV+ people's health, including CD4+ counts and viral load, can be difficult to interpret.

Ambiguous Symptoms

All people get aches and pains. HIV+ people face the uncertainty of not knowing whether these aches and pains mean that their illness is worsening. In addition, HIV+ people have many different symptoms that change often, making it difficult for them to plan for the future. HIV+ people are also likely to get opportunistic infections that take advantage of their weakened immune systems. However, they do not know which of the many infections they will eventually get, and often worry about the symptoms and consequences of the different infections.

Complex and Uncertain Treatment

Antiretroviral therapy usually requires taking three or more drugs at different times of the day according to different rules (for example, take with food vs. take on an empty stomach). These therapies also often change, so HIV+ people may worry about taking their drugs correctly. In addition, many medical treatments are experimental, and so people using them do not know their safety or effectiveness. People's bodies also vary in their responses to different therapies. It is therefore impossible to predict whether different therapies will work or what their side effects will be.

For HIV+ people, it is difficult to know which preventative measures to take against opportunistic infections and when to take them. However, they must always be vigilant about food and water safety and about being exposed to other viruses.

Unpredictable Disease Progression or Prognosis

Some HIV+ people's health quickly declines, whereas other HIV+ people's health stays stable for many years. New drugs sometimes return seriously ill people to good health, so that they have to return to planning for the future, rather than preparing for their own death.

Personal Uncertainties

Personal uncertainties include uncertainties about one's personal identities, as well as about one's financial challenges and future (Brashers et al., 2003). During the asymptomatic stage of HIV disease, people feel well but know that they are HIV-infected. This can cause them to feel tension between their roles as a sick person versus a healthy person. In addition, HIV+ people are often married to, friends with, or related to other HIV+ people, so that they often become caregivers. At the same time, these people also need care. This can cause tension between caregiver versus care-receiver roles.

Financial uncertainties are also a significant challenge for HIV+ people. Many face uncertainties about when to claim disability status. On the one hand, claiming disability means that insurance companies or social security organizations will help pay for treatment. On the other hand, however, claiming disability limits employment options. Additionally, HIV treatments are expensive. HIV+ people often feel that they are trading off their own and their family's financial well-being for their health. Finally, because of the wide variability in the course of HIV, HIV+ people have difficulty knowing how much money to budget for their treatment and for how long.

Social Uncertainties

Social uncertainties include uncertainty about how other people will react to the news that one is HIV+, how old relationships will change, and how new relationships will develop (Brashers et al., 2003). In particular, HIV/AIDS is a stigmatized illness because it has been associated with homosexuality, drug use, and promiscuity. When people let others know that they are HIV+, they often do not know whether they will be accepted or rejected. In addition, HIV+ people face the prospect of social isolation, since families and loved ones may not react well to their illness. HIV+ people also face much uncertainty in dating and long-term relationships, especially because they run the risk of infecting others.

HIV/AIDS-RELATED GRIEF

Most people living with HIV/AIDS have lost a family member, friend, or associate to HIV disease (Sikkema et al., 2000). Coping with a loss as a result of HIV/AIDS may differ from coping with losses to other diseases in several ways (Sikkema, Kochman, DiFranceisco, Kelley, & Hoffman, 2003). First, many people who die from complications of HIV disease die at a relatively young age (Kain, 2004). Although survivors may have anticipated an HIV+ person's death, they still find it difficult to reconcile the fact that the life of a young person was cut short (Walker, 1991). In addition, the stigma associated with HIV may prevent those who survive from freely mourning or acknowledging the cause of a friend or loved one's death (Mallinson, 1997). Moreover, in the United States, HIV has been highly concentrated within specific populations, including gay men and injection drug users (CDC, 2001). People in these communities have lost many more friends and loved ones to HIV/AIDS than people in less affected communities, and have watched their social networks dwindle (Sikkema et al., 2003). "Survivor's guilt" may also prevent those who have lost loved ones from fully grieving and recovering (Kain, 2004). Particularly in the gay community, survivors may feel guilty about being HIV– in light of the suffering of their peers (Boykin, 1991; Schwartzberg, 1992).

The AIDS Memorial Quilt

During the 1985 annual march in memory of assassinated gay San Francisco Supervisor Harvey Milk and Mayor George Moscone, gay activist Cleve Jones asked marchers to write the names of loved ones who had died of AIDS on placards. These were later taped to the walls of the San Francisco Federal Building. To Jones, the wall of names looked like a quilt, inspiring him to later make the first quilt panel in honor of a friend who had died of AIDS. Jones later formed the NAMES Project Foundation with friends.

The quilt has been displayed in its entirety only five times—in 1987, 1988, 1989, 1992, and 1996—each time on the National Mall in Washington, DC. The last display of the entire quilt (October 1996) covered the entire expanse of the National Mall, from the Capitol to the Washington Monument. Portions of the quilt continue to be displayed around the country (NAMES Project Foundation, 2006b). (For summary statistics on the quilt as of June 2006, see Figure 13-1.) The quilt was nominated for a Nobel Peace Prize in 1989 and remains the largest community art project in the world.

"Founded in 1987, the AIDS Memorial Quilt is a poignant memorial, a powerful tool for use in preventing new HIV infections, and it's the largest ongoing community arts project in the world. . . . Virtually every one of the more than 40,000 colorful panels that make up the Quilt memorializes the life of a person lost to AIDS" (NAMES Project Foundation, 2006a).

- Number of visitors to the quilt: 15,200,000
- Number of panels in the quilt: approximately 46,000
- Number of names on the quilt: over 83,900
- Percent of all U.S. AIDS deaths represented by the names on the quilt: approximately 17.5%
- Miles of fabric: 52.25 miles, if all 3' x 6' panels were laid end-to-end
- Total weight: more than 54 tons

Figure 13-1 AIDS Memorial Quilt facts, as of June 2006 (NAMES Project Foundation, 2006c).

The NAMES Project Foundation also manages the AIDS Memorial Quilt Archive project, which preserves the "powerful images and stories contained within The Quilt while expanding our AIDS awareness and HIV prevention education efforts" by offering a searchable database of digitized photographs and accompanying documentary materials (such as letters and biographies) on all Quilt panels (NAMES Project Foundation, 1996d).

Hospice-Based Organizations

Hospice care comprises programs for people who are dying and their caregivers. A number of AIDS-related organizations focus on providing compassionate hospice care to AIDS patients and their loved ones. One hospice-based organization, Maitri (of San Francisco, California), is highlighted in Figure 13-2.

> "Responding to AIDS with blame or abuse towards people living with AIDS simply forces the epidemic underground, creating the ideal conditions for HIV to spread."
>
> —Peter Piot
> Plenary of the World Conference against Racism, Racial Discrimination, Xenophobia, and Related Intolerance, Durban, South Africa, September 5, 2001 (WHO, 2002)

HIV/AIDS-RELATED STIGMA AND DISCRIMINATION

Originally, the word *stigma* meant a visible mark, such as a brand or tattoo, which was used to disgrace, shame, condemn, or ostracize a person. Now, stigma is used to mean a quality or condition that reduces a person who has it from a valued, respected person to a tainted, discounted one. In some cultures, being female, or black, are considered stigmatizing. Many cultures, which do not understand the biological origins of mental illness, stigmatize the mentally ill.

HIV/AIDS is one of the most stigmatizing medical conditions in modern history (Kalichman, 2004). Many communities direct unfavorable attitudes, beliefs, and policies toward people who have or who are associated with HIV/AIDS, including their loved ones, family members, close associates, and social groups (Brimlow, Cook, & Seaton, 2003). Some communities are less prejudiced toward people with HIV/AIDS than others.

Erving Goffman was a sociologist who originally developed the idea of social stigma (Goffman, 1963). In his work, he identified six dimensions that influence

Maitri (pronounced "MY-tree") is a Sanskrit word that means "compassionate friendship." This San Francisco–based nonprofit organization (http://www.maitrisf.org) provides HIV+ residents and their loved ones with comprehensive support in a peaceful home-like environment. In addition to providing nursing and personal care, the staff draws on emotional and spiritual resources to help meet the special needs of their residents. Maitri focuses especially on those who might otherwise be without access to needed resources and care.

Maitri also provides both residents and those who love them with time and space to process their grief in the final days of a resident's life, as well as during the first few days after the resident's death. Parents, spouses, partners, siblings, and friends can use these days as a time for highly personalized goodbye rituals, prayers, meditation, and the like. A remembrance book stands on a small table in Maitri's entryway, its pages filled with the words of those who have said goodbye to someone who died of AIDS.

Figure 13-2 Maitri.

13-1 | Dimensions of HIV/AIDS-Related Stigma

DIMENSIONS OF STIGMA (GOFFMAN, 1963)	DIMENSIONS OF HIV/AIDS-RELATED STIGMA (HEREK, 1990)
Concealability Can the condition be hidden from others? The less concealable a condition, the more stigmatizing it is.	Although concealable early in its course, later stages of HIV disease are rarely hidden from others.
Disruptiveness Does the condition interfere with social interactions and relationships?	HIV/AIDS disrupts social relationships.
Aesthetics Do others react to the condition's appearance with dislike or disgust?	HIV/AIDS physically disables and disfigures people, and is therefore aesthetically displeasing.
Origin Is the person responsible for having this condition in the first place?	The origin of HIV/AIDS is often, although not always, blamed on personal behaviors and choices.
Course What is the course of this condition? Can the outcome be altered?	The course of HIV/AIDS is degenerative, and the final outcome is not alterable.
Peril Can the person with the condition physically, socially, or morally contaminate others?	HIV is a high-peril condition, in that it poses physical risks to others.

whether a personal quality or condition is stigmatizing. These are summarized in Table 13-1.

Because HIV/AIDS is a stigmatizing condition, and because people do not want to be discriminated against, many people are hesitant to find out their serostatus or to seek treatment for HIV disease.

REFERENCES

Boykin, F. F. (1991). The AIDS crisis and gay male survivor guilt. *Smith College Studies in Social Work, 61*(3), 247–259.

Brashers, D. E., Neidig, J. L., Cardillo, L. W., Dobbs, L. K., Russell, J. A., & Haas, S. M. (1999). "In an important way I did die": Uncertainty and revival in persons living with HIV or AIDS. *AIDS Care, 11*(2), 201–219.

Brashers, D. E., Neidig, J. L., Reynolds, N. R., & Haas, S. M. (1998). Uncertainty in illness across the HIV/AIDS trajectory. *Journal of the Association of Nurses in AIDS Care, 9*(1), 66–77.

Brashers, D. E., Neidig, J. L., Russell, J. A., Cardillo, L. W., Haas, S. M., Dobbs, L. K., et al. (2003). The medical, social, and personal causes of uncertainty in HIV illness. *Issues in Mental Health Nursing, 24*(5), 497–522.

Brimlow, D. L., Cook, J. S., & Seaton, R. (Eds.). (2003). *Stigma and HIV/AIDS: A review of the literature*. Rockville, MD: U.S. Department of Health and Human Services.

Brooks, R. A., & Klosinski, L. E. (1999). Assisting persons living with HIV/AIDS to return to work: Programmatic steps for AIDS service organizations. *AIDS Education and Prevention, 11*(3), 212–223.

Centers for Disease Control and Prevention (CDC). (2001). HIV/AIDS—United States, 1981–2000. *Morbidity and Mortality Weekly Report, 50*, 430–434.

Chesney, M. A., Chambers, D. B., Taylor, J. M., Johnson, L. M., & Folkman, S. (2003). Coping effectiveness training for men living with HIV: Results from a randomized clinical trial testing a group-based intervention. *Psychosomatic Medicine, 65*(6), 1038–1046.

Cline, D. J. (1990). The psychosocial impact of HIV infection—what clinicians can do to help. *Journal of American Academy of Dermatology, 22*(6 Pt 2), 1299–1302.

De Gagne, D. (1994). People living with HIV/AIDS: Promoting health through partnership. *AIDS Health Promotion Exchange, 3*, 1–3.

Demmer, C. (2001). Dealing with AIDS-related loss and grief in a time of treatment advances.

American Journal of Hospice and Palliative Care, 18(1), 35–41.

Eller, L. S. (1999). Effects of cognitive-behavioral interventions on quality of life in persons with HIV. *International Journal of Nursing Studies, 36*(3), 223–233.

Goffman, E. (1963). *Stigma: Notes on the management of spoiled identity*. New York: Simon & Schuster.

Green, G., & Smith, R. (2004). The psychosocial and health care needs of HIV-positive people in the United Kingdom: A review. *HIV Medicine, 5*(Suppl 1), 5–46.

Herek, G. (1990). Illness, stigma, and AIDS. In G. M. Herek, S. M. Levy, S. Maddi, S. Taylor, & D. Wertlieb (Eds.), *Psychological aspects of chronic illness: Chronic conditions, fatal diseases, and clinical care* (pp. 107–150). Washington, DC: American Psychological Association.

Horwath, E. (2003). Psychiatric and neuropsychiatric manifestations of HIV infection. *Journal of the International Association of Physicians in AIDS Care, Supplement 1*, S1–15.

Kain, C. (2004). Teaching tip sheet: Multiple loss and AIDS-related bereavement. *American Psychological Association Online.* Retrieved June 13, 2004, from http://www.apa.org/pi/aids/tiploss.html

Kalichman, S. C. (2004). Teaching tip sheet: Stigma and prejudice. *American Psychological Association Online*. Retrieved June 13, 2004, from http://www.apa.org/pi/aids/tipstigma.html

Kalichman, S. C., Sikkema, K., & Somlai, A. (1996). People living with HIV infection who attend and do not attend support groups: A pilot study of needs, characteristics, and experiences. *AIDS Care, 8*(5), 589–599.

Kelly, J. A., & Kalichman, S. C. (2002). Behavioral research in HIV/AIDS primary and secondary prevention: Recent advances and future directions. *Journal of Consulting and Clinical Psychology, 70*(3), 626–639.

Kelly, J. A., Murphy, D. A., Bahr, G. R., Kalichman, S. C., Morgan, M. G., Stevenson, L. Y., et al. (1993a). Outcome of cognitive-behavioral and support group brief therapies for depressed, HIV infected persons. *American Journal of Psychiatry, 150*(11), 1679–1686.

Kelly, J. A., Murphy, D. A., Bahr, G. R., Koob, J. J., Morgan, M. G., Kalichman, S. C., et al. (1993b). Factors associated with severity of depression and high-risk sexual behavior among persons diagnosed with human immunodeficiency virus (HIV) infection. *Health Psychology, 12*(3), 215–219.

Low-Beer, S., Chan, K., Wood, E., Yip, B., Montaner, J. S., O'Shaughnessy, M. V., et al. (2000). Health related quality of life among persons with HIV after the use of protease inhibitors. *Quality of Life Research, 9*(8), 941–949.

Mallinson, R. K. (1997). Addressing AIDS-related grief. In *HIV Report November 1997*. Johns Hopkins AIDS Service.

McCain, N. L., & Cella, D. F. (1995). Correlates of stress in HIV disease. *Western Journal of Nursing Research, 17*, 141–155.

Murdaugh, C. (1998). Health-related quality of life in HIV disease: Achieving a balance. *Journal of the Association of Nurses in AIDS Care, 9*(6), 59–71.

NAMES Project Foundation. (2006a). *About the quilt.* Retrieved September 7, 2006, from http://www.aidsquilt.org/about.htm

NAMES Project Foundation. (2006b). *History of the quilt*. Retrieved September 7, 2006, from http://www.aidsquilt.org/history.htm

NAMES Project Foundation. (2006c). *Quilt facts*. Retrieved September 7, 2006, from http://www.aidsquilt.org/quiltfacts.htm

NAMES Project Foundation. (2006d). *The Quilt Archive Project*. Retrieved September 7, 2006, from http://www.aidsquilt.org/archive.htm

Rabkin, J. G., & Ferrando, S. (1997). A "second life" agenda: Psychiatric research issues raised by protease inhibitor treatments for people with human immunodeficiency virus or the acquired immunodeficiency syndrome. *Archives of General Psychiatry, 54*(11), 1049–1053.

Regan-Kubinski, M., & Sharts-Hopko, N. (1995). Illness cognition of HIV-infected mothers. *Issues in Mental Health Nursing, 16*, 327–344.

Schwartzberg, S. S. (1992). AIDS-related bereavement among gay men: The inadequacy of current theories of grief. *Psychotherapy, 29*(3), 422–429.

Sikkema, K. J., Kalichman, S. C., Hoffman, R. G., Koob, J. J., Kelly, J. A., & Heckman, T. G. (2000). Coping strategies and emotional wellbeing among HIV-infected men and women experiencing AIDS-related bereavement. *AIDS Care, 12*(5), 613–624.

Sikkema, K. J., Kochman, A., DiFranceisco, W., Kelley, J. A., & Hoffman, R. G. (2003). AIDS-related grief and coping with loss among HIV-positive men and women. *Journal of Behavioral Medicine, 26*(2), 165–181.

Stone, V. E., & Smith, K. Y. (2004). Improving adherence to HAART. *Journal of the National Medical Association, 96*(2), 275–295.

Taylor, S. E., Kemeny, M. E., Reed, G. M., Bower, J. E., & Gruenewald, T. L. (2000). Psychological resources, positive illusions, and health. *American Psychologist*, *55*(1), 99–109.

Walker, G. (1991). *In the midst of winter: Systemic therapy with families, couples, and individuals with AIDS infection*. New York: W.W. Norton.

Weitz, R. (1989). Uncertainty and the lives of persons with AIDS. *Journal of Health and Social Behavior*, *30*, 270–281.

World Health Organization (WHO) (Speaker). (2002). *Regional Office for the Eastern Mediterranean*. World AIDS Campaign 2002: Regional advocacy kit. Geneva, Switzerland: WHO.

Instructor Resources

LEARNING ACTIVITIES

ACTIVITY 1:

Group Activity: The NAMES Project: AIDS-Related Grief

Objective: To discuss AIDS-related grief.

Minimum Time: 45 minutes

View a detailed guide for this activity on the CD-ROM.

ACTIVITY 2:

Group Activity: The Scarlet HIV+: Social Stigma and HIV/AIDS

Objective: To illustrate the basic principles of social stigma and to demonstrate ways to reduce negative perceptions of stigmatized groups.

Minimum Time: 1 hour

View a detailed guide for this activity on the CD-ROM.

DISCUSSION QUESTIONS

1. Discuss the medical, personal, and social uncertainties that arise from a diagnosis of HIV/AIDS. How can individual and societal responses either worsen or lessen these uncertainties?
2. What can be done to reduce or eliminate HIV/AIDS-related stigma?

QUIZ

1. Forgetfulness, apathy, difficulty concentrating, and speech problems may be symptoms of:
   a) Minor cognitive-motor disorder (MCMD)
   b) Chronic somatic precoccupation
   c) Survivor's guilt
   d) HIV-associated dementia
2. What percentage of people do not improve with antiretroviral therapy?
   a) 0–10%
   b) 5–15%
   c) 15–35%
   d) 25–40%
3. True or False: Once HIV is diagnosed, CD4+ counts will consistently fall.

ANSWERS

1. **D.** Psychological disorders associated with HIV include *HIV-associated dementia* (HAD), which includes symptoms such as forgetfulness, apathy, difficulty concentrating, speech problems, tremors, and delusions.
2. **C.** Although antiretroviral therapy makes many HIV+ people healthier, between 15% and 35% of research participants in antiviral therapy studies do not improve with antiretroviral therapy.
3. **False.** CD4+ counts rise and fall, so that people diagnosed with AIDS in the past, based on their low CD4+ counts, can recover and have CD4+ counts that do not meet the CDC's diagnostic criteria for AIDS. This can be confusing for HIV+ people, both psychologically and financially. In addition, the various numbers used to monitor HIV+ people's health, including CD4+ counts and viral load, can be difficult to interpret.

WEB RESOURCES

Psychological Aspects of HIV/AIDS

The American Psychological Association's Office on AIDS

http://www.apa.org/pi/aids/about.html

Provides information, training, and technical assistance on HIV/AIDS-related coping, mental health services, prevention, technology transfer, community collaboration, public policy, and ethics.

HIV/AIDS-Related Stigma

Sexual Orientation: Science, Education, and Policy

http://www.AIDSstigma.net

Features work by Dr. Gregory M. Herek, an internationally recognized authority on sexual prejudice, hate crimes, and AIDS stigma; promotes the use of scientific knowledge for education and enlightened public policy.

RECOMMENDED READING

Psychological and Social Aspects of Living With HIV/AIDS

Spirituality, Psychological Well-Being, and HIV (Coleman, 1999)

Coleman, C. (1999). Spirituality, psychological well-being, and HIV symptoms for African Americans living with HIV disease. Journal of Association of Nurses in AIDS Care, 10*(1), 42–50.*

Explores the contribution of spiritual well-being and human immunodeficiency virus (HIV) symptoms to psychological well-being, as measured by depression, hope, and state-trait anxiety in a sample of African American men and women. Results show that existential well-being and HIV symptoms are related to psychological well-being.

Social Support for People With HIV (Serovich, Bruckner, & Kimberly, 2000)

Serovich, J., Bruckner, P., & Kimberly, J. (2000). Barriers to social support for persons living with HIV/AIDS. AIDS Care, 12*(5), 651–662.*

Shows that barriers to social support (availability, intimacy, and disclosure) diminished HIV+ gay men's acquisition of social support, and that lack of social support, in turn, affected HIV+ gay men's physical health.

Living With HIV (Klitzman, 1997)

Klitzman, R. (1997). Being positive: The lives of men and women with HIV. *Chicago: Ivan R. Dee.*

Documents six patterns of how people deal with their HIV+ status: participating in the alternative culture of HIV social organizations, deepening spirituality, focusing on work and volunteerism, turning to family, minimizing or denying illness, and seeking relief from stress through drugs and alcohol.

HIV/AIDS-Related Grief

Grief and AIDS (Bigelow & Hollinger, 1996)

Bigelow, G., & Hollinger, J. (1996). Grief and AIDS: Surviving catastrophic multiple loss. Hospice Journal, 11*(4), 83–96.*

Examines the grief brought about by multiple losses to AIDS, including trauma, survivor guilt, posttraumatic stress disorder; also discusses other historic examples of multiple loss (holocausts) and maintaining hope.

Group Intervention for Grieving HIV-Positive Men and Women (Sikkema et al., 2004)

Sikkema, K. J., Hansen, N. B., Kochman, A., Tate, D. C., & DiFranceisco, W. (2004). Outcomes from a randomized controlled trial of a group intervention for HIV positive men and women coping with AIDS-related loss and bereavement. Death Studies 28, *187–209.*

Demonstrates that brief cognitive-behavioral group interventions for coping with grief have a positive impact on the psychiatric functioning of HIV+ participants, especially HIV+ women.

HIV/AIDS-Related Stigma

Stigma and Knowledge (Herek, Capitanio, & Widaman, 2002)

Herek, G. M., Capitanio, J. P., & Widaman, K. F. (2002). HIV-related stigma and knowledge in the United States: Prevalence and trends, 1991–1999. American Journal of Public Health, 92*(3), 371–377.*

Finds that although support for extremely punitive policies toward people with AIDS has declined, AIDS remains a stigmatized condition in the United States.

POWERPOINT SLIDES

(Note: A full-color version of these slides, with graphics, is also available on the CD-ROM.)

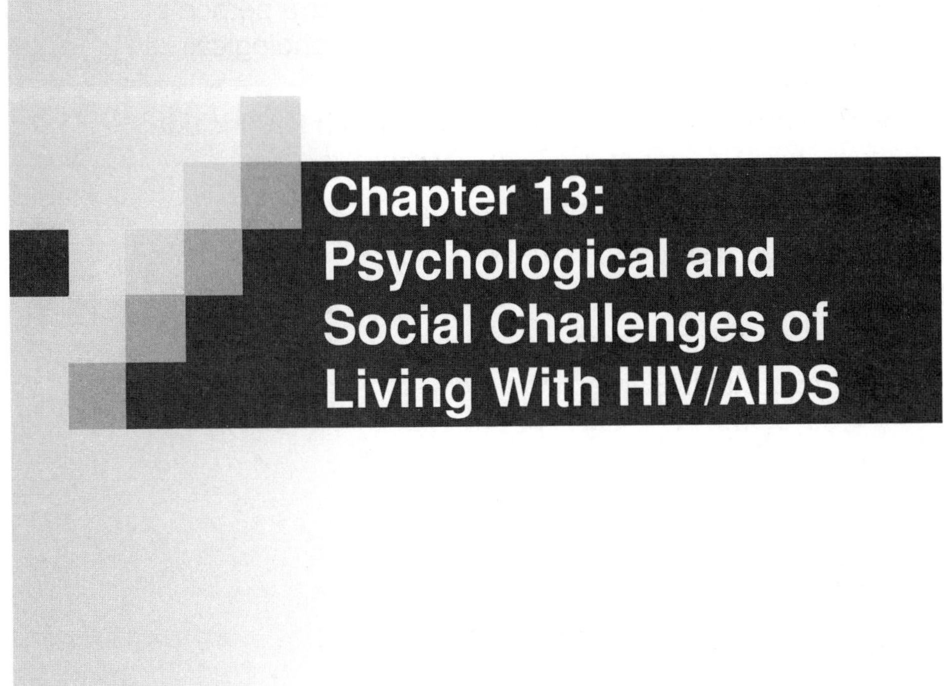

Psychological and Social Challenges of Living With HIV/AIDS

- People living with HIV/AIDS face unique psychological and social challenges:
  - from HIV disease itself
  - from anti-HIV treatment
  - from HIV/AIDS-related stress and uncertainty
  - from grieving the loss of HIV+ loved ones
  - as well as stigma and discrimination

HIV/AIDS-Related Psychological Disorders

- HIV and opportunistic diseases can alter a person's brain and nervous system, causing psychological disorders.
- Psychological disorders associated with HIV include:
  - HIV-associated dementia (HAD);
  - minor cognitive-motor disorder (MCMD);
  - mood disorders, like depression;
  - anxiety disorders;
  - brain tumors; and
  - opportunistic infections of the brain and nervous system.

Other HIV/AIDS-Related Psychological Concerns

- Psychological Side Effects of Anti-HIV Drugs
  - Can range from moodiness and aggressive behavior to severe depression, suicidal thoughts, paranoia, delusions, and hallucinations

Other HIV/AIDS-Related Psychological Concerns (continued)

- HIV/AIDS-related psychological distress
  - Chronic physical pain
  - Physical disfigurement
  - Possibility of infecting other people
  - Changes to lifestyle to accommodate illness and financial burdens of treatment
  - Possible discrimination, abuse, and loss of human rights
  - Guilt about burdening friends and family
  - Loss of independence
  - Physical, social, and emotional isolation
  - Uncertainty in the medical, personal, and social domains
  - Hopelessness, frustration, and self-blame related to not responding to treatment

Meeting the Psychological Needs of Persons Living With HIV/AIDS

- HAART gives hope and optimism to HIV+ people, which improves physical health, decreases depression, and prolongs life span.
- Providing psychological services for HIV+ persons helps the general public as well, as high levels of depression and maladaptive coping with HIV infection have been associated with substance use and risky sexual behavior, which puts others at risk for acquiring HIV.
- The stress of HIV/AIDS can be buffered by the social support provided by support groups.
- Coping and stress management programs positively affect the mental health of people living with HIV/AIDS.

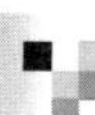

Living With the Uncertainties of HIV/AIDS

People who live with HIV/AIDS often face uncertainty. Such uncertainty is stressful and can impair HIV+ people's quality of life.

- Medical Uncertainties
  - Not enough information about diagnoses
  - Ambiguous symptoms
  - Complex and uncertain treatment
  - Unpredictable disease progression or prognosis

- Personal Uncertainties
  - Identity dilemmas

Living With the Uncertainties of HIV/AIDS (continued)

- Financial Uncertainties
  - Claiming disability status
  - Amount of money needed for treatment is unknown

- Social Uncertainties
  - Unpredictable interpersonal reactions
  - Unclear relational implications

HIV/AIDS-Related Grief

- Most people living with HIV/AIDS have lost someone to HIV disease.
- As a result, HIV+ people commonly have high levels of HIV/AIDS loss-related psychological distress.
- Coping with a loss due to HIV/AIDS may differ from coping with losses to other diseases in several ways:
  - Many people who die from complications of HIV disease die at a relatively young age.
  - The stigma associated with HIV may prevent those who survive from freely mourning or acknowledging the cause of death.
  - In the United States, HIV has been highly concentrated within specific populations. People in these communities have lost many to HIV/AIDS and have watched their social networks dwindle.
  - "Survivor's guilt" may prevent those who have lost loved ones from fully grieving and recovering.

Community-Based Responses to HIV Loss

The AIDS Memorial Quilt

- In 1985, gay activist Cleave Jones asked marchers to write the names of loved ones who had died of AIDS on placards. These were later taped to the walls of the Federal Building.
- To Jones, the names looked like a quilt, inspiring him to make the first quilt panel in honor of a friend who had died from AIDS. Jones later formed the NAMES Project Foundation with friends.
- The quilt has been displayed in its entirety only five times. The last display of the entire quilt (October 1996) covered the expanse of the National Mall from the Capitol to the Washington Monument.
- As of 2004, there are approximately 46,000 panels on the quilt, representing over 82,000 people who have lost their battle to AIDS.
- As of 2004, if all the quilt's panels were laid end to end, they would extend more than 51 miles in length.

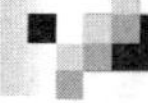

HIV/AIDS-Related Stigma and Discrimination

- HIV/AIDS is one of the most stigmatizing medical conditions in modern history.
- Many communities direct unfavorable attitudes, beliefs, and policies toward people who have or who are associated with HIV/AIDS, including their loved ones, family members, close associates, and social groups.

Effects of HIV/AIDS-Related Stigma and Discrimination

HIV/AIDS-related stigma affects HIV/AIDS diagnosis and treatment.

- Many people are hesitant to find out their serostatus or to seek treatment for HIV disease.

The stigma of HIV/AIDS is combined for many with the stigma of homosexuality and illicit drug use.

- Fear of discrimination may compel men who have sex with men to keep their sexual behavior secret and deny their sexual risk.
- Stigma from drug use restricts effective HIV/AIDS prevention and treatment.

Learning Objectives

- Understand the need for positive prevention
- List and explain positive prevention strategies
- Understand how antiretroviral therapy plays a role in positive prevention

Key Terms

beneficial disclosure
nonoccupational exposure
occupational exposure
positive prevention
postexposure prophylaxis
superinfection

14

Prevention for People With HIV/AIDS

In the early years of the HIV/AIDS epidemic, public health organizations focused on keeping uninfected people from getting HIV. Now, these organizations increasingly try to keep HIV+ people from giving HIV to others, in efforts that are called *positive prevention*. This chapter explains why HIV+ and HIV– people need positive prevention, outlines positive prevention strategies, and describes how antiretroviral therapies are used in positive prevention.

THE NEED FOR POSITIVE PREVENTION

For the first 2 decades of the HIV/AIDS epidemic, HIV prevention interventions mostly encouraged uninfected people to adopt safer-sex and drug-using behaviors, so that they would not get HIV (Office of AIDS, 2003). HIV+ people were not a focus of prevention efforts for several reasons. Among the public, there was reluctance to acknowledge that HIV+ people have sex. There also was a perception that it was contradictory to try to prevent a disease among people who already had it. In addition, there was concern that such a focus would be perceived as blaming HIV+ people for the epidemic. More recently, researchers, governments, and health care providers are recognizing that HIV+ people need prevention interventions, too (Kelly & Kalichman, 2002). These secondary prevention interventions are sometimes called positive prevention. Positive prevention is important because:

HIV is transmitted by HIV+ people. From an epidemiological and public health perspective, HIV+ people make up the most important group to address with HIV prevention strategies (DiClemente, Wingood, Del Rio, & Crosby, 2002; International HIV/AIDS Alliance, 2003). A change in the risk behavior of an HIV+ person will, on average and in almost all affected populations, have a much bigger impact on the spread of the virus than the same behavioral change in an HIV– person (King-Spooner, 1999; Vernazza, Eron, Fiscus, & Cohen, 1999).

Some people living with HIV continue to engage in risky behaviors. Following their diagnosis, many HIV+ people use condoms more regularly and adopt other safer sex and drug use practices. Over time, however, many revert back to risky sex and drug use. Prevention interventions for positives may help HIV+ people sustain healthy behavior changes (DiClemente et al., 2002; Wolitski, Janssen, Onorato, Purcell, & Crepaz, 2005).

HIV+ people have the right to live well with HIV. Living well with HIV includes having a healthy sex life. This means protecting HIV+ people against superinfection (i.e., reinfection with a different strain of HIV) and against new STIs/STDs (International HIV/AIDS Alliance, 2003; Wolitski et al., 2005).

POSITIVE PREVENTION TARGET POPULATIONS AND GOALS

Who can benefit the most from positive prevention? HIV+ individuals who are sexually active or who use injection drugs can transmit the virus to others. Thus, they are logical targets of positive prevention efforts. Successful positive prevention efforts are comprehensive, combining prevention with HIV testing, treatment, and support.

HIV+ and Sexually Active

Over 70% of HIV+ people continue to be sexually active after they learn that they are infected (Office of AIDS, 2003). Although many engage in safer-sex practices, empirical evidence suggests that some HIV+ people continue to have risky sex (Collins, Morin, Shriver, & Coates, 2000; De Cock, Mbori-Ngacha, & Marum, 2002; King-Spooner, 1999; Remien, Senterfitt, & Decarlo, 2000).

According to the Office of AIDS, HIV+ people who have unprotected sex tend to:

- Know less about HIV/AIDS, its transmission, and its effects on health
- Believe that safer sex is less pleasurable than unsafe sex
- Lack commitment to practicing safer sex
- Lack confidence in their ability to practice safer sex
- Perceive that they have little control over whether condoms are used
- Have problems communicating with partners about safer sex
- Perceive more barriers to condom use

Unprotected sex not only can transmit infection to uninfected partners; it also increases HIV+ people's risk of getting STIs/STDs. STIs/STDs are serious health conditions that may accelerate HIV disease in HIV+ people. They also can make HIV transmission to uninfected people more likely because STIs/STDs can increase the number of CD4+ cells near the genitals. Because HIV attaches to CD4+ cells, people with both STIs/STDs and HIV often have more HIV particles in their semen, vaginal secretions, anal mucus, and in the blood circulating near their genitals. They are also more likely to have open sores or easily injured skin, making direct transmission of HIV through blood more likely.

Even more serious than the threat of STIs/STDs is the threat of superinfection, which happens when an HIV+ person becomes infected with a second strain of HIV. Increasingly, second infections are resistant to antiretroviral therapy (Collins et al., 2000; De Cock, et al., 2002). This is because many HIV+ people take their antiretroviral drugs incorrectly, which allows the HIV to mutate into drug-resistant strains (International HIV/AIDS Alliance, 2002, 2003; Vernazza et al., 1999). Indeed, even recently infected people who have never taken antiretroviral therapy themselves sometimes already have drug-resistant strains of HIV, which they acquired from people who did not adhere to their antiretroviral regimens (CDC, 2003b). Moreover, research shows that people who have unprotected sex are less likely to take their antiretroviral drugs correctly (CDC, 2001, 2003b; Del Rio, 2003; International HIV/AIDS Alliance, 2002).

HIV+ and Using Injection Drugs

HIV+ injection drug users are an especially important target for HIV prevention efforts, as they may engage in both drug use and sexual behaviors that can transmit HIV to others. These behaviors also can put themselves at risk of infection with another strain of HIV, as well as other diseases that can be transmitted through unprotected sex and use of nonsterile drug paraphernalia (Wilkinson et al., 2006).

The Interrelatedness of Testing, Treatment, and Prevention

HIV prevention, testing, treatment, and support are interrelated. People living with HIV need medical treatment, psychological care, and social support, not just for their own disease but also to prevent spreading HIV to others (DiClemente et al., 2002; International HIV/AIDS Alliance, 2003). Combining HIV prevention with testing and treatment services has a number of advantages. According to the International HIV/AIDS Alliance (2002), in particular, providers can:

- Screen HIV+ patients for behavioral risk factors and address them through counseling and referrals.
- Screen HIV+ patients for clinical risk factors, such as STIs/STDs, and administer treatments and vaccinations.
- Teach recently diagnosed HIV+ people how to protect their sex and drug use partners.
- Teach HIV+ mothers how to reduce their chances of giving HIV to their children.

Positive Prevention: Goals and Barriers

In the United States, public health initiatives for people already infected with HIV aim to increase (CDC, 2003a, 2003b; Del Rio, 2003; Institute of Medicine, 2001; Janssen et al., 2001):

- Access to HIV testing
- Access to quality medical care
- Use of quality medical care
- Adherence to HIV therapy
- The adoption and maintenance of HIV risk-reduction behaviors

Despite these efforts, HIV+ individuals still face unique challenges in preventing the transmission of HIV. First, they face embarrassment, discomfort, and fear of rejection surrounding disclosure of their HIV serostatus to sexual and drug-use partners. In some cases, the desire for trusting sexual relationships outweighs fears of transmission, and thus reduces condom use.

Another challenge is conflicting messages about the state of the epidemic: Optimistic advertising of highly active antiretroviral therapy (HAART) conflicts with frightening public health warnings about HIV/AIDS. Finally, even in the United States, many misconceptions about how HIV is transmitted remain, including misconceptions about the effects of HAART on HIV transmission risk.

POSITIVE PREVENTION STRATEGIES

HIV transmission is influenced by a myriad of individual, community, and societal factors. Thus, like prevention efforts for HIV– persons, prevention efforts for HIV+ individuals must be deployed at multiple levels (DiClemente et al., 2002). Over the past decade, an increasing number of individual- and small group–level behavioral interventions have been shown to reduce HIV risk behaviors among HIV+ persons (Kalichman, 2005). In particular:

- Several interventions that targeted HIV+ men and/or women have improved their consistency of condom use, increased their perceptions of the advantages of condom use, and increased their confidence that they can use condoms consistently and correctly (Fogarty et al., 2001; Kalichman et al., 2001; Wingood et al., 2004).
- Several interventions for HIV+ injection drug users have reduced their instances of needle-sharing and unprotected sex (Margolin, Avants, Warburton, Hawkins, & Shi, 2003; Sterk, Theall, Elifson, & Kidder, 2003).
- Some social support and mental health counseling programs have reduced the number of HIV+ men's sexual partners (Coates, McKusick, Kuno, & Stites, 1989) and unsafe sexual acts (Kelly et al., 1993).
- A number of brief safer-sex counseling interventions have decreased the number of unprotected sexual acts among HIV+ people, increased consistent condom use, and increased sexual abstinence (DiScenza, Nies, & Jordan, 1996; Padian, O'Brien, Chang, Glass, & Francis, 1993; Patterson & Semple, 2003; Patterson, Shaw, & Semple, 2003).

Prevention strategies for positives focus on improving treatment and care for HIV- and AIDS-associated opportunistic infections, mobilizing communities to help reduce risk factors for HIV transmission, and changing policies that affect HIV+ persons' access to and use of prevention and treatment services (International HIV/AIDS Alliance, 2003).

Individual-Level Behavioral Interventions

Individual-level interventions strategies include voluntary counseling and testing for persons whose HIV status is unknown and post-test and ongoing counseling for HIV+ people (see Figure 14-1 for an example). Counseling efforts are designed to build the knowledge, skills, self-efficacy, and motivation needed to reduce or eliminate risky behaviors that can lead to HIV transmission. According to the International HIV/AIDS Alliance (2003), these strategies also may:

- *Encourage beneficial disclosure,* which involves the voluntary and often confidential disclosure of HIV+ people's serostatus to other people and organizations, so that the HIV-infected person will feel comfortable accessing HIV services. Beneficial disclosure also reduces the secrecy and stigma surrounding HIV/AIDS.
- *Encourage ethical partner notification,* which involves the voluntary and often confidential notification of HIV+ people's sexual and drug-use partners, so that they will get tested and take precautions.

Clinics are a key setting for such interventions, as HIV+ people need frequent medical care to monitor antiretroviral effects and to treat opportunistic infections as HIV disease progresses. A study of 839 HIV+ men and women at six public HIV clinics in California found that 50% had never discussed disclosure with a provider at their clinic, and 29% had never spoken with a provider at their clinic about

A multiagency collaboration led by Dr. Jean Richardson of the University of California Keck School of Medicine developed and implemented a brief intervention in which medical providers provided counseling and written information to HIV+ patients. This brief intervention successfully reduced unprotected anal or vaginal intercourse among participants with two or more partners. First, clinic staff were trained in the background and rationale for the intervention, behavioral change theories, communication skill building, and how to conduct a brief counseling session and make appropriate referrals. Once the intervention was initiated, providers counseled each HIV+ patient for 3–5 minutes, at each patient visit, about the patient–provider team approach to helping patients stay healthy, safer-sex goals, and risk-reduction behaviors. Providers also gave patients written materials that supported the intervention messages. The intervention counseling and written materials emphasized the negative consequences of unsafe sex for oneself and others.

Figure 14-1 Brief provider safer-sex counseling for HIV-positive patients (Richardson et al., 2004).

safer sex (Marks et al., 2002). Thus, training clinic staff to deliver individual-level prevention interventions effectively should be a prevention priority.

Small Group-Level Interventions

Like small group interventions for HIV–, effective small group programs for HIV+ are theory-based and build the knowledge, skills, motivations, and intentions needed to change risky sex and drug use behaviors. Many of the effective small group interventions for HIV negative adults given in Figure 9-2 can be adapted for use with HIV+ people.

Improved Treatment and Care

Improving treatment of and health care for HIV+ persons may include making available voluntary counseling and testing programs, integrating behavioral prevention counseling with HIV/AIDS treatment in clinical settings, and providing antiretroviral treatment as prevention for further transmission, including parent-to-child transmission. It also may involve reducing stigma and discrimination toward HIV+ persons in health care settings (International HIV/AIDS Alliance, 2003).

Community Mobilization

People living with HIV are a part of broader communities and also influence those communities. They need the support of those communities and their broader environments to implement the risk reduction behaviors promoted by individual health promotion strategies. Community mobilization efforts may have a variety of positive prevention objectives. Some seek to involve communities in positive prevention by developing peer support groups for HIV+ persons. Others have trained people with HIV as peer outreach workers, to increase the visibility of positives and reduce HIV/AIDS stigma (International HIV/AIDS Alliance, 2003). Other community-level interventions implement focused communication campaigns that raise awareness of the important role of HIV+ people in reducing transmission (see Figure 14-2 for an example).

Advocacy and Policy Change

The success of positive prevention efforts depends crucially on laws and policies, such as those concerning HIV/AIDS-related prevention and treatment funding;

HIV STOPS WITH ME is a social marketing campaign that aims to reduce the stigma associated with HIV and to acknowledge the powerful role that positives have in ending the epidemic. The campaign deals directly with sex and condom use, while raising themes of responsibility, communication, and disclosure of status. Each participating city (Boston, Buffalo, Los Angeles, Long Beach, New York, Portland, San Francisco, and Seattle) has its own Web site and several spokespeople who reflect the local demographic makeup. Spokespersons tell their own stories on the Web site and engage in online dialogue with other members of the community. The Web site also contain articles, resource lists, and an events calendar. *HIV STOPS WITH ME* further promotes its messages via billboards, print ads, posters in bars and clubs, outreach postcards, and television commercials.

In 2003 and 2005, *HIV STOPS WITH ME* was awarded with a People's Voice Webby award for Best Health Care Web site by the International Academy of Digital Artists.

Figure 14-2 HIV stops with me: A social marketing campaign (HIV STOPS WITH ME, n.d.).

informed consent and confidentiality laws for HIV testing; and restrictions on school-based sexuality education curricula. Advocacy and policy change strategies involve HIV+ people in the development of HIV-related policies and programs, including those that target HIV+ people for prevention efforts, address stigma and discrimination against positives, and increase access to treatment among all HIV+ people (International HIV/AIDS Alliance, 2003).

USING ANTIRETROVIRAL THERAPY FOR POSITIVE PREVENTION

As discussed in chapter 12, antiretroviral therapy, when properly taken, dramatically lengthens the life spans and improves the physical well-being of people living with HIV/AIDS. Although it is true that living longer and healthier lives gives HIV+ people more chances of transmitting the virus, antiretroviral therapy also lowers the amount of HIV shed through blood, genital, and anal secretions. With less virus in their body fluids, HIV+ people are less likely to transmit HIV (Center for AIDS Prevention Studies, 2003; Vernazza et al., 1999).

Preventing Vertical Transmission

Antiretroviral therapy is particularly crucial for preventing parent-to-child transmission, the primary route of transmission to children under the age of 10 years (WHO, 2001). HIV can be transmitted from an infected mother to her child during pregnancy, labor, delivery, or breast-feeding. Without intervention, the risk of transmission from an HIV+ mother to her child before or during birth is 15–25%. Breast-feeding by an HIV+ mother raises the risk to a total risk of 20–45% (Newell, 2004).

Antiretroviral treatment for HIV+ women and their infants during pregnancy, labor, delivery, and the neonatal period has been shown to reduce parent-to-child transmission significantly (Connor et al., 1994; Ferrazin et al., 1997)—to as low as 1.5% in one large research study (Stiehm et al., 1999). Guidelines that represent the official U.S. treatment standards for the use of antiretroviral therapy to reduce vertical transmission are made available by the National Institute on Allergy and Infectious Diseases (NIAID) (Public Health Service Task Force, 2006).

Postexposure Prophylaxis

Postexposure prophylaxis (PEP) is the giving of antiretroviral therapy to people after they have been exposed to HIV, in an attempt to prevent HIV infection. Studies have shown some success with postexposure prophylaxis in the following domains:

- *Occupational Exposure*: Among health care workers exposed to HIV through needle-stick injuries or other accidental contact with body fluids, those taking antiretroviral postexposure prophylaxis (PEP) were less likely to become infected than were those who did not receive PEP (Cardo et al., 1997).
- *Nonoccupational Exposure*: A growing body of evidence suggests that PEP following nonoccupational exposures (including consensual sex, nonconsensual sex, exposure to mother's body fluids, and injection drug use) may reduce HIV transmission (Roland, 2004).

NIAID makes available PEP guidelines for the treatment of both occupational (Panlilio, Cardo, Grohskopf, Heneine, & Ross, 2005) and nonoccupational exposure (Smith et al., 2005) to HIV. Unfortunately, antiretroviral therapy often has severe side effects, ranging from fatigue and nausea to diabetes and permanent liver damage. PEP is therefore not a simple "morning-after" approach to HIV prevention (Roland, 2004).

REFERENCES

Cardo, D. M., Culver, D. H., Ciesielski, C. A., Srivastava, P. U., Marcus, R., Abiteboul, D., et al. (1997). A case-control study of HIV seroconversion in health care workers after percutaneous exposure. Centers for Disease Control and Prevention Needlestick Surveillance Group. *New England Journal of Medicine, 337*(21), 1485–1490.

Center for AIDS Prevention Studies (CAPS). (2003). *What is the effect of HIV treatment on HIV prevention?* San Francisco: University of California, San Francisco.

Centers for Disease Control and Prevention (CDC). (2001). *HIV Prevention Strategic Plan through 2005.* Atlanta, GA: CDC.

Centers for Disease Control and Prevention (CDC). (2003a). Advancing HIV prevention: New strategies for a changing epidemic—United States, 2003. *Morbidity and Mortality Weekly Report, 52*(15), 329–332.

Centers for Disease Control and Prevention (CDC). (2003b). *Advancing HIV prevention: The science behind the new initiative.* Atlanta, GA: CDC.

Coates, T., McKusick, L., Kuno, R., & Stites, D. (1989). Stress reduction training changed number of sexual partners but not immune function in men with HIV. *American Journal of Public Health, 79*(7), 885–886.

Collins, C., Morin, S. F., Shriver, M. D., & Coates, T. J. (2000). *Designing primary prevention for people living with HIV.* Policy Monograph Series. University of California, San Francisco: AIDS Research Institute, AIDS Policy Research Center & Center for AIDS Prevention Studies.

Connor, E. M., Sperling, R. S., Gelber, R., Kiselev, P., Scott, G., O'Sullivan, M. J., et al. (1994). Reduction of maternal-infant transmission of human immunodeficiency virus type 1 with zidovudine treatment. Pediatric AIDS Clinical Trials Group Protocol 076 Study Group. *New England Journal of Medicine, 331*(18), 1173–1180.

De Cock, K., Mbori-Ngacha, D., & Marum, E. (2002). Shadow on the continent: Public health and HIV/AIDS in Africa in the 21st century. *The Lancet, 360*(9326), 67–72.

Del Rio, C. (2003). New challenges in HIV care: Prevention among HIV infected patients. *Topics in HIV Medicine, 11*(4), 140–144.

DiClemente, R. J., Wingood, G. M., Del Rio, C., & Crosby, R. A. (2002). Prevention interventions for HIV positive individuals. *Sexually Transmitted Infections, 78*(6), 393–395.

DiScenza, S., Nies, M., & Jordan, C. (1996). Effectiveness of counseling in the health promotion of HIV-positive clients in the community. *Public Health Nursing, 13*(3), 209–216.

Ferrazin, A., De Maria, A., Gotta, C., Mazzarello, G., Canessa, A., Ciravegna, B., et al. (1997). Zidovudine therapy of HIV-1 infection during pregnancy: Assessment of the effect on the newborns. *Journal of Acquired Immune Deficiency Syndromes, 6*(4), 376–379.

Fogarty, L. A., Heilig, C. M., Armstrong, K., Cabral, R., Galavotti, C., Gielen, A. C., et al. (2001). Long-term effectiveness of a peer-based intervention to promote condom and contraceptive use among HIV-positive and at-risk women. *Public Health Reports, 116*(Suppl. 1), 103–119.

HIV STOPS WITH ME. (n.d.). *About the campaign.* Retrieved September 8, 2006, from http://hivstopswithme.org/about.aspx?t=EN&1=home

Institute of Medicine, Committee on HIV Prevention Strategies in the United States. (2001). *No time to lose: Getting more from HIV prevention.* Washington, DC: National Academy Press.

International HIV/AIDS Alliance. (2002). *Policy briefing No. 2: Participation and empowerment in HIV/AIDS programming.* Brighton, UK: International HIV/AIDS Alliance.

International HIV/AIDS Alliance. (2003). *Positive prevention: Prevention strategies for people with HIV/AIDS.* Draft background paper. Brighton, UK: International HIV/AIDS Alliance.

Janssen, R. S., Holtgrave, D. R., Valdiserri, R. O., Shepherd, M., Gayle, H. D., & De Cock, K. M. (2001). The serostatus approach to fighting the HIV epidemic: Prevention strategies for infected individuals. *American Journal of Public Health, (91)*7, 1019–1024.

Kalichman, S. C. (Ed.). (2005). *Positive prevention: Reducing transmission among people living with HIV/AIDS.* New York: Kluwer Academic/Plenum.

Kalichman, S. C., Rompa, D., Cage, M., DiFonzo, K., Simpson, D., Austin, J., et al. (2001). Effectiveness of an intervention to reduce HIV transmission risks in HIV-positive people. *American Journal of Preventive Medicine, 21*(2), 84–94.

Kelly, J. A., & Kalichman, S. C. (2002). Behavioral research in HIV/AIDS primary and secondary prevention: Recent advances and future directions. *Journal of Consulting and Clinical Psychology, 70*(3), 626–639.

Kelly, J. A., Murphy, D. A., Bahr, G. R., Kalichman, S. C., Morgan, M. G., Stevenson, L. Y., et al. (1993). Outcome of cognitive-behavioral and support group brief therapies for depressed persons diagnosed with HIV infection. *American Journal of Psychiatry, 150*(11), 1679–1686.

King-Spooner, S. (1999). HIV prevention and the positive population. *International Journal of STD and AIDS, 10*(3), 141–150.

Margolin, A., Avants, S. K., Warburton, L. A., Hawkins, K. A., & Shi, J. (2003). A randomized clinical trial of a manual-guided risk reduction intervention for HIV-positive injection drug users. *Health Psychology, 22*(2), 223–228.

Marks, G., Richardson, J. L., Crepaz, N., Stoyanoff, S., Milam, J., Kemper, C., et al. (2002). Are HIV care providers talking with patients about safer sex and disclosure? A multi-clinic assessment. *AIDS, 16*(14), 1953–1957.

Newell, M. L. (2004). *HIV transmission through breastfeeding: A review of the available evidence.* Geneva, Switzerland: WHO.

Office of AIDS. (2003). *Prevention with positives: A guide to effective programs.* Sacramento, CA: State of California Department of Health Services.

Padian, N. S., O'Brien, T. R., Chang, Y., Glass, S., & Francis, D. P. (1993). Prevention of heterosexual transmission of human immunodeficiency virus through couple counseling. *Journal of Acquired Immune Deficiency Syndromes, 6*(9), 1043–1048.

Panlilio, A. L., Cardo, D. M., Grohskopf, L. A., Heneine, W., & Ross, C. S. (2005). Updated U.S. Public Health Service guidelines for the management of occupational exposures to HIV and recommendations for postexposure prophylaxis. *Morbidity and Mortality Weekly Report, 54*(RR-9), 1–17.

Patterson, T. L., & Semple, S. J. (2003). Sexual risk reduction among HIV-positive drug-using men who have sex with men. *Journal of Urban Health, 80*(4, Suppl 3), iii77–iii87.

Patterson, T. L., Shaw, W. S., & Semple, S. J. (2003). Reducing the sexual risk behaviors of HIV+ individuals: Outcome of a randomized controlled trial. *Annals of Behavioral Medicine, 25*(2), 137–145.

Public Health Service Task Force. (2006, July 6). Recommendations for use of antiretroviral drugs in pregnant HIV-1-infected women for maternal health and interventions to reduce perinatal HIV-1 transmission in the United States. Retrieved September 8, 2006, from http://aidsinfo.nih.gov/ContentFiles/PerinatalGL.pdf

Remien, R., Senterfitt, W., & Decarlo, P. (2000). *Fact sheet #37E: What are HIV+ persons' HIV prevention needs?* University of California, San Francisco: Center for AIDS Prevention Studies.

Richardson, J. L., Milam, J., McCutchan, A., Stoyanoff, S., Bolan, R., Weiss, J., et al. (2004). Effect of brief provider safer-sex counseling of HIV-1 seropositive patients: A multi-clinic assessment. *AIDS, 18*(8), 1179–1186.

Roland, M. (2004). Prophylaxis following nonoccupational exposure to HIV. In L. Pieperl, S. Coffey, O. Bacon, & P. Volberding (Eds.), *HIV InSite knowledge base.* San Francisco: Center for HIV Information, University of California, San Francisco.

Smith, D. K., Grohskopf, L. A., Black, R. J., Auerbach, J. D., Veronese, F., Struble, K. A., et al. (2005). Antiretroviral postexposure prophylaxis after sexual, injection-drug use, or other nonoccupational exposure to HIV in the United States. Recommendations from the U.S. Department of Health and Human Services. *Morbidity and Mortality Weekly Report, 54*(RR-2), 1–19.

Sterk, C. E., Theall, K. P., Elifson, K. W., & Kidder, D. (2003). HIV risk reduction among African-American women who inject drugs: A randomized controlled trial. *AIDS and Behavior, 7*(1), 73–86.

Stiehm, E. R., Lambert, J. S., Mofenson, L. M., Bethel, J., Whitehouse, J., Nugent, R., et al. (1999). Efficacy of zidovudine and human immunodeficiency virus (HIV) hyperimmune immunoglobulin for reducing perinatal HIV transmission from HIV-infected women with advanced disease: Results of Pediatric AIDS Clinical Trials Group protocol 185. *Journal of Infectious Diseases, 179*(3), 567–575.

Vernazza, P. L., Eron, J. J., Fiscus, S. A., & Cohen, M. S. (1999). Sexual transmission of HIV: Infectiousness and prevention. *AIDS, 13*(2), 155–166.

Wilkinson, J. D., Zhao, W., Santibanez, S., Arnsten, J., Knowlton, A., et al. & the INSPIRE Study Group (2006). Providers' HIV prevention discussions with HIV-seropositive injection drug users. *AIDS and Behavior, 10*(6), 699–705.

Wingood, G. M., DiClemente, R. J., Mikhail, I., Lang, D., Hubbard McCree, D., Davies, S. L., et al. (2004). A randomized controlled trial to reduce HIV transmission risk behaviors and STDs among women living with HIV: The WiLLOW Program. *Journal of Acquired Immune Deficiency Syndromes, 37*, S58–S67.

Wolitski, R. J., Janssen, R. S., Onorato, I. M., Purcell, D. W., & Crepaz, N. (2005). An overview of prevention with people living with HIV. In S. C. Kalichman (Ed.), *Positive prevention: Reducing transmission among people living with HIV/AIDS* (pp. 1–28). New York: Kluwer Academic/Plenum.

World Health Organization (WHO). (2001). New data on the prevention of mother-to-child transmission of HIV and their policy implications: Conclusions and recommendations. WHO Technical Consultation on behalf of the UNFPA/UNICEF/WHO/UNAIDS Inter-Agency Task Team on Mother-to-Child Transmission of HIV. Geneva, Switzerland: WHO.

Instructor Resources

LEARNING ACTIVITIES

ACTIVITY 1:

Group Activity: Controversies in Positive Prevention

Objective: To teach ethical principles that guide effective positive prevention.

Minimum Time: 45 minutes

View a detailed guide for this activity on the CD-ROM.

ACTIVITY 2:

Assignment: Successful Positive Prevention

Objective: To understand the ramifications behind HIV/AIDS prevention laws.

Minimum Time: 20 minutes

Write a reaction to the following statement:

"All HIV+ people should be reported by name to their state's health department."

What sort of legal, ethical, and medical consequences would this have if it were to become law?

ACTIVITY 3:

Assignment: Successful Positive Prevention

Objective: To understand successful HIV/AIDS prevention programs.

Identify a positive prevention program that has been researched and evaluated in the HIV/AIDS prevention literature. (See, for example, the peer-reviewed journal *AIDS Education and Prevention.*) Write a summary of the prevention program's specific target population, describe the program's approaches and activities, review the methods used to evaluate the program, and report on the outcomes of the program.

DISCUSSION QUESTIONS

1. What barriers exist to beneficial disclosure? What do you think can be done to remove those barriers?

2. Why are HIV prevention, testing, treatment, and support interrelated? Why is it beneficial to offer all of them to HIV+ people?

QUIZ

1. On average, a change in risk behavior in an HIV+ person will have ___ on the spread of the virus than the same change in an HIV– person.
   a) More of an impact
   b) Less of an impact
   c) An equal impact
   d) No discernible impact
2. True or False: Unprotected sex has no impact on the health of people who are HIV+.
3. Voluntary and confidential disclosure of HIV+ status to friends and coworkers is called ______.
4. The giving of antiretroviral therapy to people after they have been exposed to HIV is known as:
   a) Occupational exposure
   b) Nonoccupational exposure
   c) Superinfection
   d) Postexposure prophylaxis

ANSWERS

1. **A.** A change in the risk behavior of an HIV+ person will, on average and in almost all affected populations, have a much bigger impact on the spread of the virus than the same behavioral change in an HIV– person.
2. **False.** Unprotected sex increases HIV+ people's risk of getting STIs/STDs, which may accelerate HIV disease in HIV+ people. It also increases the threat of superinfection, which happens when an HIV+ person becomes infected with a second strain of HIV.
3. The voluntary and often confidential disclosure of HIV+ people's serostatus to other people and organizations is called *beneficial disclosure*.
4. **D.** Postexposure prophylaxis (PEP) is the giving of antiretroviral therapy to people after they have been exposed to HIV, in an attempt to prevent HIV infection.

WEB RESOURCES

AIDS Policy Research Center: Prevention for Positives Resources

http://ari.ucsf.edu/programs/policy_pwpresources_general.aspx

Provides research resources for HIV+ people.

RECOMMENDED READING

Sexual Risk Behavior in People Living With HIV (Crepaz & Marks, 2002)

Crepaz, N., & Marks, G. (2002). Towards an understanding of sexual risk behavior in people living with HIV: A review of social, psychological, and medical findings. AIDS, 16*(2), 135–149.*

Reviews studies that have examined psychological, social, interpersonal, and medical correlates of sexual risk behavior among HIV+ people.

Reducing Sexual Transmission of HIV by HIV+ People (Marks, Burris, & Peterman, 1999)

Marks, G., Burris, S., & Peterman, T. A. (1999). Reducing sexual transmission of HIV from those who know they are infected: The need for personal and collective responsibility. AIDS, 13*, 297–306.*

Examines risk-taking among HIV+ people and discusses personal and collective responsibility for reducing HIV transmission.

Positive Prevention: Reducing HIV Transmission Among People Living With HIV/AIDS (Kalichman, 2004)

Kalichman, S. C. (Ed.). (2004). Positive prevention: Reducing HIV transmission among people living with HIV/AIDS. *New York: Plenum.*

Includes discussions of unprotected sex among HIV+ gay and bisexual men, of the role of disclosure in preventing transmission, of mental health and HIV, of the impact of HIV diagnosis on sexual risk behaviors, of community-based interventions, and of international perspectives on positive prevention.

POWERPOINT SLIDES

(Note: A full-color version of these slides, with graphics, is also available on the CD-ROM.)

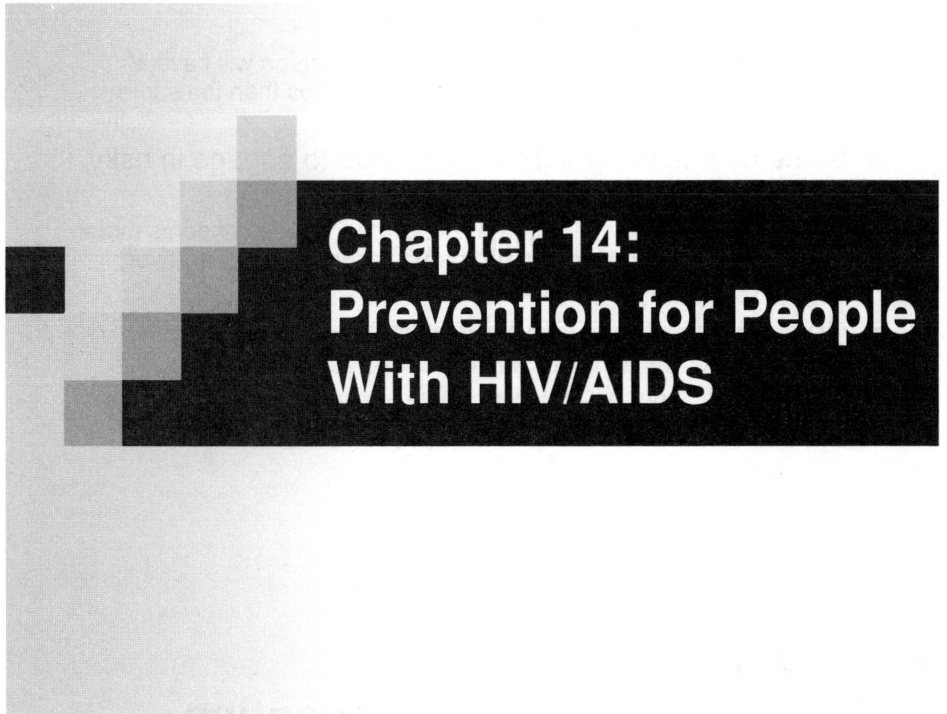

Prevention for People With HIV/AIDS

- In the earlier years of the HIV/AIDS epidemic, public health organizations focused on keeping uninfected people from getting HIV.
- Now, these organizations increasingly try to keep HIV+ people from giving HIV to others, in efforts that are called "positive prevention."

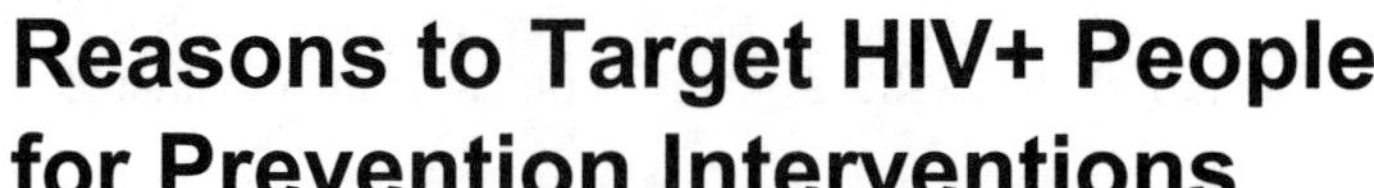

Reasons to Target HIV+ People for Prevention Interventions

- HIV is transmitted by HIV+ people.
  - A change in the risk behavior of an HIV+ person will have a much bigger impact on the spread of the virus than the same behavioral change in an HIV-person.
- Some people living with HIV continue to engage in risky behaviors.
  - Following their diagnosis, most HIV+ people use condoms more regularly and adopt other safer sex practices; however, over time, many revert back to risky sex.
- HIV+ people have the right to live well with HIV.
  - Living well with HIV includes having a healthy sex life.
  - This means protecting HIV+ people against super infection (re-infection with a different strain) and against new STDs.

Supports of Positive Prevention

In the United States, public health initiatives for people already infected with HIV aim to increase

- access to HIV testing;
- access to quality medical care;
- use of quality medical care;
- adherence to HIV therapy; and
- the adoption and maintenance of HIV risk-reduction behaviors.

Barriers to Positive Prevention

Despite outreach, HIV+ individuals still face unique challenges in preventing the transmission of HIV, such as:

- □ embarrassment, discomfort, and fear of rejection surrounding disclosure of their serostatus to sexual and drug-use partners;
- □ desires for trusting sexual relationships that outweigh fears of transmission, and thus reduce condom use;
- □ conflicting messages about the state of the epidemic; and
- □ misconceptions about how HIV is transmitted, including misconceptions about the effects of HAART on HIV transmission risk.

Positive Prevention Strategies

- **Individual Health Promotion**
  - □ Promote voluntary HIV counseling and testing
  - □ Provide post-test and ongoing counseling for HIV+ people
  - □ Encourage beneficial disclosure of HIV+ status to others, so that the HIV-infected person will feel comfortable accessing HIV services
  - □ Encourage ethical sexual and drug-use partner notification
  - □ Provide counseling for serodiscordant couples (couples where one is HIV+ and the other is HIV-)

Positive Prevention Strategies (continued)

- **Improved Treatment and Care**
  - □ Ensure availability of voluntary counseling and testing
  - □ Integrate prevention and treatment
  - □ Provide antiretroviral treatment as prevention
  - □ Reduce stigma and discrimination in the health care setting
  - □ Provide services for the prevention of parent-to-child transmission

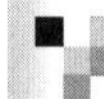

Positive Prevention Strategies (continued)

- **Community Mobilization**
  - □ Facilitate post-HIV test clubs and other peer support groups
  - □ Implement focused communication campaigns
  - □ Train people with HIV as peer outreach workers
  - □ Reinforce prevention for HIV+ people through home-based care
  - □ Address HIV-related gender-based violence

- **Advocacy and Policy Change**
  - □ Involve HIV+ people in the creation of HIV-related policies and programs
  - □ Target prevention to HIV+ people
  - □ Reform legislation to decrease stigma and discrimination
  - □ Increase access to treatment for all HIV+ people

HIV and Sex

- Over 70% of HIV+ people continue to be sexually active after they learn that they are infected.
- While many engage in safer-sex practices, evidence suggests that some HIV+ people continue to have risky sex.
- HIV+ people who have unprotected sex tend to:
    - know less about HIV/AIDS, its transmission, and its effects on health;
    - believe that safer sex is less pleasurable than unsafe sex;
    - lack commitment to practicing safer sex;
    - lack confidence in their ability to practice safer sex;
    - perceive that they have little control over whether condoms are used;
    - have problems communicating with partners about safer sex; and
    - perceive more barriers to condom use.

Risks of Unprotected Sex for HIV+ People

- Unprotected sex not only can transmit infection to uninfected partners; it also increases HIV+ people's risk of getting STIs/STDs.
    - STIs/STDs may accelerate HIV disease in HIV+ people.
    - STIs/STDs can also make HIV transmission to uninfected people more likely.
    - STIs/STDs are often accompanied by open sores or easily injured skin, making direct transmission of HIV through blood more likely.

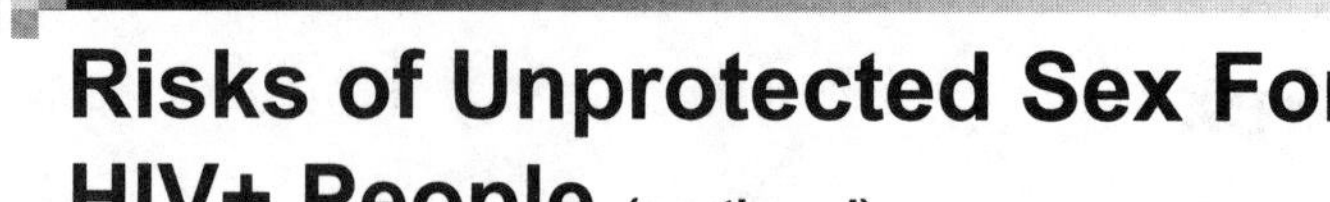

Risks of Unprotected Sex For HIV+ People (continued)

- Unprotected sex can also lead to the more serious threat of superinfection, which happens when an HIV+ person becomes infected with a second strain of HIV.
  - Increasingly, second infections are resistant to antiretroviral therapy.
  - Even recently infected people who have never taken antiretroviral therapy themselves sometimes already have drug-resistant strains of HIV, which they acquired from people who did not adhere to their antiretroviral regimens.
  - Research shows that people who have unprotected sex are less likely to take their antiretroviral drugs correctly.

Reducing HIV Transmission Among HIV+ People

- Prevention interventions improve consistency of condom use, increase perceptions of the advantages of condom use, and increase condom use self-efficacy.
- Social support and mental health counseling reduce the number of HIV+ men's sexual partners and unsafe sexual acts.
- Interventions for HIV+ injection drug users reduce their instances of needle-sharing and unprotected sex.
- Brief safer-sex counseling decreases the number of unprotected sexual acts among HIV+ people, increases consistent condom use, and increases sexual abstinence.

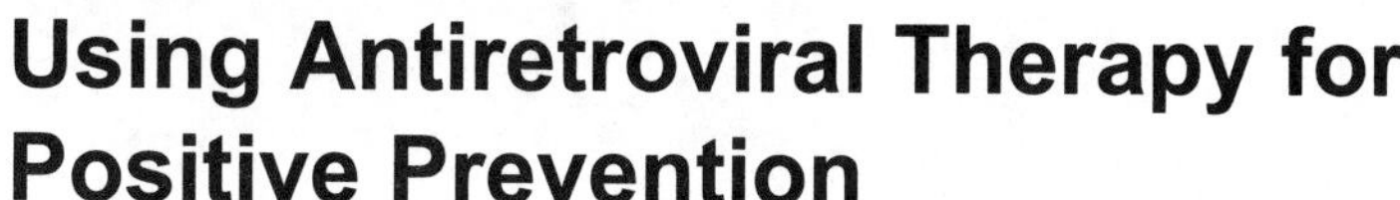

Using Antiretroviral Therapy for Positive Prevention

- Antiretroviral therapy lowers the amount of HIV shed through blood, genital, and anal secretions; with less virus in their body fluids, HIV+ people are less likely to transmit HIV.
- Antiretroviral treatment for HIV+ women and their infants during pregnancy, labor, delivery, and the neonatal period have been shown to reduce parent-to-child transmission.
- Postexposure prophylaxis (PEP) is the giving of antiretroviral therapy to people after they have been exposed to HIV, in an attempt to prevent HIV infection.

PART IV

Gender, Culture, and HIV/AIDS

When it was first reported in June 1981, the unknown disease that later came to be called AIDS seemed to infect only gay men. This has changed. The HIV infection rates and AIDS death toll are evident among people of all age, gender, sexual orientation, socioeconomic status, racial, and ethnic groups. Worldwide, approximately as many women as men have been infected with HIV. However, there are marked differences in the circumstances and implications of the disease for men and for women. Some of these result from biological differences in sex between men and women (as was discussed in Part 1), but more result from socially and culturally defined gender differences. Part 4 explores how gender-based and sociocultural factors come together to increase an individual's risk of becoming infected with HIV, and how gender and culture influence how individuals and societies are affected by AIDS.

"In addition to being a personal tragedy, AIDS has proven to be a social challenge, a cultural catharsis, a political quagmire, and a scientific puzzle. Perhaps more than any other threat to the public health in modern times, the AIDS epidemic has entangled not only individuals but also families and friends, cultures and communities, cities and nations throughout the world. It has cut across race and ethnicity, class and education, age and religion, gender and sexual orientation, challenging the compassion and ingenuity of humankind at every turn" (Smith, 1998).

Learning Objectives

- Describe how issues of sex and gender impact HIV/AIDS
- Understand how culture impacts HIV/AIDS
- Understand the impact of HIV/AIDS on women

Key Terms

culture
disparities
gender
sex

15

Introduction to Gender, Culture, and HIV/AIDS

This chapter defines the concepts of gender and culture and introduces the connection between gender, sociocultural factors, and HIV/AIDS. It also reviews the latest data on the impact of HIV/AIDS on women.

SEX, GENDER, AND HIV/AIDS

Sex versus Gender

Sex describes a biological distinction between men and women. A person's sex is defined by physical features, including a person's chromosomes (genes), internal and external anatomy, and hormones. *Gender*, by contrast, is a social categorization that is learned, rather than inherent. Gender defines the roles, responsibilities, rights, and obligations of men and women (as well as those of boys and girls). Gender roles are defined differently across cultural groups. They are a very powerful feature of social organization, as they not only describe how males and females are expected to behave but also influence power relations, decision-making authority, and individual responsibility. Gender determines to a great extent how we think, how we feel, and what we believe we can and cannot do as women and as men (Feinstein & Prentice, 2001; Lewis, 2003; Wingood & DiClemente, 2000).

Within a given culture, gender roles may differ across the life cycle of men and of women. Moreover, like other social roles and relationships, gender roles can change over time in response to shifts in educational opportunities, economic circumstances, and technology.

Sex describes a biological distinction between men and women.
Gender is a social construct that differentiates the power, roles, responsibilities, and obligations of women from that of men.

Gender influences how women and men seek out and understand information about reproduction, sexuality, and HIV risk; the sexual and drug-use behaviors and practices that foster HIV risk; and how men and women cope with HIV/AIDS-related illness once infected or affected.

Sex, Gender, and HIV/AIDS

As was discussed in Part 2, in the HIV/AIDS epidemic, sex (i.e., the biological state of being male or female) influences the degree and nature of HIV risk. For example, HIV has an easier time surviving in the vagina than it does on the surface of the penis, making it easier for HIV to be transmitted from a man to a woman than from a woman to a man during heterosexual vaginal sex. However, gender also plays a significant role in HIV risk for both men and women. Gender norms influence the psychological states, sexual and drug use behaviors, and economic circumstances that in turn determine men's and women's vulnerability to infection, access to HIV/AIDS treatment services, and ability to sustain themselves economically when they or a family member is diagnosed with or dies of AIDS (Feinstein & Prentice, 2001; Lewis, 2003; Türmen, 2003; UNAIDS, 1999; WHO, 2000, 2002).

A Gender-Based Approach to HIV/AIDS

A gender-based approach to understanding and mobilizing against HIV/AIDS considers how biological, gender, and other sociocultural factors come together to influence risks for and outcomes of HIV/AIDS. A gender-based approach promises to shed light on a number of key facets of the HIV epidemic worldwide, including:

- **Biology:** A gender-based approach helps illuminate the ways that biological differences between men and women shape their experiences with HIV/AIDS risk and transmission in critical ways.
- **Scientific Methodology:** A gender-based approach highlights the fact that clinical research on HIV/AIDS has historically been undertaken with men as research subjects, but that differences in pathology require that clinical management be tailored to women's particular symptoms, disease progression, HIV-related illnesses, and other related issues.
- **Inequality:** A gender-based approach turns a needed focus on gender inequality in its many forms. These include social and cultural attitudes, beliefs and behaviors that support different levels of power and personal control for men and women, and differential access to needed social and medical resources.
- **Oppression:** A gender-based approach requires that we assess the ways that gender-based oppression—including discrimination, stigma, and violence—increases a person's exposure to HIV/AIDS and adversely affects the lives of those living with HIV/AIDS (Feinstein & Prentice, 2001; Lewis, 2003; WHO, 2002).

CULTURE AND HIV/AIDS

What Is Culture?

Culturally determined values influence how HIV and AIDS are perceived, how attitudes toward high-risk behavior are formed, how habits that characterize high-risk behavior are developed, and how risk-reduction information is processed.

When we think about *culture*, we often think about things like foods and festivals, or costumes and customs. But cultures are more than just collections of objects and practices (although these are aspects of culture). Most definitions of culture include the following elements:

- Culture comprises a widely shared set of values, institutions, practices, and beliefs that emerges—and changes—as a group adapts to its environment.
- Culture is learned through social interactions that provide contexts for behavior and influence behavior.
- Cultural traditions are passed down through generations.

People never have just one cultural background. Instead, people are defined by a wide variety of cultural categories. Examples of cultural categories include ethnicity, race, national origin, religion, geographic region, political orientation, sexual orientation, age cohort (e.g., "Generation X"), and disability status. Gender is also an example of a cultural category.

Cultural identity varies both within cultural groups and individuals. For example, Asian American is an extremely broad term that can refer to both third-generation Vietnamese Americans and recent immigrants from Pakistan. Yet, these two groups hold extremely different cultural beliefs and practices. At the same time, each person within a group has a different sense of themselves in relation to their cultural identities (Wilson & Miller, 2003). An individual may identify more strongly with being lesbian than with being an Asian American, a third-generation immigrant, or a woman. HIV prevention programming needs to take into account diversity both across and within clients' cultural groups, as well as the multiple cultural identities of individuals in those groups (Raj, Amaro, & Reed, 2001).

The Relationship Between Culture and HIV/AIDS

People in some cultural groups become infected with HIV and develop AIDS at higher rates than people in others. For example, according to a study of U.S. Job Corps applicants, HIV prevalence among African American adolescent girls was 4.9 per 1,000, whereas rates among White and Hispanic adolescent girls were 0.7 and 0.6, and rates among White, Hispanic, and African American adolescent boys were 0.8, 1.5, and 3.2 per 1,000 (Valleroy, MacKellar, Karon, Janssen, & Hayman, 1998).

Culture plays a significant role in these disparities; it helps shape the many individual, community, and societal-level risk and protective factors for HIV infection, as well as access to HIV/AIDS-related prevention and treatment services (Wilson & Miller, 2003). In particular, cultural beliefs and norms shape definitions of health and illness, beliefs about what causes AIDS and how to prevent HIV transmission, attitudes toward communicating about HIV-related behaviors, and attitudes toward risky behaviors.

For example, to prove their "manhood," Hispanic men may seek many sexual partners (Marín, 2003; Marín, Gómez, & Hearst, 1993). Hispanic women may feel unable to insist on safer sex practices, such as condom use, with male partners (Gómez & Marín, 1996). Cultural values, including racism and sexism, also affect individuals' ability and motivation to access and use HIV prevention and treatment services (Lum, 2003; Office of Minority Health [OMH], 2001; Scott, Gilliam, & Braxton, 2005; Smedley, Adrienne, & Nelson, 2002; Wilson & Miller, 2003). In addition, culture influences the way that those living with HIV/AIDS are understood, perceived, and treated, and the way that communities respond politically, socially, and financially to the threat of further spread of HIV/AIDS (Hoban & Ward, 2003; Smedley, et al., 2002).

WOMEN AND HIV/AIDS

In most societies, girls and women face greater risk of HIV infection than men not only because of biological differences between men and women (NIAID, 2004) (see chapter 3) but also because in many societies women's diminished economic and social status compromises their ability to choose safer and healthier life strategies (UNAIDS, 2001). The epidemic's impact on women has become more pronounced over time.

Rates Among Women Worldwide

In 2005, an estimated 17.5 million women were living with HIV—1 million more than in 2004 (UNAIDS, 2005). Women also comprise an increasing share of new HIV and AIDS cases reported each year. Specifically, as of the end of 2005, women accounted for 48% of the adults ages 15 and over living with HIV/AIDS worldwide (UNAIDS, 2006); in 1997, 41% of HIV+ adults were women (UNAIDS, 2001). This trend also impacts children, as the increase in HIV infection among women of

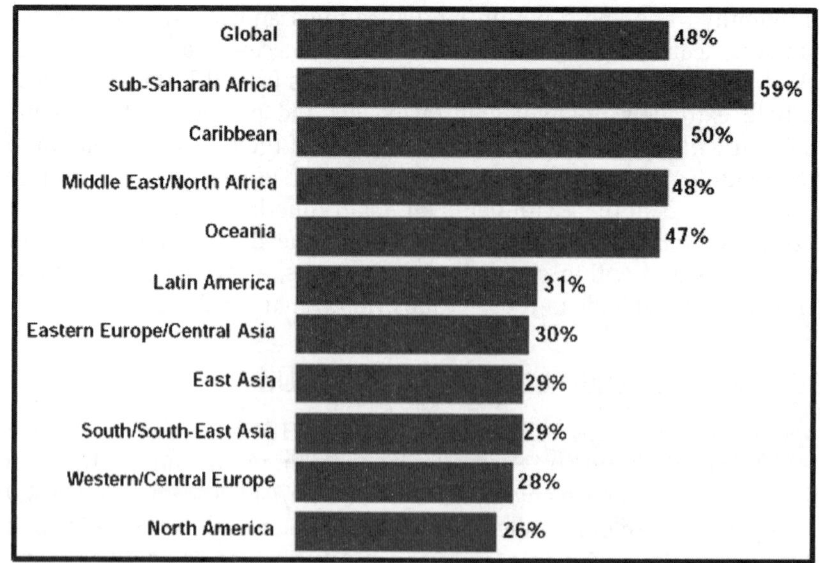

Figure 15-1 Women as a percent of adults (ages 15 and over) living with HIV/AIDS by region, 2006 (Henry J. Kaiser Foundation, 2006, Figure 2).

childbearing age increases the potential risk for vertical transmission of infection to their unborn children and infants.

In certain parts of the world, the rate of HIV/AIDS among women has come to equal or exceed that of men. Women represented at least 50% of the adults living with HIV in sub-Saharan African, Oceania, and the Caribbean as of 2005 (UNAIDS, 2006) (see Figure 15-1). Teens and young adults, particularly girls and young women ages 15–24, are particularly hard hit by the epidemic. In sub-Saharan Africa, on average, three young women are infected for every young man (UNAIDS, 2006). In the Caribbean, young women are about twice as likely to be infected as young men (UNAIDS, 2005, 2006).

Women and HIV/AIDS in the United States

In the United States, the proportion of AIDS cases among female adults and adolescents (age > 13 years) increased from 7% in 1985 to 27% in 2004 (CDC, n.d.b) (see Figure 15-2).

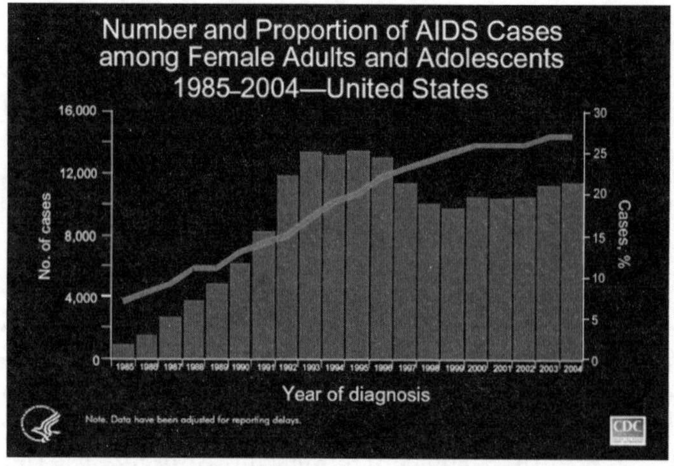

Figure 15-2 Number and proportion of AIDS cases among female adults and adolescents, 1985–2004—United States (CDC, n.d.b).

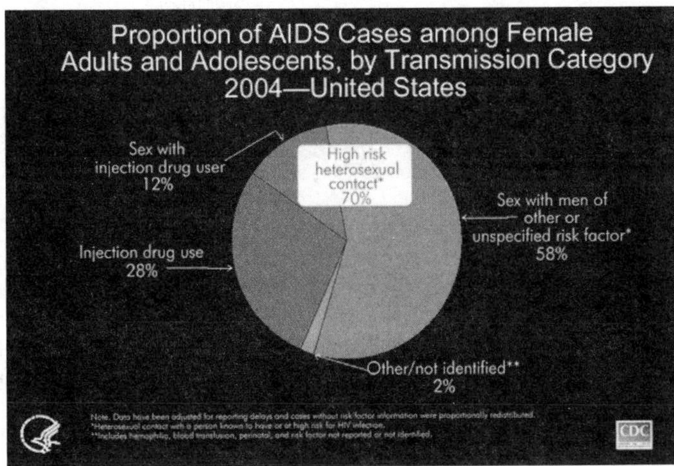

Figure 15-3 Proportion of AIDS cases among female adults and adolescents, by transmission category, 2004—United States (CDC, n.d.c).

For women diagnosed with AIDS in 2004, heterosexual contact with a person known to have HIV or to be at high risk of HIV infection accounted for 70% of cases (CDC, n.d.c) (see Figure 15-3).

The rates of HIV/AIDS across women of different ethnic groups are far from uniform. African American women have the highest rate at 67.0 per 100,000 population (CDC, n.d.a) (see Figure 15-4). This is over 20 times the rate for White women, which is 3.2. Hispanic women have the second highest rate at 16.3 per 100,000.

Frameworks for Studying the Causes and Prevention of HIV Infection in Women

Understanding the causes and reducing the incidence of HIV infection in women depends in part on the conceptual frameworks that guide data collection and interpretation, and program design and implementation. In addition to studying biomedical, lifestyle, and psychological explanations of disease causation, it is important to explore the connections between disease and inequality and between health and social justice. Table 15-1 summarizes alternative frameworks for studying the cause and prevention of HIV infection in women.

Estimated Number of HIV/AIDS Cases and Rates for Female Adults and Adolescents, by Race/Ethnicity 2004—33 States

Race/Ethnicity	Cases*	Rate (cases per 100,000 population)
White, not Hispanic	1,782	3.2
Black, not Hispanic	7,009	67.0
Hispanic	1,400	16.3
Asian/Pacific Islander	94	4.1
American Indian/ Alaska Native	57	7.7
Total**	10,391	13.2

Note. Data include persons with a diagnosis of HIV regardless of AIDS status at diagnosis. Data from 33 states with confidential name-based HIV infection reporting since at least 2000. Data have been adjusted for reporting delays.
* Data exclude persons from US dependencies, possessions and associated nations because of the lack of data by race from these areas.
** Includes 49 female adults and adolescents of unknown race or multiple races.

Figure 15-4 Estimated number of HIV/AIDS cases and rates for female adults and adolescents, by race/ethnicity, 2004—33 states (CDC, n.d.a).

Alternative Frameworks for Studying the Causes and Prevention of HIV Infection in Women (Zierler & Krieger, 2000)

Framework	Assumptions	Examples of Relevant Topics of Study
Feminist	Gender inequality affects health	■ Gender disparity in power and risk of HIV ■ Gender differences in socially sanctioned sexual expression ■ Sexual and physical violence against women as determinants of HIV risk ■ Reproductive autonomy and HIV testing among pregnant women
Sociopolitical	Economic and social relationships affect health	■ Socioeconomic status and HIV infection ■ Social welfare policy, economic dependence on men, and risk of sexual HIV transmission to women ■ Racism and onset of injection drug use in women ■ Reduction in municipal fire protection, destruction of housing, and HIV incidence
Ecosocial	Biology interacts with social, economic, and political conditions to affect health	■ Thinness of peripubescent vaginal mucosal lining and vaginal susceptibility to HIV infection among girls dependent on older men ■ Age-specific vaginal tract inflammation and HIV among women
Human Rights	Violations of human rights affect patterns of disease	■ Relationship between legal barriers to educating women and HIV incidence ■ HIV incidence among drug-using pregnant women in places that criminalize drug use during pregnancy ■ Enforcement of domestic violence and marital rape laws in relation to HIV incidence among women

REFERENCES

Centers for Disease Control and Prevention (CDC). (n.d.a). Estimated number of HIV/AIDS cases and rates for female adults and adolescents, by race/ethnicity, 2004—33 States. In *HIV/AIDS surveillance in women* [Slide series], slide 14. Atlanta, GA: CDC.

Centers for Disease Control and Prevention (CDC). (n.d.b). Number and proportion of AIDS cases among female adults and adolescents, 1985–2004—United States. In *HIV/AIDS surveillance in women* [Slide series], slide 1. Atlanta, GA: CDC.

Centers for Disease Control and Prevention (CDC). (n.d.c). Proportion of AIDS cases among female adults and adolescents, by transmission category, 2004—United States. In *HIV/AIDS surveillance in women* [Slide series], slide 3. Atlanta, GA: Centers for Disease Control and Prevention.

Feinstein, N., & Prentice, B. (2001). *The UNAIDS gender and AIDS almanac.* Los Altos, CA: Sociometrics Corporation.

Gómez, C. A., & Marín, B. V. (1996). Gender, culture, and power: Barriers to HIV prevention strategies. *Journal of Sex Research, 33*(4), 355–362.

Henry J. Kaiser Family Foundation. (2006). *HIV/AIDS policy fact sheet: The global HIV/AIDS epidemic.* Washington, DC: Henry J. Kaiser Family Foundation.

Hoban, M. T., & Ward, M. S. (2003). Building culturally competent college health programs. *Journal of American College Health, 52*(3), 137–141.

Lewis, J. (2003). *Gendering prevention practices.* Oslo, Norway: Nordic Institute for Women's Studies and Gender Research (NIKK).

Lum, D. (2003). *Culturally competent practice: A framework for understanding diverse groups and justice issues.* Pacific Grove, CA: Brooks/Cole.

Marín, B. V. (2003). HIV prevention in the Hispanic community: Sex, culture, and empowerment. *Journal of Transcultural Nursing, 14*(3), 186–192.

Marín, B. V., Gómez, C. A., & Hearst, N. (1993). Multiple heterosexual partners and condom use among Hispanics and non-Hispanic Whites. *Family Planning Perspectives, 25*(4), 170–174.

National Institute of Allergy and Infectious Diseases (NIAID). (2004). *Research on: HIV infection in women.* Bethesda, MD: National Institutes of Health.

Office of Minority Health (OMH), U.S. Department of Health and Human Services (DHSS). (2001). *National standards for culturally and linguistically appropriate services in health care: Final report.* Washington, DC: DHHS.

Raj, A., Amaro, H., & Reed, E. (2001). Culturally tailoring HIV/AIDS prevention programs: Why, when, and how. In S. S. Kazarian & D. R. Evans (Eds.), *Handbook of cultural health psychology* (pp. 195–239). San Diego, CA: Academic Press.

Scott, K. D., Gilliam, A., & Braxton, K. (2005). Culturally competent HIV prevention strategies for women of color in the United States. *Health Care for Women International, 26*(1), 17–45.

Smedley, B. D., Adrienne, Y. S., & Nelson, A. R. (Eds.). (2002). *Unequal treatment: Confronting racial and ethnic disparities in healthcare.* Washington, DC: National Academic Press.

Smith, R. A. (Ed.). (1998). Editor's note and guide to usage. In *The encyclopedia of AIDS: A social, political, cultural, and scientific record of the HIV epidemic* (pp. xxv–xxviii). Chicago: Fitzroy Dearborn.

Türmen, T. (2003). Gender and HIV/AIDS. *International Journal of Gynecology and Obstetrics, 82*(3), 411–418.

United Nations Programme on HIV/AIDS (UNAIDS). (1999). *Gender and HIV/AIDS: Taking stock of research and programmes.* UNAIDS Best Practice Collection. Geneva, Switzerland: UNAIDS.

United Nations Programme on HIV/AIDS (UNAIDS). (2001). *Fact sheet: Gender and HIV/AIDS.* Geneva, Switzerland: UNAIDS.

United Nations Programme on HIV/AIDS (UNAIDS). (2005). *AIDS epidemic update: December 2005.* Geneva, Switzerland: UNAIDS.

United Nations Programme on HIV/AIDS (UNAIDS). (2006). *2006 report on the global AIDS epidemic.* Geneva, Switzerland: UNAIDS.

Valleroy, L. A., MacKellar, D. A., Karon, J. M., Janssen, R. S., & Hayman, C. R. (1998). HIV infection in disadvantaged out-of-school youth: Prevalence for US Job Corps entrants, 1990 through 1996. *Journal of Acquired Immune Deficiency Syndromes and Human Retrovirology, 19*(1), 67–73.

Wilson, B. D. M., & Miller, R. L. (2003). Examining strategies for culturally grounded HIV prevention: A review. *AIDS Education and Prevention, 15*(2), 184–202.

Wingood, G. M., & DiClemente, R. J. (2000). Reconceptualizing women's HIV risk. *Health Education and Behavior, 27*, 570–571.

World Health Organization (WHO). (2000). *Women and HIV/AIDS (Fact sheet no. 242).* Geneva, Switzerland: WHO.

World Health Organization (WHO). (2002). *Integrating gender into HIV/AIDS programmes, review paper for expert consultation, June 3–5, 2002.* Geneva, Switzerland: WHO.

Zierler, S., & Krieger, N. (2000). Social inequality and HIV infection in women. In K. H. Mayer & H. F. Pizer (Eds.), *The emergence of AIDS: The impact on immunology, microbiology, and public health* (pp. 76–97). Washington, DC: American Public Health Association.

Instructor Resources

LEARNING ACTIVITIES

ACTIVITY 1:

Group Activity: Defining Gender and Sex: What Do They Mean?

Adapted from Exercise 1A in Gender or Sex: Who Cares? Skills-Building Resource Pack on Gender and Reproductive Health for Adolescents and Youth Workers (de Bruyn, 2001), page 20.

Objective: To enable participants to begin to distinguish the concepts of "gender" and "sex."

Minimum Time: 20 minutes

View this activity at http://www.genderandaids.org/modules.php?name=News&file=article&sid=173

ACTIVITY 2:

Group Activity: Gender Not Sex

Adapted from Exercise 3 in Gender or Sex: Who Cares? Skills-Building Resource Pack on Gender and Reproductive Health for Adolescents and Youth Workers (de Bruyn, 2001), page 26.

Objective: To improve participants' understanding of the difference between "sex" and "gender," and to learn to recognize gender stereotypes.

Minimum Time: 20 minutes

View this activity at http://www.genderandaids.org/modules.php?name=News&file=article&sid=173

ACTIVITY 3:

Group Activity: Is It Sex or Gender?

Adapted from Exercise 11 in Gender or Sex: Who Cares? Skills-Building Resource Pack on Gender and Reproductive Health for Adolescents and Youth Workers (de Bruyn, 2001), page 32.

Objective: To improve participants' understanding of the difference between gender and sex, and to create a setting in which to discuss the inequalities between men and women that affect sexuality and risk.

Minimum Time: 30 minutes

View this activity at http://www.genderandaids.org/modules.php?name=News&file=article&sid=173

ACTIVITY 4:

Assignment: Gender, Culture, and HIV/AIDS

Objective: To understand how HIV/AIDS affects particular geographic regions.

Choose a country or region in the world. Write an eight- to ten-page research paper on how gender and culture influence the transmission of or protection against HIV/AIDS in that country or region of the world.

Please include the following in your paper:

- A description of the current status of the HIV/AIDS epidemic in that part of the world
- Your definitions of "gender" and "culture"

ACTIVITY 5:

Assignment: Studying the Causes and Prevention of HIV Infection in Women

Objective: Understanding how HIV/AIDS impacts women.

Much of the literature on women and HIV has relied on biomedical, lifestyle, and psychological explanations of disease causation. Write a two- to three-page paper presenting an alternative framework for studying the causes and prevention of HIV infection in women that make connections between disease and inequality and between health and social justice. Offer examples of recent research that is based on the framework.

View Table 15-1, "Alternative Frameworks for Studying the Causes and Prevention of HIV Infection in Women."

DISCUSSION QUESTIONS

1. Describe some gender roles in your culture that might affect sexual behavior.
2. How might cultural beliefs affect rates of HIV/AIDS transmission?
3. What causes racial and ethnic disparities in health issues? Why are these causes important to understand and address?

QUIZ

1. ___ describes the biological distinction between men and women; ___ is a learned social characterization.
   a) Gender; sex
   b) Sex; gender
   c) Sex; culture
   d) Gender; culture
2. True or False: Gender roles are largely similar across different cultural groups.
3. Which of the following is not a cultural category?
   a) Gender
   b) Ethnicity

c) Race
d) Religion
e) Sexual orientation
f) Age
g) Political affiliation
h) All of the above
i) None of the above

4. Compared to Whites, HIV prevalence among African Americans is:
a) Higher
b) Lower
c) About the same
d) Impossible to measure

5. How many women were living with HIV in 2005 worldwide?
a) Nearly 5 million
b) Nearly 10 million
c) Nearly 15 million
d) Nearly 20 million

6. Compared to 1997, in 2005 the number of women living with HIV/AIDS worldwide was:
a) Higher than in 1997
b) Slightly lower than in 1997
c) Significantly lower than in 1997
d) About the same as 1997

7. In the United States, the proportion of AIDS cases among females ___ from 1985 to 2004.
a) Increased slightly
b) Increased significantly
c) Decreased slightly
d) Decreased significantly

8. What was the most common cause of HIV transmission among U.S. women diagnosed with AIDS in 2004?
a) Homosexual sex
b) Heterosexual sex
c) Intravenous drug use
d) Childbirth

ANSWERS

1. B. *Sex* describes a biological distinction between men and women. A person's sex is defined by physical features, including a person's chromosomes (genes), internal and external anatomy, and hormones. *Gender*, by contrast, is a social categorization that is learned, rather than inherent.

2. False. Gender roles are defined differently across cultural groups.

3. I. Examples of cultural categories include ethnicity, race, national origin, religion, geographic region, political orientation, sexual orientation, age cohort (e.g., "Generation X"), and disability status. Gender is also an example of a cultural category.

4. A. Culture plays a significant role in these disparities.

5. D. In 2005 an estimated 17.5 million women were living with HIV.

6. **A.** As of the end of 2005, women accounted for 48% of the adults ages 15 and over living with HIV/AIDS worldwide; in 1997, 41% of HIV-positive adults were women.
7. **B.** In the United States, the proportion of AIDS cases among female adults and adolescents increased from 7% in 1985 to 27% in 2004.
8. **B.** For women diagnosed with AIDS in 2004, heterosexual contact with a person known to have HIV or to be at a high risk of HIV infection accounted for 70% of cases.

WEB RESOURCES

Facts and Figures About HIV/AIDS

Current Worldwide HIV/AIDS Statistics—AIDS Epidemic Update (UNAIDS)

http://www.unaids.org/en/HIV_data/default.asp

This report, published annually in December by WHO and UNAIDS, contains up-to-date information and statistics about the global pandemic.

Current U.S. HIV/AIDS Statistics—HIV/AIDS Surveillance Report (CDC)

http://www.cdc.gov/hiv/topics/surveillance/resources/reports/index.htm

This report, published annually by the Centers for Disease Control, contains up-to-date information and statistics about the epidemic in the United States.

Women and HIV/AIDS in the United States: Setting an Agenda for the Future, A Policy Forum (Kaiser Family Foundation)

http://www.kff.org/hivaids/hiv102303package.cfm

This site contains links to information presented at a meeting hosted by the Kaiser Family Foundation in 2003, including fact sheets on women and HIV/AIDS in the United States and a link to a documentary film created by Rory Kennedy and Moxie Firecracker Films—*Hidden Crisis: Women and AIDS in America.*

Gender and HIV/AIDS

EngenderHealth

http://www.engenderhealth.org/

The Web site of EngenderHealth, a U.S.-based organization that works to improve reproductive health in developing countries, offers a wide range of information and resources on family planning, maternal/child health, men's health, HIV and other sexually transmitted infections, and sexuality and gender. Special "in-action" sections discuss topics such as "ensuring women's health" and "working with men." EngenderHealth also provides Web-based and CD-ROM self-instructional courses for health care providers, supervisors, students, and trainers all over the world. The courses are designed particularly for those in low-resource settings, and cover such topics as sexuality and sexual health, sexually transmitted infections, HIV and AIDS, and infection prevention. Also available are a number of professional materials, including a training package on men's reproductive health.

Gender and AIDS (UNIFEM/UNAIDS)

http://www.genderandaids.org

The United Nations Development Fund for Women (UNIFEM) and UNAIDS recently created "the first comprehensive gender and HIV/AIDS web portal." This site is committed to providing users with cutting-edge research, studies and surveys, training materials, multimedia advocacy tools, speeches and presentations, press releases and current news, best practices, e-mail updates and newsletters, online discussion forums, and links to Web sites and databases.

Culture and HIV/AIDS

A Cultural Approach to HIV/AIDS Prevention and Care (UNESCO and UNAIDS)

http://portal.unesco.org/aids

This Web site, sponsored by the United Nations Educational, Scientific, and Cultural Organization and UNAIDS, provides information and stimulates reflection and action for better application of "a cultural approach" in strategies, policies, projects, and fieldwork. This strategy engages populations in the fight against HIV/AIDS on the basis of their own cultural references and resources (ways of life, value systems, traditions, beliefs, religions, and fundamental human rights).

RECOMMENDED READING

Gender, Culture, and HIV/AIDS

Fact Sheet on HIV/AIDS Among U.S. Women (Centers for Disease Control and Prevention, 2003)

This fact sheet provides statistics and outlines the prevention needs of women in the United States.
Available online at http://www.cdc.gov/hiv/topics/women/resources/factsheets/women.htm

Fact Sheet on HIV Infection and Women (National Institute of Allergy and Infectious Diseases, 2003)

This fact sheet provides an overview of HIV/AIDS in women and reviews gender-specific manifestations of HIV infection and AIDS disease.
Available online at http://www.niaid.nih.gov/factsheets/womenhiv.htm

AIDS Action Policy Fact Sheet on Women and HIV/AIDS (AIDS Action, 2002)

This fact sheet discusses risk factors, HIV prevention and women, as well as how HIV affects women differently than men.
Available online at http://www.aidsaction.org/

United Nations Development Programme (UNDP) HIV/AIDS Publications

A series of papers exploring specific areas of the relationship between the epidemic and gender, including adolescent sexuality, violence, and the involvement of men.
Available online at http://www.undp.org/dpa/publications/hiv.html

Key Facts: Women and HIV/AIDS (Kaiser Family Foundation, 2003)

Kates, J., Ruiz, S., Ranji, U., Salganikoff, A., & Pontius, C. O. (2003). Key facts: Women and HIV/AIDS (report #6093). *Menlo Park, CA: Kaiser Family Foundation.*

Key Facts: Women and HIV/AIDS provides comprehensive data on the impact of HIV/AIDS epidemic on women in the United States. Based on the most recent data and research on the epidemiology of HIV/AIDS among women, the report includes an overview of the epidemic profile, a profile of women living with HIV/AIDS, data on access to and use of health services, and women's perceptions of HIV/AIDS.
Available online at http://www.kff.org/hivaids/hiv6093report.cfm

Integrating Gender Into HIV/AIDS Programs (WHO, 2002)

WHO. (2002). Integrating gender into HIV/AIDS programmes, review paper for expert consultation 3–5 June 2002. Geneva, Switzerland:WHO.

This review paper was prepared for an Expert Consultation organized by the World Health Organization that brought together experts from the field of HIV/AIDS, gender, health and development, as well as program managers who implement HIV/AIDS programs at the national level. This paper provided participants to the Expert Consultation with background information and a suggested framework for considering the issues and challenges of integrating gender into programmatic and policy action. It also offers some programmatic examples of successful HIV/AIDS interventions that have addressed gender in a meaningful and significant way.
Available online at http://www.who.int/gender/hiv_aids/hivaids1103.pdf

Social Inequality and HIV Infection in Women (Zierler & Krieger, 2000)

Zierler, S., & Krieger, N. (2000). Social inequality and HIV infection in women. In K. H. Mayer & H. F. Pizer (Eds.), The emergence of AIDS: The impact on immunology, microbiology, and public health. *Washington, DC: American Public Health Association.*

Social inequality plays a significant role in HIV infection among U.S. women. To explain which women are at risk and why, this chapter reviews the epidemiology of HIV and AIDS among women in light of conceptual frameworks that link health with social justice. Specifically, data linking inequality of class, race/ethnicity, sex, and sexuality to the distribution of HIV among women are reviewed.

Gendering Prevention Practices (Nordic Institute for Women's Studies and Gender Research [NIKK], 2003)

Lewis, J. (2003). Gendering prevention practices. *Oslo, Norway: Nordic Institute for Women's Studies and Gender Research (NIKK).*

This training manual lays out eight sessions, each with an array of diverse learning activities, for capacity building to help participants grasp the implications of working with gender in HIV prevention. The session themes are: Perceptions of Gender, Ways of Understanding Gender, Key Aspects of Gender for HIV Prevention, Sex as a Gendered Activity, Gender and HIV, Embodying Change, A Sense of Working Together, Reviewing Gender Issues in Context.
Available for free download at http://www.nikk.uio.no/forskning/nikk/living/manuals_questionnaire.html

Culture and AIDS (Feldman, 1990)

Feldman, D. A. (Ed.). (1990). Culture and AIDS. *Westport, CT: Praeger.*

This collection of essays focuses on the meaning and manifestations of AIDS as a cultural phenomenon. Written almost entirely by anthropologists, the chapters of this volume look at the meaning of AIDS in Africa, how one Haitian village handles AIDS in their midst, possible cofactors in HIV transmission, social service needs of gay men with AIDS in New York City, how psychological factors influence adjustment among HIV-infected gay men in Houston, social behavior of female prostitutes in London, the social effects of AIDS on minority women, the role of AIDS-related stigma in the press, the relationship between language and AIDS, and other AIDS-related arenas.

Cultural Competence in HIV/AIDS Prevention (Vinh-Thomas, Bunch, & Card, 2003)

Vinh-Thomas, P., Bunch, M. M., & Card, J. J. (2003). A research-based tool for identifying and strengthening culturally competent and evaluation-ready HIV/AIDS prevention programs. AIDS Education and Prevention, 15*(6), 481–498.*

Recent literature on racial disparities in HIV/AIDS and effective HIV/AIDS health service delivery efforts has underscored the importance of cultural sensitivity, relevance, and competence in reducing such disparities and providing effective health service delivery. Less work has been done on the role of cultural competence in the delivery of effective HIV/AIDS prevention programs, perhaps because few such prevention programs aimed at minority populations have to date been demonstrated as effective. This paper surveys the various ways that the concept of cultural competence has been studied, extends the concept to the field of HIV/AIDS prevention, and presents a simple-to-use instrument that operationalizes the concept for use with HIV/AIDS prevention programs.

POWERPOINT SLIDES

(Note: A full-color version of these slides, with graphics, is also available on the CD-ROM.)

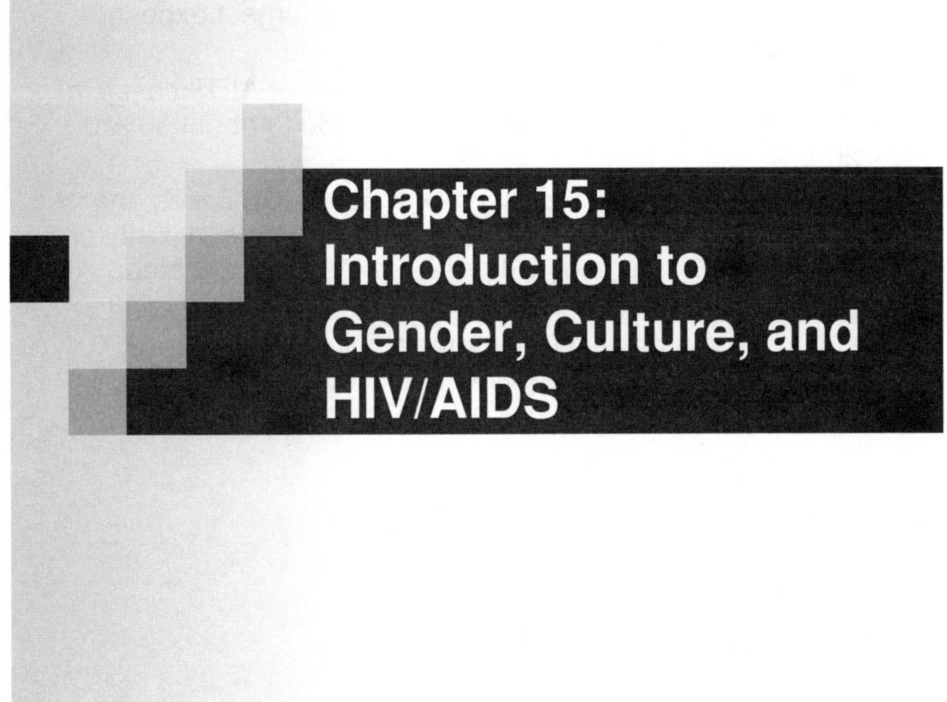

Introduction to Gender, Culture, and HIV/AIDS

- The death toll and HIV infection rates are evident among people of all ages, genders, sexual orientations, socioeconomic levels, races, and ethnicities.
- More than four in ten Americans (43%) say they know someone who is either living with HIV/AIDS or has died of AIDS.
- More than one in three Americans (37%) say they are personally concerned about becoming infected.
- There are 1 million people living with HIV in the United States.

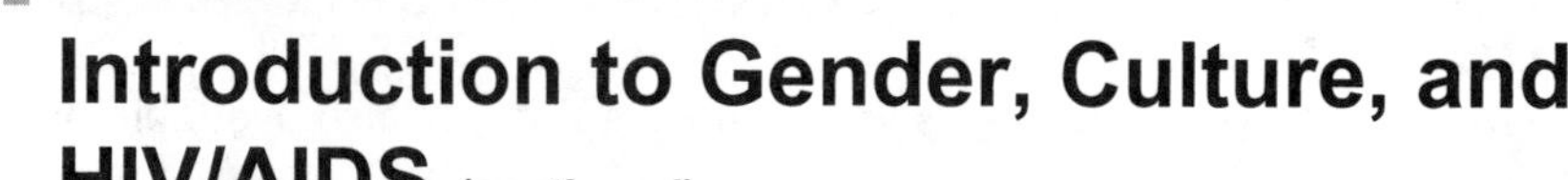

Introduction to Gender, Culture, and HIV/AIDS (continued)

- Men who have sex with men remain the largest exposure group in the United States.
- Women account for a growing proportion of AIDS cases in the United States, rising from 7% in 1986 to about 30% in 2002.
- Minorities represent the majority of new AIDS cases, the majority of Americans living with AIDS, and the majority of deaths among persons with AIDS in the United States.
- HIV/AIDS is more concentrated in the developing world and in the marginalized communities in industrialized countries. HIV/AIDS flourishes in conditions of poverty, conflict, and inequality.

Sex, Gender, and Biology

Biological differences between men and women account for differences in vulnerability to HIV transmission and infection.

The Connection Between Gender and HIV/AIDS

- A gender-based approach to understanding HIV/AIDS involves understanding how biological and gender factors increase an individual's risk of becoming infected and ability to access treatment and care once infected.
- For example:
  - □ Looking critically at how the gender norms and expectations within a culture inform and affect sexual behaviors promotes key understandings about what perpetuates heterosexual risk behaviors
  - □ Highlighting how gender stereotypes and expectations affect both women and men, and supporting work to improve gender equality and equity in relationships and in the public spheres

Biological Factors Correlated With HIV Infection

Biological risk factors that are correlated with HIV infection include:

- increased accessibility of HIV to infectable cells (through cuts, tears, or exposed sensitive skin like in the vagina or anus);
- infection with another STI/STD (especially ulcerative ones);
- stage of the illness (higher concentrations of HIV are found in blood and semen during the first few months and at later phases of infection); and
- history of antiretroviral medication (antiretroviral medications lower concentrations of HIV in blood, which may potentially reduce infectivity).

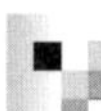

The Connection Between Culture and HIV/AIDS

- Culture is the process of sharing language and utilizing symbols to organize and give meaning to behavior.
- Culture influences:
  - the way people think about gender, sexuality, health, and illness;
  - the way people perceive HIV/AIDS;
  - the choices we make in relation to HIV/AIDS risk behaviors;
  - the ways that those with HIV/AIDS are perceived and treated; and
  - social, educational, political, religious, institutional, and community responses to HIV/AIDS.
- Culturally competent programs are tailored to fit the linguistic, socioeconomic, and functional needs of a given population.

Women and HIV/AIDS: Global

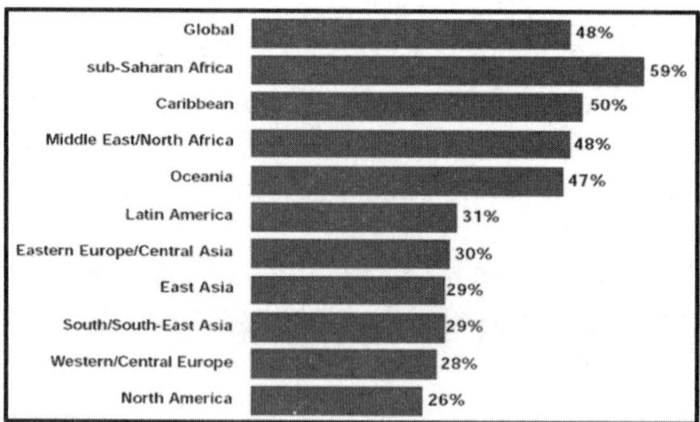

Women and HIV/AIDS: Global (continued)

- The epidemic's impact on women has become greater over time, with women comprising an increasing share of new HIV and AIDS cases reported each year.
- Girls and women face heavier risks of HIV infection than men because of biological differences and diminished economic and social status.
- In 1997, 41% of people living with HIV around the world were women; in 2006, about 48% were women.
- In 2001, AIDS ranked as one of the leading causes of death among women aged 20-40 in several cities in Europe, sub-Saharan Africa, and North America.
- At the beginning of the 21st century, women accounted for over 50% of adults who have died of AIDS since the epidemic began.

Women and HIV/AIDS: United States

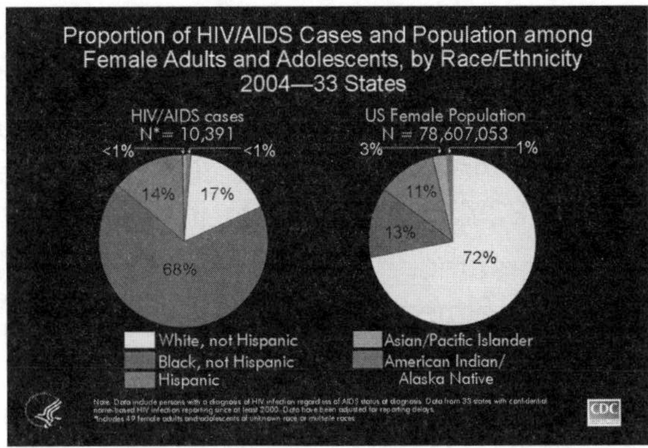

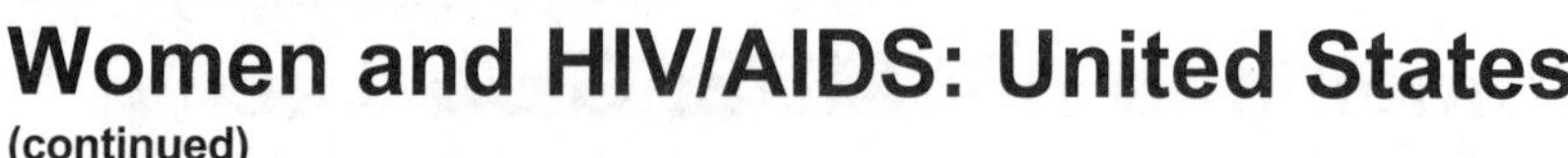

Women and HIV/AIDS: United States
(continued)

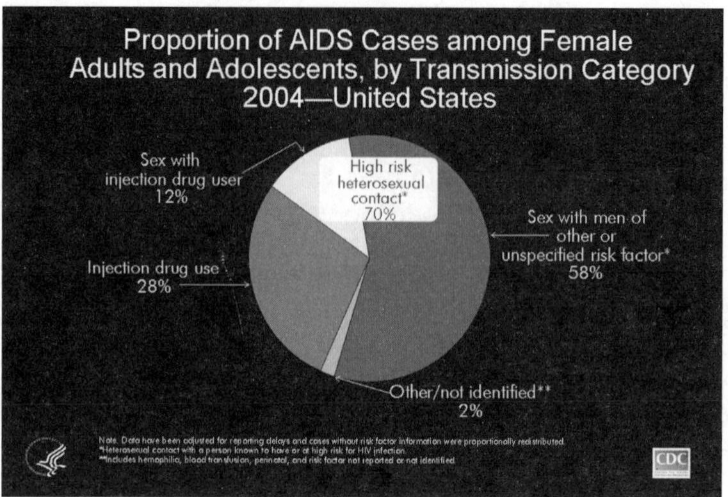

Women and HIV/AIDS: United States
(continued)

- In the United States, HIV infection disproportionately affects African American and Hispanic women. Together they represent less than 25% of all U.S. women, yet they account for about 82% of AIDS cases in women.
- The rate of infection among African American women in the United States is almost 4 times that among White women.
- The most common sources of infections for women remain heterosexual intercourse with an injection drug user and injection drug use.

Studying HIV Infection in Women

- Understanding and reducing HIV infection in women depends, in part, on conceptual frameworks that guide data collection and interpretation, and program design and implementation.
- It is important to explore the connections between disease and inequality and between health and social justice.
- Some alternative frameworks for studying HIV infection in women include:
  - Feminist – focusing on how gender inequality affects health
  - Sociopolitical – focusing on how economic and social relationships affect health
  - Ecosocial – focusing on how biology interacts with social, economic, and political conditions to affect health
  - Human Rights – focusing on how violations of human rights affect patterns of disease

Learning Objectives

- Understand how gender norms influence the risk of HIV/AIDS for both men and women

Key Terms

dry sex
female circumcision
female genital mutilation
gender norms
wife inheritance

16

Gender-Based Cultural Expectations and Traditions

A culture's gender norms influence the behavior that is expected of men and women, boys and girls. Culturally defined "masculine" and "feminine" roles are a powerful feature of social organization that also influence power relations, decision-making authority, and individual responsibility. This chapter explores how gender-based expectations and selected cultural practices intersect to influence risk for, and responses to, HIV/AIDS.

It is important to bear in mind that although the gender norms presented are common worldwide, in every society there are many kinds of masculinity and femininity that may vary by social class, ethnicity, sexuality, and age. Gender roles are learned, rather than inherent, and vary from culture to culture. They can change over time as a result of evolving economic, educational, political, religious, and technological circumstances and opportunities.

The social status and cultural expectations of both men and women can increase the risk of HIV infection.

GENDER NORMS FOR WOMEN

The dominant ideology of femininity in most societies dictates that women should be subordinate, dependent, and passive. Key virtues of the ideal woman include virginity (if she is not married), chastity, motherhood, moral superiority, and obedience to men (WHO, 2002). (See Figure 16-1 for an example.) These beliefs may be magnified in the context of poverty or limited formal education (Lewis, 2003).

Traditional norms concerning femininity tend to encourage women to be:

- **Sexually Ignorant**—Many cultures consider female ignorance of sexual matters a sign of purity. Conversely, knowledge of sexual matters and reproductive physiology is a sign of promiscuity. Young women are hesitant to seek information on sexual health for fear of appearing sexually active. Even when a woman does know about HIV/AIDS, its transmission, and how to protect herself, she is usually not empowered to use that knowledge to change the risky sexual situation.
- **Sexually Passive**—This means that women are not supposed to initiate sexual encounters, and that within sexual encounters, women should defer to the sexual pleasure of men. This leaves women and girls with little control

Marianismo and *machismo* refer to traditional values that govern how Hispanic men and women should behave and be perceived. These roles influence many behaviors, including sexual behaviors that affect HIV risk (UNAIDS, 1999; UNFPA, 2000).

Marianismo

Marianismo is a cultural value that prescribes that a woman should be emotional, kind, passive, religiously observant, chaste, and a virgin until married. She should put her family's needs above her own and obey her father or (once married) her husband ("The Marianismo Ideal"). Women who appear to deviate from this ideal by talking about sex, acting like they enjoy sex, or initiating discussion about condoms may be considered promiscuous (Faulkner, 2003). Because of *marianismo*, women may have difficulty refusing sex or negotiating condom use, as it is considered the man's role to know about sex and make these decisions (HIV/AIDS Bureau, 1999).

Machismo

Machismo is a Hispanic cultural value that prescribes that a man should be strong and a protector of his family. However, machismo also entails that a man constantly "prove" his masculinity. This may lead men to have multiple sex partners, engage in other risky sexual behaviors, and avoid discussing the consequences of those risks with partners. Men also may sexually coerce women to show their strength and exhibit homophobia to show their disdain of men who do not conform to traditional macho standards (Marín, 2003).

Figure 16-1 Example of traditional gender roles: Marianismo and machismo.

over when, where, whether, and how sexual activities occur, including the use of condoms.

- **Sexually Innocent**—In societies that place a high value on virginity and sexual inexperience among young, unmarried women, some young women practice anal sex in order to "protect" their virginity (UNAIDS, 1999). In addition, in areas of high seroprevalence, it has been reported that older men seek out younger girls in the belief that, as virgins, they are free from HIV. In some areas, men believe they can rid themselves of HIV or STDs/STIs by having sex with a virgin.

As a result of traditional gender values, women tend to have less power than men to decide with whom, how, when and whether they have sex. The state of women's lower sexual status is reflected in the following statistics: Each year worldwide, there are an estimated 80 million unwanted pregnancies, 20 million unsafe abortions, and 500,000 maternal deaths (including 78,000 as a result of unsafe abortions) (UNFPA, 2000).

GENDER NORMS FOR MEN

In contrast to the prevalent ideology of femininity, the dominant ideology of masculinity characterizes men as independent, dominant, invulnerable aggressors, and providers whose key virtues are strength, virility, and courage. (See Figure 16-1 for an example.) Most cultures socialize men to believe that it is integral to being a man to take risks—particularly sexual risks, including having sex with multiple partners. Men are also often expected to display dominant, sometimes violent, behavior toward women and toward men perceived to be weak or effeminate, and to be the breadwinners for their families. These cultural beliefs and expectations heighten men's vulnerability to HIV infection, as they encourage men to be:

- **Sexually Knowledgeable**—Men and boys in many cultures are expected to know about sex and sexuality. This expectation that they should "know what to do" in regard to sex may deter them from seeking information about

HIV/AIDS for fear of appearing ignorant about sexual matters and therefore unmasculine.

- **Sexually Aggressive**—Stereotypical characteristics of men include dominance, physical strength, virility, and risk-taking. The pressure to exhibit these characteristics can encourage men to engage in unsafe sex practices. In addition, sexual aggression implies pursuing a number of sexual partners and being "in control" of sexual interactions.
- **Sexually Experienced**—There is often an underlying belief that men "need" multiple sexual partners. Having multiple partners, particularly high-risk partners such as commercial sex workers, and engaging in unprotected sex increase the risk of contracting HIV.

GENDER, TRADITIONAL PRACTICES, AND RISK

Traditional cultural practices reflect values and beliefs held by members of a community that are often passed down from generation to generation. Every social grouping in the world has specific traditional cultural practices and beliefs, some of which are beneficial to all members, while others are harmful to a specific group, such as women (Office of the High Commissioner for Human Rights [OHCHR], n.d.). Several of these harmful traditional practices include *female genital mutilation (FGM)*, child marriage, the practice of *dry sex*, and the practice of *wife inheritance* (Human Rights Watch, 2003; OHCHR, n.d.).

Examples of gender-based traditional customs and practices that promote the risk of acquiring and transmitting HIV/AIDS include:

- Female Genital Mutilation
- Child Marriage
- Dry Sex
- Wife Inheritance and Ritual Cleansing

Female Genital Mutilation

Female genital mutilation (FGM), often referred to as *female circumcision*, is a culturally motivated practice that involves partial or complete removal of the external female genitalia, or other injury to the female genitals (WHO, 2000). FGM is usually performed in childhood or adolescence (Human Rights Watch, 2003; WHO, 2000). Most of the estimated 100–140 million girls and women worldwide who have undergone FGM live in Africa, although some live in Asia and the Middle East. An increasing number are living in Europe, Australia, Canada, and the United States, primarily as a result of immigration (WHO, 2000).

The immediate and long-term health consequences of the procedure can include hemorrhage, infection, urinary incontinence, sexual dysfunction, complications in childbirth, anxiety and depression, and death (WHO, 2003). Although few clinical studies have been conducted, it is clear that FGM also may increase the HIV transmission risk faced by women and girls, as instruments used in the cutting may be shared, facilitating HIV infection via the blood on non-sterile instruments. In addition, some types of FGM are associated with chronic genital injury and tearing, ulceration and delayed healing of injuries, all of which may increase HIV risk through sexual contact (Brady, 1999).

As was described in chapter 3, male circumcision (surgical removal or partial removal of the foreskin of the penis), a common practice in many cultures, can reduce the risk of a man's acquiring or transmitting HIV both directly and indirectly. It reduces risk directly by removing cells that are particularly susceptible to HIV infection. It reduces risk indirectly by making it less likely that a man will acquire or transmit other STIs/STDs that can increase HIV infection and transmission risk. However, as in the case of FGM, when circumcision is performed using non-sterile instruments, HIV transmission risk may be increased (Feinstein & Prentice, 2001).

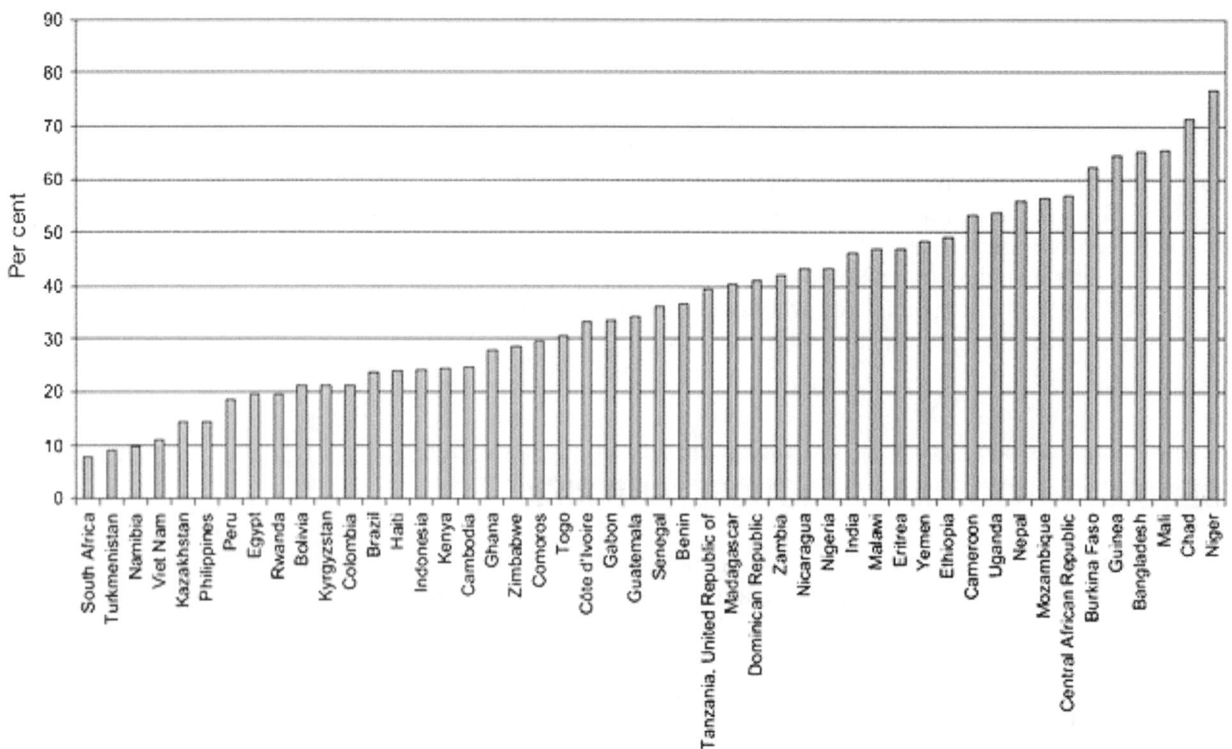

Figure 16-2 Proportion of women aged 20–24 married by the age of 18 (UNICEF, 2006).

Child Marriage

Instead of being viewed as youth with potential and opportunities in their lives, girls are often defined by social customs and gender norms solely as wives and mothers. As a result, although many countries have national laws and signed international agreements forbidding early marriage, millions of young girls, particularly in the developing world, are married when they are still children (see Figure 16-2). Married adolescent girls typically are much younger and more sexually inexperienced than their husbands, have limited educational attainment and social support, experience intense pressure to become pregnant, have limited access to modern media (e.g., television, radio), and lack viable work skills (UNFPA, n.d.). These factors make it difficult for adolescent wives to access HIV prevention education and treatment services, negotiate safer sex with their husbands, and leave husbands who are violent or substance-using or who engage in risky sexual practices with other women. Studies have shown that girls who are married before age 18 are less likely than women who marry at older ages to know how to prevent HIV infection (UNICEF, 2006).

Dry Sex

The use of herbs and other substances to reduce vaginal fluids and tighten the vagina for increased friction during sexual intercourse is known as "dry sex." Dry sex practices has been identified in South Africa, Senegal, Zaire, Cameroon, Malawi, Zambia, Kenya, Zimbabwe, Nigeria, Saudi Arabia, Indonesia, Malaysia, Haiti, and Costa Rica (Kun, 1998). In one study of sexual practices in Zimbabwe, some women reported that they practiced dry sex to enhance male pleasure, in order to keep their male partners from leaving, and/or to minimize the number of girlfriends they may seek. Men corroborated this sentiment (Van de Wijgert et al., 1999). In some cultures, dry sex is practiced because vaginal secretions are associated with infidelity, infection, or dirtiness (Access Working Group, 2002).

Dry sex has important implications for women's vulnerability to HIV. First, dry sex increases risk of HIV infection because it increases the likelihood of tears and lacerations in the vaginal wall, especially among adolescent girls (Human Rights Watch, 2003). In addition, the practice of dry sex may deter women from using microbicides, substances that women can insert into the vagina or rectum to help prevent sexual transmission of HIV by killing or inactivating the virus (Van de Wijgert et al., 1999).

Wife Inheritance and Ritual Cleansing

Wife inheritance is a traditional practice in many parts of Africa whereby a young widow is inherited by a brother in-law or any other suitor chosen by the village elders (Muthengi, 2003). If the widow's husband died of AIDS, it is likely that she is also infected and may transmit the virus to her new husband. A widow who is not HIV+ is likewise at risk for acquiring HIV from her new husband. Ritual cleansing is a traditional practice whereby widows are obliged to have sex (usually unprotected) one time or over a short period with a man who is a social outcast and who is paid for this purpose (Human Rights Watch, 2003). These traditional practices have the intent and effect of perpetuating women's dependence on men and undercutting their social and economic status, which in turn further increases women's risk for acquiring HIV. In Western Kenya, where these practices are most common, the HIV infection rate in girls and young women is 6 times higher than that of their male counterparts (Human Rights Watch, 2003).

REFERENCES

Access Working Group, Microbicide Initiative. (2002). *Preparing for microbicide access and use.* New York: The Rockefeller Foundation.

Brady, M. (1999). Female genital mutilation: Complications and risk of HIV transmission. *AIDS Patient Care and STDs, 13*(12), 709–716.

Faulkner, S. L. (2003). Good girl or flirt girl: Latinas' definition of sex and sexual relationships. *Hispanic Journal of Behavioral Sciences, 25*(2), 174–200.

Feinstein, N., & Prentice, B. (2001). *The UNAIDS gender and AIDS almanac.* Los Altos, CA: Sociometrics Corporation.

HIV/AIDS Bureau, Health Resources and Services Administration (HRSA). (1999). *Hispanics with HIV disease: Barriers to care.* Washington, DC: Department of Health and Human Services (DHSS).

Human Rights Watch. (2003). *Policy paralysis: A call for action on HIV/AIDS-related human rights abuses against women and girls in Africa.* Chicago, IL: Human Rights Watch.

Kun, K. (1998). Vaginal drying agents and HIV transmission. *International Family Planning Perspectives, 24*(2), 93–94.

Lewis, M. (2003). *Gendering AIDS: Women, men, empowerment, mobilisation.* London: VSO.

Marín, B. V. (2003). HIV prevention in the Hispanic community: Sex, culture, and empowerment. *Journal of Transcultural Nursing, 14*(3), 186–192.

Muthengi, A. (2003, November 18). Kenyan women fight wife inheritance. *BBC News* [Television broadcast].

Office of the High Commissioner for Human Rights (OHCHR). (n.d.). *Fact sheet 23: Harmful traditional practices affecting the health of women and children.* Geneva, Switzerland: OHCHR.

The marianismo ideal. (n.d). Retrieved September 18, 2006, from http://web.grinnell.edu/LatinAmericanStudies/this.html

United Nations Children's Fund (UNICEF). (2006). *Early marriage: A harmful traditional practice.* Retrieved September 19, 2006, from http://www.unicef.org/publications/files/Early_Marriage_12.lo.pdf

United Nations Population Fund (UNFPA). (2000). *The state of the world's population—Lives together, worlds apart: Men and women in a time of change.* New York: UNFPA.

United Nations Population Fund (UNFPA). (n.d.). Child marriage fact sheet. In *State of the World Population 2005: Journalists' Press Kit.* New York: UNFPA.

United Nations Programme on HIV/AIDS (UNAIDS). (1999). *Gender and HIV/AIDS: Taking stock of research and programmes*. UNAIDS Best Practice Collection. Geneva, Switzerland: UNAIDS.

Van de Wijgert, J., Khumalo-Sakutukwa, G. N., Coggins, C., Dube, S. E., Nyamapfeni, P., Mwale, M., et al. (1999). Men's attitudes toward vaginal microbicides and microbicide trials in Zimbabwe. *International Family Planning Perspectives, 25*(1), 115–120.

World Health Organization (WHO). (2000). *Female genital mutilation*. Geneva, Switzerland: WHO.

Instructor Resources

LEARNING ACTIVITIES

ACTIVITY 1:

Group Activity: The Game

Developed by Donnovan Somera Yisrael and Carolyn Laub for the MidPeninsula YWCA, 1998. Used with permission.

Objective: To enable participants to first see and then become critical of the complex system of values and rules (most of which are gender-based) which regulate our sexual behavior.

Minimum Time: 45 minutes

View a detailed guide for this activity on the CD-ROM.

ACTIVITY 2:

Group Activity: Gender Role Play: What's Going On?

Adapted from Exercise 11 in Gender or Sex: Who Cares? Skills-Building Resource Pack on Gender and Reproductive Health for Adolescents and Youth Workers (de Bruyn, 2001).

Objective: To guide participants through an analysis of situations involving gender norms, relationships, and sex, and to encourage them to think of ways to reduce possible risks.

Minimum Time: 30 minutes

View this activity at
http://www.genderandaids.org/modules.php?name=News&file=article&sid=173

ACTIVITY 3:

Group Activity: Creating Sexual Situations

Adapted from Exercise 4.6 in Gendering Prevention Practices (Lewis, 2003).

Objective: To guide participants in a discussion about the diversity of situations created around sex, and to highlight issues of gender and power.

Minimum Time: 30 minutes

View this activity at
http://www.nikk.uio.no/forskning/nikk/living/manuals_questionnaire.html

ACTIVITY 4:

Assignment: Gender in the Real World

Objective: To understand how gender stereotypes can influence HIV/AIDS risk.

Collect examples of gender bias or stereotypes about women's and men's roles from the following sources:

- Proverbs and sayings
- Words to popular songs
- Newspaper and magazine articles

Collect examples from the same sources that show gender equality or positive expectations concerning women's and men's roles in the society.

Answer the following questions:

1. What negative ideas are reinforced by the gender-stereotype and gender-equality examples?
2. How can such negative ideas contribute to increased HIV/AIDS risk?
3. What positive ideas are reinforced by the gender-stereotype and gender-equality examples?
4. How can such positive ideas help individuals and communities reduce risks for HIV/AIDS?

DISCUSSION QUESTIONS

1. Are there gender norms in your culture or community that dictate how women and girls should behave? How might these norms influence risk of HIV/AIDS?
2. Are there gender norms in your culture or community that dictate how men and boys should behave? How might these norms influence risk of HIV/AIDS?

QUIZ

1. True or False: A culture's ideas about gender roles, once set, rarely change.
2. Some cultures discourage women from understanding sexual and reproductive issues because such knowledge is considered a sign of:
   a) Virginity
   b) Passivity
   c) Aggression
   d) Promiscuity
3. Every year, worldwide, there are an estimated ____ unwanted pregnancies.
   a) 20 million
   b) 50 million
   c) 80 million
   d) 120 million

4. In some cultures men are expected to be sexually ___, which may deter them from seeking information about HIV/AIDS.
   a) Knowledgeable
   b) Aggressive
   c) Experienced
   d) All of the above

5. The number of girls and women worldwide who have undergone female genital mutilation is estimated to be:
   a) 10–40 million
   b) 50–90 million
   c) 100–140 million
   d) 200–220 million

6. True or False: The practices of male and female circumcision have no impact on HIV/AIDS risk.

ANSWERS

1. False. Gender roles can change over time as a result of evolving economic, educational, political, religious, and technological circumstances and opportunities.

2. D. Many cultures consider female ignorance of sexual matters a sign of purity. Conversely, knowledge of sexual matters and reproductive physiology is a sign of promiscuity.

3. C. The state of women's lower sexual status is reflected in the following statistics: Each year worldwide, there are an estimated 80 million unwanted pregnancies, 20 million unsafe abortions, and 500,000 maternal deaths (including 78,000 as a result of unsafe abortions).

4. D. Men and boys in many cultures are expected to know about sex and sexuality. This expectation that they should "know what to do" in regard to sex may deter them from seeking information about HIV/AIDS for fear of appearing ignorant about sexual matters (and therefore unmasculine).

5. C. Most of the estimated 100–140 million girls and women worldwide who have undergone FGM live in Africa, although some live in Asia and the Middle East. An increasing number are living in Europe, Australia, Canada, and the United States, primarily as a result of immigration.

6. False. Although few clinical studies have been conducted, it is clear that FGM also may increase the HIV transmission risk faced by women and girls, since instruments used in the cutting may be shared, facilitating HIV infection via the blood on non-sterile instruments. In addition, some types of FGM are associated with chronic genital injury and tearing, ulceration, and delayed healing of injuries, all of which may increase HIV risk through sexual contact. Male circumcision can reduce the risk of a man's acquiring or transmitting HIV. It also can reduce the likelihood that he will acquire or transmit other STIs/STDs, which can in turn increase HIV risk. However, as in the case of FGM, when circumcision is performed using non-sterile instruments, HIV transmission risk may be increased.

WEB RESOURCES

More Information About Gender Roles and Gender-based Traditions

Sex Roles: A Journal of Research

http://www.springerlink.com/content/1573–2762/

On this Web site, Springer Netherlands, an academic publisher, provides the tables of contents for *Sex Roles: A Journal of Research.* Articles are available for download and purchase, and select articles are available to download for free.

Traditional Practices Affecting the Health of Women and Girls

http://www.unhchr.ch/Huridocda/Huridoca.nsf/70ef163b25b2333fc1256991004de370/aa473b2f9071ea17c12569700050c785?OpenDocument

A page within the "Women's Rights and Human Rights" Web site sponsored by the United Nations' Office of the High Commissioner for Human Rights (OHCHR), this site gives details on the background of, and policy approaches to, traditional practices that affect the health of women and girls around the world.

RECOMMENDED READING

Men, Women, and Gender Roles

Gender Differences in Sexuality (Oliver & Hyde, 1993)

Oliver, M. B., & Hyde, J. S. (1993). Gender differences in sexuality: A meta-analysis. Psychological Bulletin, 114, *29–51.*

This meta-analysis surveyed 177 usable sources that reported data on gender differences on 21 different measures of sexual attitudes and behaviors.

An Exploratory Analysis of Relationship Scripts, Sexual Scripts, and Condom Use Among African American Women (Bowleg, Lucas, & Tschann, 2004)

Bowleg, L., Lucas, K. J., & Tschann, J. M. (2004). "The ball was always in his court": An exploratory analysis of relationship scripts, sexual scripts, and condom use among African American women. Psychology of Women Quarterly, 28*(1), 70–82.*

This qualitative study explored the association between African American women's interpersonal relationship and sexual scripts and condom use with their primary sex partners. Interpersonal scripts are discussed within the context of sociocultural factors relevant to African American women, heterosexual relationships, and communities.

Good Girl or Flirt Girl: Latinas' Definitions of Sex and Sexual Relationships (Faulkner, 2003)

Faulkner, S. L. (2003). Good girl or flirt girl: Latinas' definitions of sex and sexual relationships. Hispanic Journal of Behavioral Sciences, 25*(2), 174–200.*

This study provides theoretical understanding of 31 young adult Latinas' experiences and understandings of sexuality through in-depth interviews. The grounded theory analysis of defining sex and sexual relationships revealed similar descriptions of processes within Latinas' accounts (27 pages).

Targeting "Risky" Gender Ideologies (Laub et al., 1999)

Laub, C., Somera, D., Gowen, L., & Diaz, R. (1999). Targeting "risky" gender ideologies: Constructing a community-driven, theory-based HIV prevention intervention for youth. Health Education and Behavior, 26*(2), 185–199.*

In this article, the authors propose that the underlying or implicit theories about young people's risk behavior that guide many prevention programs are not accurate descriptions or valid explanations of sexual risk in this population. The authors articulate the theories underlying HIV prevention activities that are typically found in prevention curricula, discuss increased awareness of the role of gender ideologies and sexual scripts in the lives of youth, and describe a prevention activity ("The Game") that addresses the critical role of gender-based ideologies and sexual scripts in young people's sexual risk behavior.

An abstract of this article is available online at http://heb.sagepub.com/cgi/content/abstract/26/2/185

Gender-Based Traditional Practices and Risk

Harmful Traditional Practices Affecting the Health of Women and Children (OHCHR)

This fact sheet identifies and analyzes the background to harmful traditional practices, their causes, and their consequences for the health of women and the girl child. It also reviews the action taken by United Nations organs and agencies, governments and organizations (NGOs).
Available online at: http://www.unhchr.ch/html/menu6/2/fs23.htm

Too Young to Wed: The Lives, Rights, and Health of Young Married Girls (ICRW, 2003)

Mathur, S., Greene, M., & Malhotra, A. (2003). Too young to wed: The lives, rights, and health of young married girls. *Washington, DC: International Center for Research on Women.*

The report examines international findings of research on child marriage, and offers policy and programmatic recommendations to end early marriage.
Available online at http://www.icrw.org/docs/tooyoungtowed_1003.pdf

Vaginal Drying Agents and HIV Transmission (Kun, 1998)

Kun, K. (1998). Vaginal drying agents and HIV transmission. International Family Planning Perspectives 24*(2), 93–94.*

Kun provides a basic overview of vaginal drying agents, their use, research findings on HIV transmission, and programming implication. The author notes the complex nature of vaginal drying agent practices and the need for more qualitative data on the topic. The author reports on an evaluation of sex workers in Zaire, who were examined before and after inserting drying agents. Of the seven participants, only one was left with intact vagina mucosa. All others had vaginal inflammation resembling a chemical burn or allergic reaction.
Available online at: http://www.guttmacher.org/pubs/journals/2409398.html

POWERPOINT SLIDES

(Note: A full-color version of these slides, with graphics, is also available on the CD-ROM.)

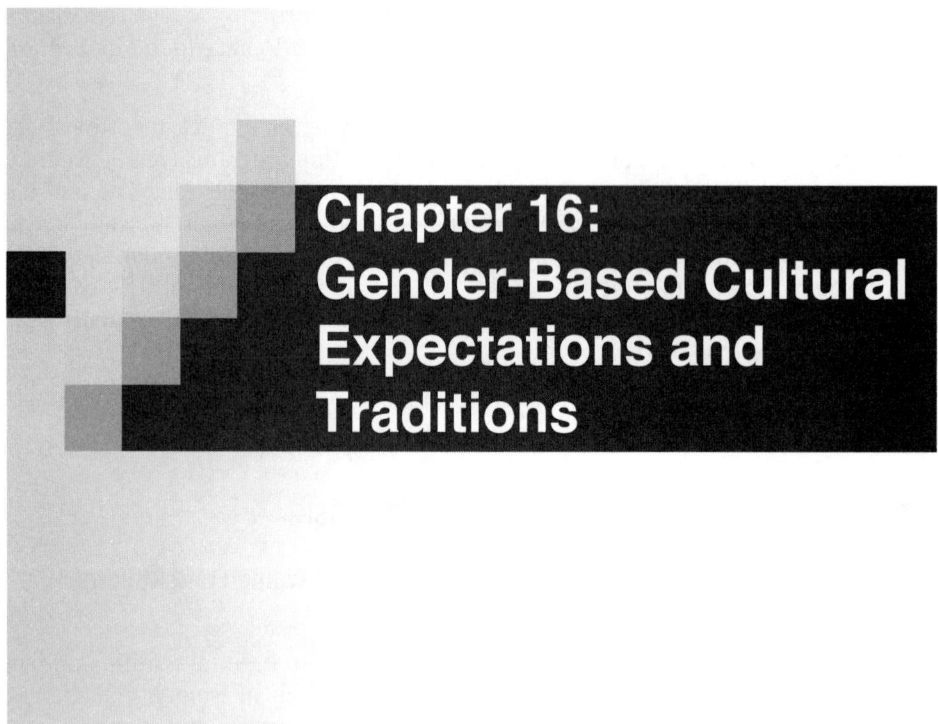

Gender-Based Cultural Expectations and Traditions

- The social status and cultural expectations of both men and women are influenced by a culture's gender norms and can increase the risk of HIV infection.
- Gender roles based on culturally ascribed notions of "masculine" and "feminine" are a powerful feature of social organization.

Masculinity and Femininity

- In every society there are many kinds of masculinity and femininity that vary by social class, ethnicity, sexuality, and age.
- Gender roles are learned, rather than inherent, and vary from culture to culture and from generation to generation.
- "Marianismo" and "machismo" prescribe traditional gender roles of masculine and feminine behavior, including sexual behavior, for Latino men and women in the United States.

Masculinity

- The dominant ideology of masculinity characterizes men as independent, dominant, invulnerable aggressors, and providers, whose key virtues are strength, virility, and courage.
- Most cultures socialize men to believe that it is integral to being a man to take risks – particularly sexual risks—including having sex with multiple partners.

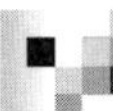

Femininity

- The dominant ideology of femininity in most societies dictates that women should be subordinate, dependent, and passive.
- Key virtues of an ideal woman include virginity (if unmarried), chastity, motherhood, moral superiority, and obedience.
- In many cultures, these beliefs dictate that women generally have less power than men do to decide with whom, how, and when they have sex.

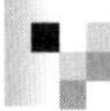

Gender Norms for Men and Women

Gender Norms for Men

- Sexual knowledge
- Sexual aggression
- Sexual experience

Gender Norms for Women

- Sexual ignorance
- Sexual passivity
- Sexual innocence

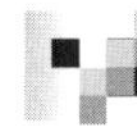

Gender, Traditional Practices, and Risk

Gender-based traditional customs and practices that promote the risk of acquiring and transmitting HIV/AIDS include:

- **Child marriage**
  - Girls' husbands are usually more sexually experienced
  - Girls are economically and socially dependent on husbands

- **Female genital mutilation**
  - Nonsterile tools are used
  - Causes tearing, ulceration, and delayed healing

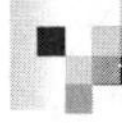

Gender, Traditional Practices, and Risk (continued)

Gender-based traditional customs and practices that promote the risk of acquiring and transmitting HIV/AIDS include:

- **Wife inheritance and ritual cleansing**
  - Perpetuates women's dependence on men and undercuts their social and economic status

- **Dry sex**
  - Increases the likelihood of tears and lacerations in the vaginal wall, especially among adolescent girls
  - May deter women from using microbicides

Learning Objectives

- Understand how poverty, economic inequality, and HIV/AIDS are interrelated
- Understand how educational inequality impacts HIV/AIDS
- Describe the connection between gender-based violence and HIV/AIDS
- Discuss how women's unequal legal and socioeconomic status affects their risk of HIV/AIDS
- List the key ways in which the HIV/AIDS crisis among women is being addressed

Key Terms

AIDS orphans
gender-based violence
zero tolerance

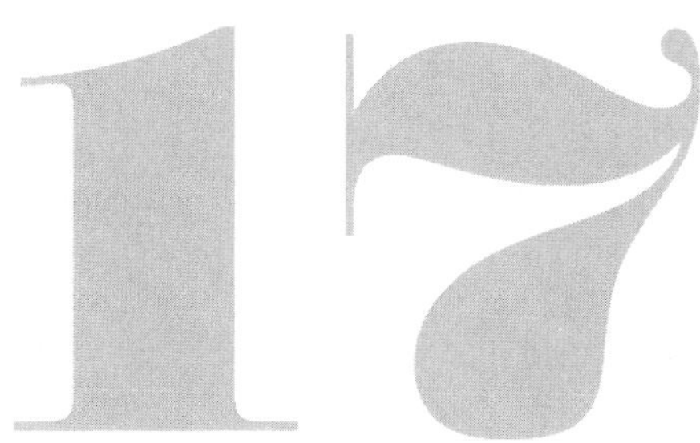

Gender, Culture, and Inequality

This chapter explores gender and related social and cultural inequalities that are causally linked to the spread of HIV and AIDS and that compound the impact of the epidemic on women and men.

Research conducted by the World Bank shows that the more unequal gender relationships are in a country, the higher its HIV prevalence rate (World Bank, 2001). Gender relationships affect risk factors for HIV/AIDS in many complex ways because gender norms influence people's attitudes, behaviors, and opportunities in the social, personal, and economic realms.

> "The concentration of HIV/AIDS in the developing world and in the marginalized communities of the first world confirm that the HIV/AIDS epidemic mirrors the conditions of global inequality. Tracking the path of least resistance, HIV/AIDS flourishes in conditions of poverty, conflict and inequality, and in states with weak resources and capacity" (Albertyn, 2000).

POVERTY, ECONOMIC INEQUALITY, AND HIV/AIDS

HIV/AIDS flourishes under conditions of poverty. The vicious cycle of poverty providing a breeding ground for HIV/AIDS, and HIV/AIDS then furthering poverty among families and communities struck by HIV/AIDS, is important to understand and address.

Global Inequality, the Cycle of Poverty, and HIV/AIDS

The world's economic resources are concentrated in a few places—for example, the United States. However, illnesses such as HIV/AIDS flourish in places with few economic resources. Currently, rates of HIV mortality are declining in the United States, in part because many (although not all) Americans have access to adequate health care and risk information. Also, the United States has enough educated people, technology, and money to discover and manufacture anti-HIV drugs. In other parts of the world that do not have access to adequate knowledge, resources, and technology, however, rates of HIV/AIDS are climbing.

Many communities worldwide are locked in a vicious cycle in which poverty helps to drive the HIV/AIDS epidemic, and the epidemic in turn forces the community into greater poverty. Poverty contributes to rising HIV/AIDS rates by fueling migration by men, women, and children to areas with greater economic opportunities. Migration disrupts marital and familial ties and leads to sexual networks in urban areas where there is an unequal ratio of men to women and seroprevalence is likely to be high (UNFPA, 2000; WHO, 2002a). Migrating men are more likely to visit sex workers, putting themselves and their families at risk when they return home (Brummer, 2002). Migrating women often have sex with multiple partners for economic gain or protection. The risk of infection for migrating women is further increased when they are forced to submit to unwanted sex, for example, at border crossings or in exchange for physical protection (UNFPA, 2000; WHO, 2002a).

In addition, people who live in poverty are also less likely to have information about how HIV/AIDS is transmitted and how to protect themselves than those from higher income levels (WHO, 2002a). They are more likely to focus on day-to-day survival, and not on the reduction of risk for diseases that may not manifest themselves for years (UNAIDS, 1999; UNFPA, 2000). Once people do become ill from HIV/AIDS, insufficient resources often prevent them from obtaining medical care.

At the same time, HIV/AIDS also contributes to poverty in various ways. In particular, when the primary household breadwinner becomes ill with AIDS and can no longer work, household income drops. In countries where women cannot own or inherit land, the wife and children of a man who has died from AIDS may lose access to their only source of livelihood (Lewis, 2003). The number of AIDS orphans is expected to reach 25 million by 2010 (Global AIDS Alliance, 2005). On the death of one or both parents from AIDS, these children are left in the care of already overburdened relatives or in overcrowded orphanages, or they must fend for themselves in child-headed households or in the streets (AVERT, 2005).

The cost of HIV/AIDS treatments and treatment for opportunistic infections also can bankrupt those who are ill and their friends and extended family who try to assist them. At the national level, the impact of HIV/AIDS could cut the wealth of some less developed countries by as much as 20%, deepening existing poverty and drying up resources needed to fight the pandemic (BBC, 2000).

The Feminization of Poverty

Seventy percent of the 1.2 billion people worldwide who live in poverty are female.

Women and girls are disproportionately impacted by poverty, representing 70% of the 1.2 billion people who live in poverty worldwide (Amnesty International, 2005). Worldwide, women receive an average of 30–40% less pay than men for the same work (WHO, 2000a). This economic inequality may influence their ability to control the timing and safety of sexual intercourse. Specifically, economic dependence on men forces some women to remain silent about HIV risk issues and to stay with partners who refuse to engage in safer-sex practices. For example, a study of African American women in Los Angeles found that women who depended on their male partners for financial assistance for housing were more likely to have sex without condoms than women who did not depend on men for economic reasons (Wyatt & Dunn, 1991). International research shows that women in monogamous relationships who are vulnerable to HIV infection perceive the negative economic and potentially violent consequences of leaving high-risk relationships to be far more serious than the health risks of staying in the relationship (UNAIDS, 1999).

Poverty also leads to greater HIV risk among women by leading women to barter sex for economic gain or survival (Weiss, Whelan, & Gupta, 1996). Commercial sex work is the most well-known way for women to exchange sex for money, but many women exchange sex for comfort or goods as a rational means of making ends meet. In addition, there is evidence that girls and young women may willingly initiate relationships with "sugar daddies," much older, relatively well-off (usually married) men who support them in exchange for sex. Some girls also may exchange sex for money for school fees or to help their families. Once in these relationships with teachers, drivers, shopkeepers, or even policemen, girls have little power to negotiate the use of condoms (UNFPA, 2003).

EDUCATIONAL INEQUALITY AND HIV/AIDS

Women make up almost two-thirds of the world's 876 million illiterates (United Nations [UN], 2000). Worldwide, there are 90 young women in secondary school for every 100 young men, although in some countries, including Bangladesh, Yemen, Cambodia, Chad, and Niger, there are fewer than 60 young women in secondary school for every 100 young men (Population Reference Bureau, 2000). In some societies, girls are not able to continue with their education because they are taken out of school by their families to care for sick family members or to perform other household tasks.

In some parts of the world, the low social value placed on educating girls and women increases the risk of HIV infection.

Educational inequality contributes to a woman's HIV risk directly, by making information on HIV/AIDS less accessible to her, and indirectly, by increasing her economic dependence on a male partner. In particular, studies show that more educated women are more likely to know how to prevent HIV transmission, delay sexual activity, to use health care services, and take other steps to prevent the spread of HIV (UNAIDS, UNFPA, & UNIFEM, 2004). Education also reduces poverty and affords women greater decision-making power (Global Campaign for Education, 2004).

Because many cultures value ignorance about sex as a feature of femininity, many young women are prevented by husbands, fathers, or other family members from obtaining education about HIV/AIDS. Others decline to seek such information out of fear for their reputations, and those who do learn about HIV/AIDS may hide HIV-related knowledge (Feinstein & Prentice, 2001). Lack of education about the causes, prevention, and treatment of HIV/AIDS contributes to high transmission rates and low treatment-seeking and adherence, and perpetrates stigma and discrimination toward people with HIV/AIDS.

GENDER-BASED VIOLENCE AND HIV/AIDS

Gender-based violence is rooted in the historically unequal power relations (social, economic, cultural, and political) between males and females. Such violence increases women's vulnerability to HIV/AIDS.

Gender-based violence is causally linked to HIV and AIDS transmission through rape and intimate partner violence, and also may be a reaction to a positive HIV diagnosis within a relationship. Violence and the threat of violence increase women's vulnerability to HIV/AIDS and can compound the barriers to HIV+ women's access to care.

Gender-Based Violence

Gender-based violence takes many forms and can include physical, emotional, economic, and sexual abuse. These abuses may include such acts as use of coercion and threats to get one's way (such as threatening to leave a relationship, to take the children away, to commit suicide, or to report the victim to welfare authorities); destruction of personal property; displaying of weapons; abuse of pets; making the victim feel guilty, worthless, or humiliated; isolating the victim from sources of social support; denying the abuse or blaming the victim for it; and keeping the victim economically dependent by blocking employment opportunities or access to family income.

Although both males and females can suffer from gender violence, studies show that women, young women, and children of both sexes are most often the victims of such violence, particularly sexual violence. Available data suggest that at least one in five of the world's female population has been physically or sexually abused at some time in their lives (Gordon & Crehan, 1999), and reported rates of physical assault by a male partner among adult women have ranged from 16% (in Cambodia) to 67% in Papua New Guinea, according to one review of studies (UNFPA, 2000) (see Figure 17-1). Sexual violence does not have to include direct physical contact between perpetrator and victim: Sexual threats, humiliation, and intimidation may

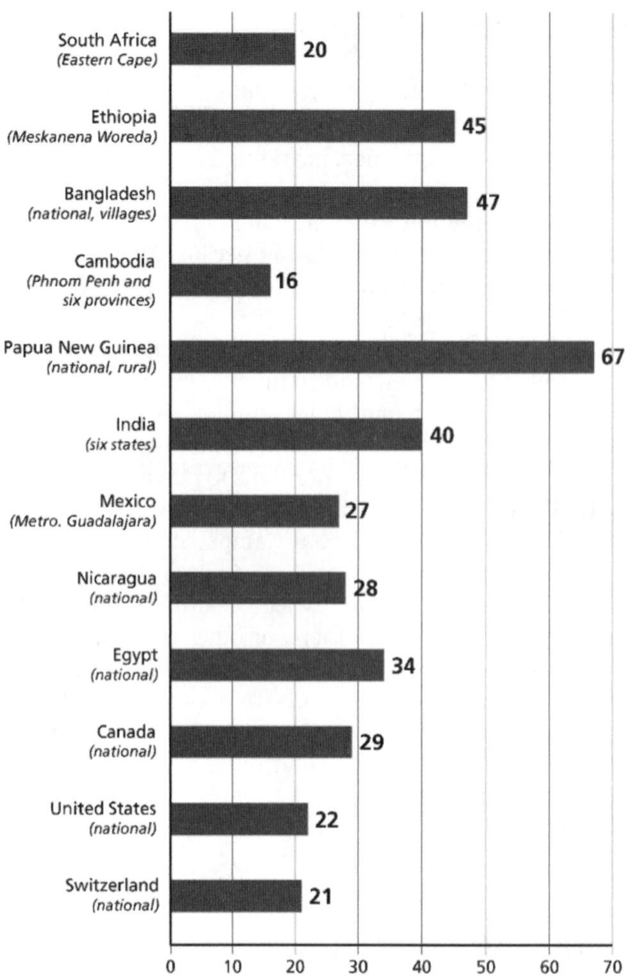

Figure 17-1 Percentage of adult women by country reporting physical assault by a male partner (in any intimate relationship; selected studies) (UNFPA, 2000, Figure 5).

be considered sexual violence when they are used to demonstrate power over, or inflict pain and humiliation on, another person (Gordon & Crehan, 1999).

Violence against women, in particular forced or coerced sex (rape), increases a woman's vulnerability to HIV/AIDS. The proportion of HIV infections around the world that are attributable, directly or indirectly, to gender-based violence is unknown. But, existing evidence suggests that it is likely to be significant (Gordon & Crehan, 1999). South African women, for example, who have been physically abused, or whose partner has excessive control in the relationship, have a 50% higher rate of HIV infection than other women (Dunkle et al., 2004). Gender-based violence also can compound the barriers to HIV+ women obtaining medical care.

Conversations about safer sex, HIV status, or HIV risk reduction are unlikely to take place in situations of rape, particularly when the rapist has a weapon. Violence between intimate partners often contributes to HIV transmission by harming the ability of partners to communicate openly with each other about safe sex, their HIV status, or ways to reduce the risk of infection (Feinstein & Prentice, 2001; Wingood & DiClemente, 1997b).

Nonconsensual Sex

Although some forms of gender-based violence are region-specific (e.g., female genital mutilation), most are universal (UNAIDS, 1999). One ubiquitous manifestation of violence toward women is nonconsensual sex, which research has shown to be a pervasive reality of adolescent girls' and women's lives worldwide (Feinstein & Prentice, 2001). Studies show that in many countries, a young girl's first act of intercourse is often forced (Feinstein & Prentice, 2001). A study by the Pan American Health Organization (PAHO), for example, found that half of all young women in the Caribbean reported that their first sexual encounter was forced or coerced (Halcón, Beuhring, Blum, & WHO Collaborating Centre, 2000). In the United States, 24% of those who had intercourse before age 14 reported having been forced (Abma, Driscoll, & Moore, 1998). According to the Youth Risk Behavior Surveillance Survey (YRBSS), a national survey of high school students in the United States, 7.7% of students have been forced to have sexual intercourse when they did not want to. Female students (10%) were significantly more likely than male students (5%) to have been forced to have sexual intercourse (CDC, 2002).

In situations of rape or coerced sex, a woman is more likely to experience bleeding and tearing of the genital area. This can create passageways for HIV to enter the bloodstream. In addition, conversations about HIV status, HIV risk reduction, and condom use are unlikely to take place in forced sex situations. These problems are especially acute in conflict, postconflict, and refugee situations, where women and girls are subjected to high rates of sexual assault (UNIFEM, 2001). A number of studies have also shown that women who experienced childhood sexual abuse are more likely to engage in sexual risk-taking behavior as adolescents and adults (Wingood & DiClemente, 1997a).

Other Gender-Based Violence

The range of physical, emotional, and economic abuses that comprise gender-based violence increases HIV risk for women in a number of ways. Research conducted in countries as diverse as Guatemala, India, Jamaica, Papua New Guinea, and Tanzania shows that women often avoid discussing safer sex or bringing up condom use for fear of triggering a violent response from their intimate partners (Türmen, 2003; UNAIDS, 1999).

Women with HIV are already at increased risk for violence relative to the general population, perhaps because demographic and behavioral factors associated with HIV (e.g., poverty, drug use, bartering sex) also increase a woman's exposure to violence (Koenig et al., 2002). Research also has shown that some HIV-infected women are at additional risk for violence when their positive serostatus is disclosed (Gielen, McDonnell, Burke, & O'Campo, 2000). For example, more than half of the women surveyed by Kenya's Population Council who knew they were HIV infected said that they had not disclosed their HIV status to their partners because they feared violence or being abandoned (Türmen, 2003). This threat of violence may affect women's use of services such as HIV testing and counseling.

THE UNEQUAL LEGAL STATUS OF WOMEN

Around the world, men and women have different status in society, which usually limits women's access to productive resources such as land, property, credit, employment, training, and education (UNAIDS, 1999). Women's subordinate roles are often reinforced by laws and policies that, for example, prohibit women from owning land, inheriting property, asking for a divorce, participating in democratic processes, protecting themselves from forced marriages, and making decisions about their children's education (Ofosu-Amaah, n.d.; UNAIDS, 1999). These discriminatory laws and policies not only deny equal access to resources but also fail to provide women with the opportunities to realize the full benefits of economic and social development (UNAIDS, 1999). Such legal inequalities increase women's vulnerability to HIV/AIDS in a number of ways.

> Legal restrictions promote economic and social conditions that contribute to women's vulnerability to HIV/AIDS.

Property Rights

In many countries, women's rights to land and property are attained primarily through marriage. If marriage ends, women's rights to land or home may end as well. Unequal rights and access to property perpetuate women's dependence on men and undercut their social and economic status. Studies from all over the world, developed and developing countries alike, have found that some women believe that the economic consequences of leaving a high-risk relationship are far worse than the health consequences of staying with their partners (WHO, 2002a; Zierler & Krieger, 2000). In addition, a woman who has been widowed by HIV and AIDS risks losing her land and all her belongings to her husband's family (Lewis, 2003). This can leave her economically destitute and force her into commercial sex work or a risky sexual relationship with another man so that she can feed herself and her children.

Rape, Sexual Harassment, and Coerced Sex

Narrow definitions for these offenses in some legal systems, coupled with the associated stigma and blame, can transform a rape victim into a suspect, deny rights if the victim is married to the offender, or decriminalize many kinds of unwanted sexual advances (Ofosu-Amaah, n.d.). In some cases, rape victims can be legally executed for having tarnished the honor of their families. These legal circumstances often force women to remain in abusive relationships and to avoid seeking treatment for injuries, STIs/STDs, and HIV sustained as a result of rape or sexual abuse.

Reproductive Rights

Some laws deny women, especially young women, the right to control their fertility via contraception or abortion (Ofosu-Amaah, n.d.). Laws or policies also may prevent young people from obtaining information and treatment pertaining to sexuality, STIs/STDs, and HIV.

GENDER AND THE STIGMA OF HIV/AIDS

HIV-related stigma refers to all unfavorable attitudes, beliefs, and policies directed toward people perceived to have HIV/AIDS, as well as toward their significant others and loved ones, close associates, social groups, and communities (Brimlow, Cook, & Seaton, 2003). HIV/AIDS is associated with sex, disease, and death, and with behaviors that may be illegal, forbidden, or taboo, such as sex work, sex between men, and injection drug use. This encourages and perpetuates stigmatization of persons perceived to have HIV/AIDS. This stigma often translates into discriminatory practices that deny employment, housing, education, medical care, and health insurance to persons who have—or who have even been tested for—HIV/AIDS. Fear of such stigma and discrimination prevents people from finding out their HIV serostatus and from seeking treatment for HIV/AIDS (Aggleton & Parker, 2002).

> "HIV/AIDS related stigma and discrimination comes from the powerful combination of shame and fear—shame because the sex or drug injecting behavior that transmit HIV are surrounded by taboo and moral judgment, and fear because AIDS is relatively new, and considered deadly. Responding to AIDS with blame or abuse towards people living with AIDS simply forces the epidemic underground, creating the ideal conditions for HIV to spread. The only way of making progress against the epidemic is to replace shame with solidarity and fears with hope."
>
> —Statement by Peter Piot to Plenary of the World Conference against Racism. Racial Discrimination, Xenophobia and Related Intolerance, Durban, South Africa, September 5, 2001 (WHO, 2002b)

The Scarlet HIV+: Stigma Against Women

Stigma against HIV+ women is particularly strong. HIV/AIDS is misperceived in many parts of the world as a "promiscuous woman's disease" or a "prostitute's disease." Women are often blamed for the spread of HIV/AIDS to their families because they were the first ones in their families to be tested, as testing during pregnancy or just after childbirth is common. In reality, most HIV+ women in the world contracted HIV from their husbands. HIV+ women may be expelled from their households, fired from their jobs, and shunned by their communities. Some advocates of women's rights point out that a vestige of the blame and stigma against women is manifest in the fact that infection of newborn babies is still often termed "mother-to-child-transmission" and not "parent-to-child-transmission" (GENDER-AIDS eFORUM, 2003). The stigma of being HIV+ and the social and economic consequences of being labeled HIV+ cause some women to refrain from being tested for HIV and seeking out care (Albertyn, 2000).

Stigma Against Men Who Have Sex With Men

In many industrialized nations and developing nations alike, homosexual intercourse is highly stigmatized and in some cases illegal, forcing men who have sex with men to keep their relationships secret. Men who have sex with men are often targets of intolerance and hate crimes. As a result of these norms and legal circumstances, government officials and the general public may refuse to admit that homosexual transmission occurs and allocate no funds for HIV/AIDS prevention among men who have sex with men. Men who have sex with men may, in turn, feel compelled to keep their sexual behavior secret, deny their sexual risk, and avoid HIV testing and treatment (Aggleton, Khan, & Parker, 1999; McKenna, 1999). This increases their own risk as well as the risk of their partners, female or male.

UNEQUAL ACCESS TO TREATMENT: WOMEN'S STATUS IN THE FAMILY

In an analysis of several studies involving more than 4,500 people with HIV infection, women were 33% more likely than men to die within the study period (NIAID, 2006). This disparity appears largely because of differing access to and use of treatment services, along with domestic violence, homelessness, and lack of social support among women, rather than to biological differences between men and women. In many countries, women with HIV/AIDS are also more likely than men to suffer from malnourishment, which accelerates disease progression (Solomon, 1998). Women whose HIV infections are detected early and receive appropriate treatment have been shown to survive as long as infected men (WHO, 2000b).

Even in areas where high-quality HIV/AIDS care is available to women, there is evidence that they wait longer than men before seeking care and are less likely to seek care at all (Solomon, 1998). As was discussed in the previous section, stigma is one factor in women's decision not to seek treatment. A second factor is women's role and status in the family.

Women are traditionally responsible for the well-being and health of their families. When a husband or children are sick, women are expected to care for them. This often leaves little time for women to attend to their own health needs. In addition, within a family, men's illnesses are often perceived as more important because they tend to have a greater impact on wage-earning. "Women's work" is usually undervalued, and women's illnesses may be ignored until women are unable to perform daily tasks (World Bank, 1999). When a woman is unable to care for her family because of her own illness, she may experience feelings of failure and decreased self-esteem. This low self-esteem is another factor that makes a woman less likely to seek out care for herself (NIAID, 2006; Ziegler & Krieger, 2000).

ADDRESSING THE HIV/AIDS CRISIS AMONG WOMEN

> Involvement of multiple sectors of society, including public health, education, and the legal system, is essential to addressing the HIV/AIDS crisis among women.

A joint report by the Joint United Nations Programme on HIV/AIDS (UNAIDS), the United Nations Population Fund (UNFPA), and the United Nations Development Fund for Women (UNIFEM) has made a set of research-based recommendations

Shaping the Health of Adolescents in Zimbabwe (SHAZ) is a multicomponent HIV prevention intervention that combines life skills training and economic development strategies. It has been described as "a financial prophylactic aimed at shielding young girls from sexual liaisons that transmit the virus." Extreme poverty often leads teenage girls in Zimbabwe to trade sex for food and gifts from much older, more sexually experienced men who serve as their "sugar daddies." In such relationships, the girls are often powerless to negotiate condom use. SHAZ seeks to counteract the draw of the sugar daddies and empower young women to engage in safer-sex practices. The program provides participants with life skills training, including HIV education and practice in negotiating condom use, and vocational skills training. Participants also develop business plans and receive a microcredit loan to start a small business enterprise that can afford them greater economic self-sufficiency. Each participant has a mentor who is a local businesswoman.

Figure 17-2 Shaping the health of adolescents in Zimbabwe (SHAZ) (Chase, 2004).

concerning how best to address the current HIV/AIDS crisis among women. These recommendations collectively stress the importance of working through multiple sectors simultaneously (e.g., public health, education, the legal system) and actively involving men and boys in efforts that will ultimately benefit both genders.

1. Support positive women and their organizations and networks. Include women who are living with HIV/AIDS in policy and programming efforts at the local, regional, and national levels.

2. Make AIDS money work for women. Ensure that sufficient resources are provided to programs that address women's needs in the areas of prevention, treatment, education, community-based care, violence, and human rights. Ensure that gender analysis is undertaken at every stage of program and policy design, implementation, and evaluation, to ensure that gender discrimination is eliminated and human rights are promoted.

Economic independence and access to education, information, and skills increase a woman's ability to protect herself from HIV/AIDS.

3. Promote girls' primary and secondary education and women's literacy. Eliminate school fees to help keep girls in school. Promote school policies that do not tolerate violence against or sexual harassment of female students. Implement curricula that promote mutual respect and equality between the sexes, promote girls' leadership and self-esteem, and provide age-appropriate sex and HIV education. Ensure that women of all ages have access to literacy classes.

4. Ensure that adolescent girls and women have the knowledge and means to prevent HIV infection. Institute community-wide gender-sensitive media and advocacy campaigns that convey basic, accurate information about HIV/AIDS, dispel harmful stereotypes about gender roles, provide a warning that marriage does not necessarily afford protection from HIV/AIDS, and involve both men and women in promoting positive reproductive and sexual health among their peers. Empower women and girls economically with access to job training, banking services, and credit to break the cycle of poverty, gender inequality, and HIV/AIDS (for an example, see Figure 17-2 on the Shaping the Health of Adolescents in Zimbabwe program). Increase access among women to methods of HIV prevention such as male and female condoms. Female condoms have demonstrated rising rates of acceptability in developing countries (Bala Nath, 2000; FHI, n.d.), and their availability has been increasing as their cost has been dropping. Push forward development of vaginal microbicide gels, lubricants, or suppositories that kill or disable the HIV virus promise to afford women even greater opportunities to protect themselves against HIV. Offer harm-reduction programs and needle exchange for male and female injection drug users, and provide HIV prevention services in all health care settings.

5. Ensure equal and universal access to treatment. Provide mobile health centers, reduce or eliminate health care fees, provide child care at health centers, and offer family-focused care so that no one family member is treated at the expense of others. Increase availability of voluntary, confidential testing and counseling that

South Africa's Men as Partners (MaP) program (http://www.engenderhealth.org/ia/wwm/index.html), initiated by the New York–based nonprofit organization EngenderHealth, trains men to be peer leaders in addressing gender roles. MaP has expanded throughout South Africa and is now used in trade unions and the South African National Defence Force. The program encourages men to challenge traditional gender roles and relationships in their households.

One MaP peer leader has said, "I realized it was impossible to work around issues of gender when you haven't started with yourself. I started becoming a counselor to abusive men when I was actually getting assistance for myself. It is impossible to talk about HIV/AIDS when you are not talking about domestic and sexual violence."

Figure 17-3 South Africa's Men as Partners (MaP) program (UNAIDS, 2004).

addresses HIV-related stigma and discrimination and gender-based violence. For persons who are HIV+, make antiretroviral therapies widely available, along with counseling and social services to support adherence to prescribed treatment. Conduct and disseminate further research on the effects of antiretroviral therapies used to prevent vertical transmission.

6. Recognize and support home-based caregivers of AIDS patients and orphans. Provide training, counseling, and social support to home-based caregivers who caring for sick and dying family members and orphans, Implement campaigns that raise awareness of the burden and importance of the care that women provide, and encourage more equitable sharing of caregiving responsibilities within the household. Strengthen public health services and community activities that can relieve the burden of care that is currently on individual households.

7. Promote zero tolerance of all forms of violence against women and girls. Involve multiple sectors and stakeholders—health care, education, the legal system, religious institutions, and community groups—in efforts to reduce violence against women and girls. Implement community-wide media campaigns promoting zero tolerance for gender-based violence. Provide counseling services to victims of gender-based violence, and offer prompt postexposure prophylaxis to rape victims to reduce the likelihood of infection with HIV and other STIs/STDs. Ensure that humanitarian responses to crisis situations include sexual and reproductive health services. Involve men and boys in efforts that address the gender-based norms and behaviors that put both males and females at risk of HIV infection (for an example, see Figure 17-3 on South Africa's Men as Partners program).

8. Promote and protect the human rights of women and girls. Codify and revise laws and policies that protect and promote women's rights in alignment with the United Nations Convention on the Elimination of All Forms of Discrimination Against women (CEDAW), and ensure their implementation. Document human rights violations and responses and report on them to the United Nations committee that monitors CEDAW. Promote and protect women's property and inheritance rights, and support free or low-cost legal services that protect the rights of women and girls who are affected with HIV/AIDS.

REFERENCES

Abma, J., Driscoll, A., & Moore, K. (1998). Young women's degree of control over first intercourse: An exploratory analysis. *Family Planning Perspectives, 30*(1), 12–18.

Aggleton, P., & Parker, R. (2002). HIV/AIDS: stigma, discrimination and human rights abuses. Geneva, Switzerland: Joint United Nations Programme on HIV/AIDS (UNAIDS).

Aggleton, P., Khan, S., & Parker, R. (1999). Men who have sex with men. In L. Gibney, R. DiClemente, & S. Vermund (Eds.), *Preventing HIV in developing countries: Biomedical and behavioural approaches* (pp. 313–330). New York: Kluwer Academic/Plenum.

Albertyn, C. (2000). *Prevention, Treatment and Care in the Context of Human Rights: Expert Group Meeting on "The HIV/AIDS Pandemic and Its Gender Implications."* EGM/HIV-AIDS/2000/WP1, Windhoek, Namibia, November 13-17 (2000), Windhoek, Namibia.

Amnesty International. (2005). *Economic, social and cultural rights (ESCR) and women: A fact sheet*. Retrieved September 19, 2006, from http://www.amnestyusa.org/women/economicrights.html

Bala Nath, M. (2000). *How to empower women to negotiate safer sex: A resource guide for NGOs*. New Delhi: Har-Anand.

Brimlow, D. L., Cook, J. S., & Seaton, R. (Eds.). (2003). *Stigma and HIV/AIDS: A review of the literature*. Rockville, MD: U.S. Department of Health and Human Services.

British Broadcasting Corporation (BBC). (2000, August 12). AIDS tops African agenda. *BBC Online*. Retrieved from http://news.bbc.co.uk/1/hi/health/878042.stm

Brummer, D. (2002). *Labour migration and HIV/AIDS in South Africa*. Pretoria, South Africa: International Organization for Migration (IOM).

Centers for Disease Control and Prevention (CDC). (2002).Youth risk behavior surveillance—United States, 2001. *Morbidity and Mortality Weekly Report Surveillance Summaries 2002, 51*(SS-04), 1–64.

Chase, M. (2004, February 25). African girls taught to say no to "sugar daddies." *The Wall Street Journal*.

Dunkle, K. L, Jewkes, R. K., Brown, H. C., Gray, G. E., McIntryre, J. A., & Harlow, S. D. (2004). Gender-based violence, relationship power, and risk of HIV infection in women attending antenatal clinics in South Africa. *Lancet, 363*(9419), 1415–1421.

Family Health International. (n.d.). Female condom acceptability and sustained use. In *FHI Research Briefs on the Female Condom No. 4*. Arlington, VA: Family Health International.

Feinstein, N., & Prentice, B. (2001). *The UNAIDS gender and AIDS almanac*. Los Altos, CA: Sociometrics Corporation.

Fredriksson, J., & Kanabus, A. (2005). *AIDS orphans*. West Sussex, UK: AVERT.org. Retrieved September 19, 2006, from http://www.avert.org/aidsorphans.htm

GENDER-AIDS eForum. (2003). Women "often blamed" for virus. *AEGiS Digest, 1159*(7). Retrieved October 10, 2003, from http://www.aegis.com/news/bp/2003/ BP031003.html

Gielen, A. C., McDonnell, K., Burke, J., & O'Campo, P. (2000). Women's lives after an HIV positive diagnosis: Disclosure and violence. *Maternal and Child Health Journal, 4*, 111–120.

Global AIDS Alliance (GAA). (2005). *An overview of the epidemic*. Washington, DC: GAA.

Global Campaign for Education. (2004). *Learning to survive: How education for all would save millions of young people*. Brussels: Global Campaign for Education.

Gordon, P., & Crehan, K. (1999). *Dying of sadness: Gender, sexual violence, and the HIV epidemic*. New York: United Nations Development Program.

Halcón, L. T., Beuhring, T., Blum, R. W., & The WHO Collaborating Centre on Adolescent Health. (2000). *A portrait of adolescent health in the Caribbean*. Minneapolis, MN: The Who Collaborating Centre on Adolescent Health.

Koenig, L., Whitaker, D., Royce, R., Wilson, T., Callahan, M., & Fernandez, M. (2002). Violence during pregnancy among women with or at risk for HIV infection. *American Journal of Public Health, 92*(3), 367–370.

Lewis, M. (2003). *Gendering AIDS: Women, men, empowerment, mobilisation*. London: VSO.

McKenna, N. (1999). *The silent epidemic: HIV/AIDS and men who have sex with men in the developing world*. London: Panos Institute.

National Institute of Allergy and Infectious Diseases (NIAID). (2006). *HIV infection in women*. Bethesda, MD: NIAID.

Ofosu-Amaah, A. (n.d.). *Unprotected women: Gender and the legal dimensions of HIV/AIDS*. The World Bank Development Outreach Special Report.

Population Reference Bureau. (2000). *World population data sheet*. Washington, DC: Population Reference Bureau.

Rivers, K., & Aggleton, P. (1999). *Adolescent sexuality, gender and the HIV epidemic*. New York: United Nations Development Programme.

Solomon, S. (1998). *Women and HIV/AIDS concerns—A focus on Thailand, Philippines, India and Nepal*. Discussion paper from expert group meeting on Women and health: Mainstreaming the gender perspective into the health sector. Tunis, Tunisia.

Türmen, T. (2003). Gender and HIV/AIDS. *International Journal of Gynecology and Obstetrics, 82*(3), 411–418.

United Nations (UN). (2000). *The world's women 2000: Trends and statistics*. New York: UN.

United Nations Development Fund for Women (UNIFEM). (2001). *Turning the tide: CEDAW and the gender dimensions of the HIV/AIDS pandemic*. New York: UNIFEM.

United Nations Population Fund (UNFPA). (2000). *Lives together, worlds apart: Men and women in a time of change. The state of the world's population*. New York: UNFPA.

United Nations Population Fund (UNFPA). (2003). *State of world population 2003: Making 1 billion count: Investing in adolescents' health and rights*. New York: UNFPA.

United Nations Population Fund (UNFPA). (n.d.). The state of the world population 2000. Citing L. Heise, M. Ellsberg, & M. Gottemoeller (1999). *Ending violence against women. Population Reports, Series L, no. 11*. Baltimore: Johns Hopkins School of Public Health, Population Information Program.

United Nations Programme on HIV/AIDS (UNAIDS). (1999). *Gender and HIV/AIDS: Taking stock of research and programmes*. UNAIDS Best Practice Collection. Geneva, Switzerland: UNAIDS.

United Nations Programme on HIV/AIDS (UNAIDS), the United Nations Population Fund(UNFPA), and the United Nations Development Fund for Women (UNIFEM). (2004). *Women and HIV/AIDS: Confronting the crisis*. Geneva, Switzerland; New York: UNAIDS, UNFPA, UNIFEM.

Weiss, E., Whelan, D., & Gupta, G. (1996). *Vulnerability and opportunity: Adolescents and HIV/AIDS in the developing world*. Washington, DC: International Center for Research on Women.

Wingood, G. M., & DiClemente, R. J. (1997a). Child sexual abuse, HIV sexual risk and gender relations of African-American women. *American Journal of Preventive Medicine, 13*(5), 380–384.

Wingood, G. M., & DiClemente, R. J. (1997b). Consequences of having a physically abusive partner on condom use and sexual negotiation of young adult African-American women. *American Journal of Public Health, 87*(6), 1016–1018.

World Bank. (1999). *Confronting AIDS: Public priorities in a global epidemic*. New York: Oxford University Press.

World Bank. (2001). *Policy research report: Engendering development through gender equality in rights, resources and voice*. Washington, DC: Oxford University Press.

World Health Organization (WHO). (2000a). *Gender, health and poverty (Fact sheet no. 251)*. Geneva, Switzerland: WHO.

World Health Organization (WHO). (2000b). *Women and HIV/AIDS (Fact sheet no. 242)*. Geneva, Switzerland: WHO.

World Health Organization (WHO). (2002a). *Integrating gender into HIV/AIDS programmes. Review paper for expert consultation, June 3–5, 2002*. Geneva, Switzerland: WHO.

World Health Organization (WHO). (2002b). Regional Office for the Eastern Mediterranean. *World AIDS Campaign 2002: Regional advocacy kit*. Geneva, Switzerland: WHO.

Wyatt, G. E., & Dunn, K. M. (1991). Examining predictors of sex guilt in multiethnic samples of women. *Archive of Sexual Behavior, 20*, 471–485.

Zierler, S., & Krieger, N. (2000). Social inequality and HIV infection in women. In K. H. Mayer & H. F. Pizer (Eds.), *The emergence of AIDS: The impact on immunology, microbiology, and public health* (pp. 76–97). Washington, DC: American Public Health Association.

Instructor Resources

LEARNING ACTIVITIES

ACTIVITY 1:

Group Activity: What Is Violence?

Adapted from Exercise 8 in Gender or Sex: Who Cares? Skills-Building Resource Pack on Gender and Reproductive Health for Adolescents and Youth Workers (de Bruyn, 2001).

Objective: To help participants develop definitions of violence and to explore how these relate to their lives.

Minimum Time: 45 minutes

View this activity at www.genderandaids.org/modules.php?name=News&file=article&sid=173

ACTIVITY 2:

Group Activity: Experiencing Violence

Adapted from Exercise 9 in Gender or Sex: Who Cares? Skills-Building Resource Pack on Gender and Reproductive Health for Adolescents and Youth Workers (de Bruyn, 2001).

Objective: To help participants identify some ways in which men and women mistreat each other and how this can affect sexual and reproductive health.

Minimum Time: 30 minutes

View this activity at www.genderandaids.org/modules.php?name=News&file=article&sid=173

ACTIVITY 3:

Assignment: The Tension Between Autonomy and Vulnerability

Objective: To understand the connection between gender and HIV/AIDS.

Write a five- to six-page paper examining the tensions between approaches that emphasize women's vulnerabilities versus women's agency in responding to HIV/AIDS. Refer to issues such as sexual violence, drug use, and transactional sex.

ACTIVITY 4:

Assignment: Gender Inequality and HIV/AIDS

Objective: To understand the relationship between gender inequality and risk of HIV/AIDS.

Write a five- to six-page paper describing one manifestation of gender inequality that increases a man or a woman's vulnerability for acquiring HIV. Report on at least one instance in which this form of inequality has been or is being addressed successfully to reduce the burden or the risk of HIV/AIDS.

DISCUSSION QUESTIONS

1. Discuss the link between poverty and HIV/AIDS. Do you think they need to be addressed simultaneously?
2. Why is educational equality an important component of HIV/AIDS prevention?
3. How can improvements in a woman's legal rights increase her protection against HIV/AIDS?

QUIZ

1. True or False: Unequal gender relationships are associated with HIV prevalence.
2. List any three ways in which poverty can lead to higher HIV/AIDS prevalence.
3. List any three ways in which HIV/AIDS prevalence can contribute to poverty.
4. The number of AIDS orphans is expected to reach _____ by 2010.
   a) 1 million
   b) 15 million
   c) 25 million
   d) 45 million
5. Women and girls represent ____% of people who live in poverty worldwide.
   a) 80%
   b) 70%
   c) 60%
   d) 50%
6. List any three ways in which gender-based violence can lead to increased risk for HIV/AIDS.
7. True or False: On average, women with HIV/AIDS die more quickly than men with HIV/AIDS because of a biological difference between women and men.

ANSWERS

1. **True.** Research conducted by the World Bank shows that the more unequal gender relationships are in a country, the higher its HIV prevalence rate. Gender relationships affect risk factors for HIV/AIDS in many complex ways because gender norms influence people's attitudes, behaviors, and opportunities in the social, personal, and economic realms.

2. Poverty contributes to rising HIV/AIDS rates by fueling migration by men, women, and children to areas with greater economic opportunities. Migrating men are more likely to visit sex workers, and migrating women often have sex with multiple partners for economic gain or protection. The risk of infection for migrating women is further increased when they are forced to submit to unwanted sex. People who live in poverty are also less likely to have information about how HIV/AIDS is transmitted and how to protect themselves than those from higher income levels. They are more likely to focus on day-to-day survival, and not on the reduction of risk for diseases that may not manifest themselves for years. Once people do become ill from HIV/AIDS, insufficient resources often prevent them from obtaining medical care.

3. HIV/AIDS contributes to poverty in various ways. In particular, when the primary household breadwinner becomes ill with AIDS and can no longer work, household income drops. In countries where women cannot own or inherit land, the wife and children of a man who has died from AIDS may lose access to their only source of livelihood. On the death of one or both parents from AIDS, AIDS orphans are left in the care of already overburdened relatives or in overcrowded orphanages, or they must fend for themselves. The cost of HIV/AIDS treatments and other medical treatments can also bankrupt those who are ill and their friends and extended family who try to assist them.

4. **C.** The number of AIDS orphans is expected to reach 25 million by 2010.

5. **B.** Women and girls are disproportionately impacted by poverty, representing 70% of the 1.2 billion people who live in poverty worldwide.

6. Violence against women, in particular forced or coerced sex (rape), increases a woman's vulnerability to HIV/AIDS. Gender-based violence also can compound the barriers to HIV+ women obtaining medical care. Conversations about safer sex, HIV status, or HIV risk reduction are unlikely to take place in situations of rape, particularly when the rapist has a weapon. Violence between intimate partners often contributes to HIV transmission by harming the ability of partners to communicate openly with each other about safe sex, their HIV status, or ways to reduce the risk of infection. In situations of rape or coerced sex, a woman is more likely to experience bleeding and tearing of the genital area. This can create passageways for HIV to enter the bloodstream. A number of studies also have shown that women who experienced childhood sexual abuse are more likely to engage in sexual risk-taking behavior as adolescents and adults.

7. **False.** Women's shorter survival time appears to be the result of social and economic factors, including differing access to health care and quality of care, as well as domestic violence, homelessness, and lack of social support.

WEB RESOURCES

Human Rights and Gender Inequality

Human Rights Watch International—Women's Rights

http://hrw.org/doc/?t=women_hivaids

Research and information on the relationship between abuses of women's rights and their vulnerability to AIDS.

International Center for Research on Women

http://www.icrw.org

The International Center for Research on Women is a private nonprofit organization founded in 1976 and based in Washington, DC, with an office in India. ICRW's mission is to improve the lives of women in poverty, advance women's equality and human rights, and contribute to their broader economic and social well-being. ICRW accomplishes this, in partnership with others, through research, capacity building, and advocacy on issues affecting women's economic, health, and social status in low- and middle-income countries.

HIV/AIDS and Human Rights-Related Resources (HIV InSite Knowledge Base)

http://hivinsite.ucsf.edu/InSite?page=kbr-08-01-07#S1X

The HIV InSite Knowledge Base is a "hypertextbook" that organizes and provides access to related materials. The related materials for the topic *HIV/AIDS and Human Rights* include links to organizations and projects that focus on the intersection between HIV/AIDS and human rights.

UNFPA Interactive Population Center: Working to Empower Women (UNFPA)

http://www.unfpa.org/intercenter/beijing/index.htm

A United Nations Population Fund Interactive Population Center site that highlights the following specific areas in which women need to be empowered, and ways to ensure their human rights: women and poverty, education and training of women, women and health, violence against women, women and armed conflict, women and the economy, women in power and decision making, institutional mechanisms for the advancement of women, human rights of women, women and the media, women and the environment, and the girl-child.

UNFPA Interactive Population Center: Women's Empowerment and Reproductive Health (UNFPA)

http://www.unfpa.org/intercenter/cycle/

A United Nations Population Fund Interactive Population Center site that describes the international consensus reached at the Fourth World Conference on Women (FWCW) in Beijing in 1995 about empowering women and ending gender inequality. The site defines key human rights concepts, and examines key issues related to reproductive health and rights that affect women throughout their lives.

UNFPA Interactive Population Center: Violence Against Girls and Women (UNFPA)

http://www.unfpa.org/intercenter/violence/index.htm

A United Nations Population Fund Interactive Population Center site that reviews the forms of gender-based violence and their consequences, the effects of violence on sexual and reproductive health decision making, the effects of violence on the economics of reproductive health, and efforts to reform policy to address violence in societies around the world.

RECOMMENDED READING

Gender Inequality, Human Rights, and Development

Engendering Development—Through Gender Equality in Rights, Resources, and Voice (World Bank, 2001)

"Engendering Development—Through Gender Equality in Rights, Resources, and Voice" is a Policy Research Report by the World Bank focusing on gender issues and their broad economic and social implications in developing and transitional countries. The report examines the conceptual and empirical links between gender, public policy, and development outcomes and demonstrates the value of applying a gender perspective to the design of development policies. The evidence presented shows that societies that discriminate by gender pay a high price in terms of their ability to develop and to reduce poverty. To promote gender equality, the report proposes a three-part strategy emphasizing institutional reforms, based on a foundation of equal rights for women and men; policies for sustained economic development; and active measures to redress persistent gender disparities.

To order this report, go to http://publications.worldbank.org/ecommerce/catalog/product?item_id=217246

For a 40-page summary of the report, go to http://www.worldbank.org/gender/prr/module7ekam.pdf

Gender, HIV and Human Rights: A Training Manual (UNIFEM, 2000)

UNIFEM. (2000). Gender, HIV and human rights: A training manual. *New York:UNIFEM.*

HIV/AIDS is increasingly affecting women around the globe, partly as a result of gender inequality. "Gender, HIV and Human Rights: A Training Manual" addresses HIV as a gender issue and a human rights issue. It aims to help teachers and practitioners enhance their understanding about the gender dimensions of HIV/AIDS, so that they can then effectively influence a critical mass of change makers in their "spheres of influence" to undertake appropriate responses to the challenges posed by the epidemic. Includes information and activities addressing gender inequality and legal and ethical concerns in the context of HIV/AIDS.

The manual also contains two training modules and a section on lessons learned. http://www.unifem.org/resources/item_detail.php?ProductID=5

Gendering AIDS: Women, Men, Empowerment, Mobilisation (VSO, 2003)

Lewis, M. (2003). Gendering AIDS: Women, men, empowerment, mobilisation. *London: VSO.*

This report was published at the launch of VSO's campaign, AIDS Agenda, which focuses attention on the need for more equality between women and men as part of an effective response to HIV and AIDS. Research for Gendering AIDS was carried out in South Africa, India, Namibia, and Cambodia and reflects the priorities of the organizations VSO works with in those countries. In particular, it examines how national and international policies designed to protect women's rights can be put into practice, and how men can be more constructively involved in HIV and AIDS work at the grassroots.

Empowering Men in Prevention

It Takes 2: Partnering With Men in Reproductive and Sexual Health (UNFPA, 2003)

UNFPA. (2003). It takes 2: Partnering with men in reproductive and sexual health. *New York: UNFPA.*

Partnering with men is emerging as an important strategy for improving reproductive health. This new publication offers guidance on effective and gender-sensitive ways to engage men in reproductive and sexual health and their partners. It includes examples of successful strategies and programming as well as lessons learned.
Available online at http://www.unfpa.org/upload/lib_pub_file/153_filename_ItTakes2.pdf

Men and AIDS: A Gendered Approach (UNAIDS, 2000)

UNAIDS. (2000). Men and AIDS: A gendered approach. *Geneva, Switzerland: Joint United Nations Programme on HIV/AIDS (UNAIDS).*

Produced for the 2000 World AIDS Campaign, this thorough document maintains that women are at particular risk of HIV infection as a result of their "lack of power to determine where, when and whether sex takes place." At the same time, the report underscores the need to establish a balance between acknowledging how the behavior of some men fuels the HIV/AIDS pandemic and blaming—thereby perhaps alienating—all men. Men and AIDS also discusses in detail such topics as the roots of masculinity, reaching adolescent boys, men's relations with women, sex between men, preventing sexual transmission of HIV, violence and HIV, substance use, special settings (such as prisons, mines, the military, areas of migrant workers and long-distance truck drivers, and zones frequented by sex workers and people who live on the street), men's health needs and health-seeking behavior, and how men interact with their families. The document concludes with a series of points for action aimed at increasing gender awareness, improving sexual communication and negotiations, reducing violence and sexual violence, and promoting support and care.
Available online at http://www.thebody.com/unaids/men/contents.html

The State of the World's Population—Lives Together, Worlds Apart: Men and Women in a Time of Change (UNFPA, 2000)

UNFPA. (2000). The state of the world's population—Lives together, worlds apart: Men and women in a time of change. *New York: UNFPA.*

The report examines a broad range of evidence from around the world showing that systematic discrimination against women and girls causes extensive suffering and lost opportunities for both women and men, and holds back efforts to reduce poverty, improve health, stem the spread of HIV/AIDS, and slow rapid population growth.
Available online at http://www.unfpa.org/swp/2000/english/

Gender Inequality and Violence

Dying of Sadness: Gender, Sexual Violence, and the HIV Epidemic (UNDP, 1999)

Gordon, P., & Crehan, K. (1999). Dying of sadness: Gender, sexual violence, and the HIV epidemic. *New York: United Nations Development Program* (UNDP).

An overview of multiple determinants, consequences, and manifestations of sexual violence in the context of gender and the HIV epidemic.
This document is available on the CD-ROM.

Policy Paralysis: A Call for Action on HIV/AIDS-Related Human Rights Abuses Against Women and Girls in Africa (Human Rights Watch International, 2003)

This 40-page report documents human rights abuses that women and girls suffer at each stage of their lives and that increase their risk for HIV infection. Girls face sexual abuse and violence, in and out of school. Women in long-term relationships risk violence if they insist on condom use or refuse sex. Widows are discriminated against in property and inheritance rights. And, women and girls are raped in war and civil conflict, where rape is used strategically as a weapon.
Available online at http://www.hrw.org/reports/2003/africa1203/

Stigma and Discrimination

HIV/AIDS, Stigma, and Discrimination (UNAIDS, 2002)

Aggleton, P., & Parker, R. (2002). A conceptual framework and basis for action. *Geneva, Switzerland: Joint United Nations Programme on HIV/AIDS (UNAIDS).*

In this report, the authors explore definitions and relationships between stigma, discrimination, and consequent human rights abuses. In considering responses, they outline key stakeholders and describe some examples of programs around the world that have been successful in tackling stigma and discrimination. They discuss a number of interrelated strategies for success and conclude that "work has to occur simultaneously on several fronts: communication and education to encourage better understanding; action and intervention to establish a more equitable policy context; and legal challenge, where necessary, to bring to account governments, employers, institutions, and individuals."
Available online at http://data.unaids.org/Publications/IRC-pub02/JC891-WAC_Framework_en.pdf

POWERPOINT SLIDES

(Note: A full-color version of these slides, with graphics, is also available on the CD-ROM.)

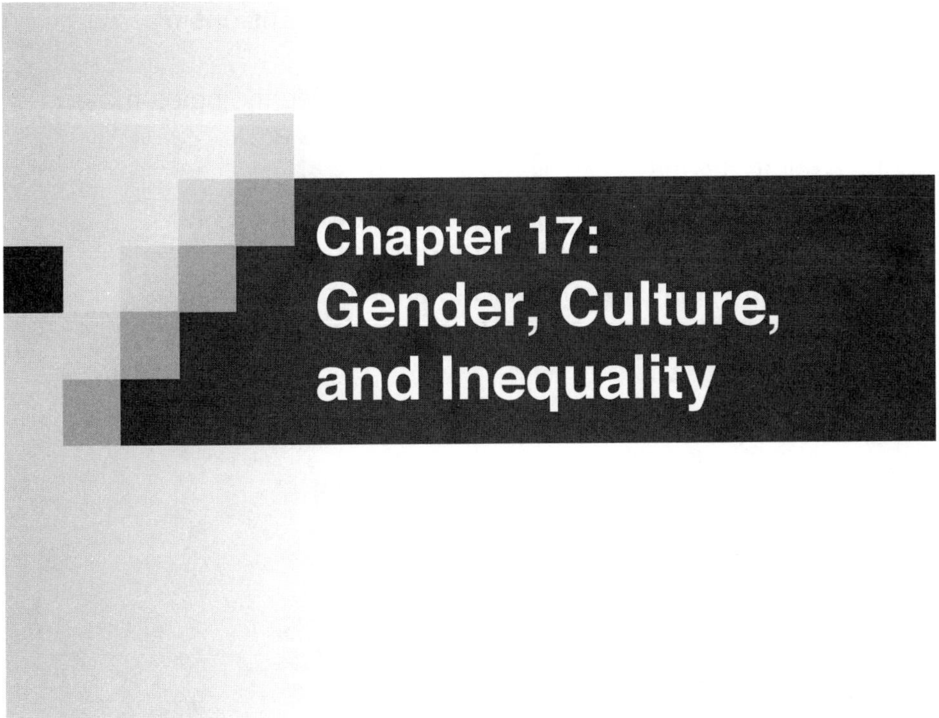

Gender, Culture, and Inequality

- The more unequal gender relationships are in a country, the higher its HIV prevalence rate.
- Gender differences affect risk and vulnerability factors for HIV/AIDS in many complex ways because gender norms influence men's and women's relative ability to protect themselves.
- Manifestations of gender inequality:
  - Gender-based violence
  - Unequal rights to property
  - The burden of caring for the sick
  - Unequal access to treatment

Strategies to Address Gender Inequality

- Promote awareness about gender dimensions of HIV/AIDS
- Provide women with HIV prevention technologies that they can control (i.e., female condoms and microbicides)
- Promote women's economic empowerment and access to education, information, and skills
- Ensure that existing policies and commitments supporting women's rights are implemented

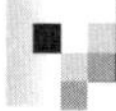

Strategies to Address Gender Inequality (continued)

- Ensure women's access to medical and social support
- Increase the constructive involvement of men and boys in activities and interventions designed to reduce gender inequalities and minimize the impact of HIV and AIDS
- Use the Gender Equality Index to guide intervention efforts
  - The Gender Equality Index lists several areas of life concerns with respect to gender inequality along with indicators to target.

Human Rights Abuses and HIV/AIDS

- Human rights abuses that increase vulnerability to HIV infection:
  - Sexual violence and coercion against women and girls
  - Confiscation of property from women whose husbands have died of AIDS
  - Stigmatization of men who have sex with men
  - Abuses against sex workers and injection drug users
  - Violations of rights of young persons to information on HIV transmission

Human Rights Abuses and HIV/AIDS
(continued)

- Human rights violations against children who have lost parents to AIDS or whose parents are living with the disease include: loss of inheritance rights; necessity to take on hazardous labor, including prostitution; and being forced to live on the streets where they are subject to police violence and other abuses.
- Human rights violations against people with HIV and AIDS include: mandatory HIV testing; restrictions on international travel; barriers to employment and housing; access to education, medical care, and/or health insurance; issues raised by names reporting, partner notification, and confidentiality.

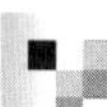

HIV/AIDS and Women's Rights

- Major issues related to the abuse of women's rights and their vulnerability to HIV/AIDS:
  - ☐ ***Lack of control*** over their own sexuality and sexual relationships
  - ☐ ***Poor reproductive and sexual health*** leads to serious morbidity and mortality.
  - ☐ ***Neglect of health needs, nutrition, medical care.*** Women's access to care and support for HIV/AIDS is much delayed (if it arrives at all) and limited. Family resources are nearly always devoted to caring for the man. Women, even when infected, are providing most, if not all of the care.
  - ☐ ***Clinical management*** of HIV/AIDS is based on research on men.
  - ☐ ***All forms of coerced sex*** from violent rape to cultural/economic obligations to have sex when it is not wanted, increase risk of microlesions and, therefore, of STI/HIV infection.

HIV/AIDS and Women's Rights (continued)

- Major issues related to the abuse of women's rights and their vulnerability to HIV/AIDS (continued):
  - ☐ ***Sexual abuse.*** This is an underestimated mode of transmission of HIV infection in children (even very small children). Adult men seek ever younger female partners (younger than 15 years of age) in order to avoid HIV infection, or if already infected, in order to be "cured."
  - ☐ ***Harmful cultural practices***, for example, genital mutilation and "dry" sex, increase a woman's vulnerability to acquiring HIV.
  - ☐ ***Stigma and discrimination*** in relation to HIV/STD is much stronger against women, who risk violence, abandonment, neglect (of health and material needs), destitution, and ostracism from family and community. Furthermore, women are often blamed for spread of disease.
  - ☐ ***Disclosure of status, partner notification, confidentiality***. These are all more difficult issues for women than for men for the reasons listed above.

Men's Roles in Gender Equality

- In order for the efforts to empower women to be successful, men's involvement and support are essential.
- Strategies that allow men to be part of the solution to the gender imbalance that fuels the HIV/AIDS epidemic focus on:
  - **Gender awareness**—challenge harmful stereotypes and promote understanding of the ways in which stereotypes affect women and men
  - **Sexual communication and negotiations**—encourage men to talk about sex, drug use, and HIV with their partners and others, and access information, support, and counseling
  - **Violence and sexual violence**—support actions to reduce male violence and sexual violence
  - **Support and care**—help men in their roles as fathers and providers of care

Gender-Based Violence and HIV/AIDS

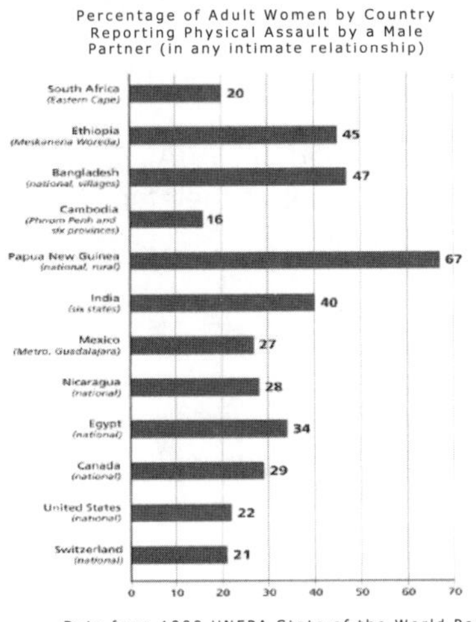

Data from 1999 UNFPA State of the World Population 2000

Gender-based violence takes many forms, and can include physical, emotional or sexual abuse.

Gender-based violence is causally linked to HIV and AIDS transmission through rape and intimate partner violence, and may also be a reaction to a positive HIV diagnosis within a relationship.

Violence and the threat of violence increases women's vulnerability to HIV/AIDS and can compound the barriers to HIV+ women's access to care.

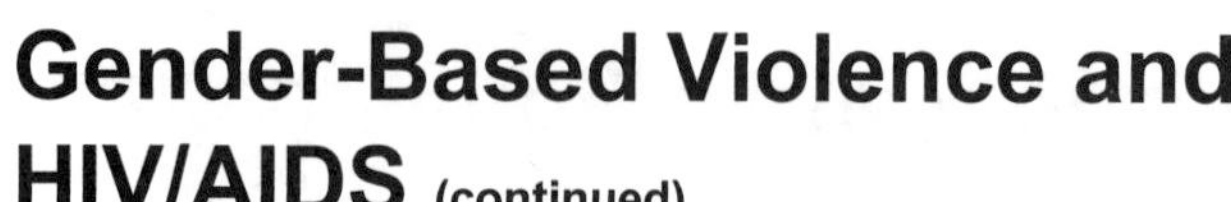

Gender-Based Violence and HIV/AIDS (continued)

- **Gender-based violence** is rooted in the historically unequal power relations (social, economic, cultural, and political) between males and females.
- Available data suggest that **at least one in five of the world's female population** has been physically or sexually abused at some time in their lives.
- **Nonconsensual sex** is a common form of sexual violence that puts women at risk for HIV/AIDS.

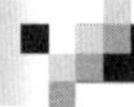

Gender, Stigma, and Discrimination

- HIV-related stigma refers to all unfavorable attitudes, beliefs, and policies directed toward people perceived to have HIV/AIDS as well as toward their significant others and loved ones, close associates, social groups, and communities.
- Discrimination prevents people from finding out their serostatus and from seeking treatment for AIDS.
- Women are often blamed for the spread of HIV/AIDS to their families because they were the first ones in their families to be tested, often during pregnancy or delivery.

Gender, Stigma, and Discrimination
(continued)

- Because of stigma, women refrain from being tested for HIV and seeking out care to avoid being ostracized, abused, and viewed as promiscuous.
- Homophobia and stigmatization compel men who have sex with men to keep their sexual behavior secret and deny their sexual risk, increasing their own risk as well as the risk of their partners, female or male.

Gender and Legal Dimensions of HIV/AIDS

Legal restrictions and social customs can prevent women from benefiting from economic and social progress, contributing to women's vulnerability to HIV/AIDS.

- Areas of legal inequality that increase vulnerability to HIV/AIDS for women include:
  - property rights;
  - rape, sexual harassment, and coerced sex;
  - reproductive rights; and
  - mixed legal traditions.

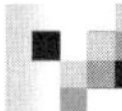

Gender and Legal Dimensions of HIV/AIDS (continued)

- Starting points to remedy women's legal inequality include:
  - □ privacy and confidentiality in voluntary-counseling and testing services;
  - □ criminalization of sexual violence, including marital rape; and
  - □ reproductive law and policy to enable women to make decisions free of coercion, violence, and discrimination.

Unequal Access to Treatment and Care

- Women are likely to die of HIV/AIDS sooner than their male counterparts; this disparity is likely to be a result of differing access to care and quality of care rather than biological differences.
- Women whose HIV infections are detected early and receive appropriate treatment survive as long as infected men.
- However, even in areas where women have good access to HIV/AIDS care, there is evidence that they wait longer than men before seeking care, and are less likely to seek care at all.
- Low self-esteem together with the higher priority placed on children's health makes women less likely to seek out care for themselves.

Poverty, Inequality, and AIDS

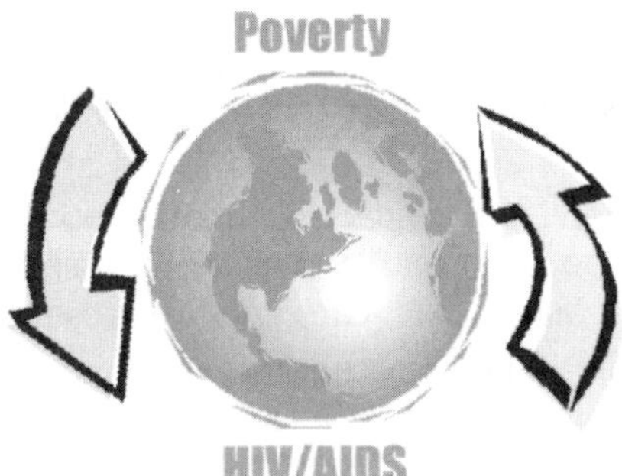

"The concentration of HIV/AIDS in the developing world and in the marginalized communities of the first world confirm that the HIV/AIDS epidemic mirrors the condition of global inequality. Tracking the path of least resistance, HIV/AIDS flourishes in conditions of poverty, conflict, and inequality, and in states with weak resources and capacity."

Albertyn, C. Prevention, treatment, and care in the context of human rights. Presentation at the Expert Group Meeting on the HIV/AIDS Pandemic and its Gender Implications, Windhoek, Namibia, 2000.

Poverty, Inequality, and AIDS (continued)

HIV/AIDS impacts poverty in several ways, including:

- When the primary breadwinner becomes ill with AIDS or dies, household income falters, leading to hardship and child labor; and in countries where women cannot own property, the wife and children may lose access to their source of livelihood.
- HIV/AIDS deepens existing poverty and dries up resources needed to fight the pandemic in less developed countries.

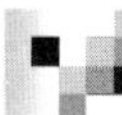

Poverty, Inequality, and AIDS (continued)

Poverty affects the risks and consequences of HIV/AIDS for women and men:

- Because women have limited economic opportunities and are considered to be lower priority than men within a family, their access to fee-based health care services is severely restricted.
- Women and men who are economically disadvantaged are less likely to have information about HIV/AIDS than those from higher income levels.
- Street youth who have to worry about day-to-day survival place less emphasis on safety from HIV/AIDS.
- Poverty often leads to migration, which increases HIV risk.

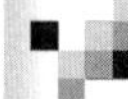

Economic Inequality and Social Disempowerment

- Poverty is overwhelmingly the root cause of women bartering sex for economic gain or survival—giving them less power in their sexual relationships and leaving them vulnerable for HIV infection.
- Some examples:
  - Commercial sex work
  - Sex with "sugar daddies"
  - Trading sex for school fees or other goods and services

Educational Inequality

- Educational inequality compounds a woman's dependence on a man, and the risk of being rejected from her boyfriend/husband may be more compelling than the risk of becoming ill.
- Indicators representing literacy, income, and education point to women's and girls' unequal status.
- Inequality in education or knowledge about sex affects a woman's ability to make informed decisions to protect herself.

Empowering Women

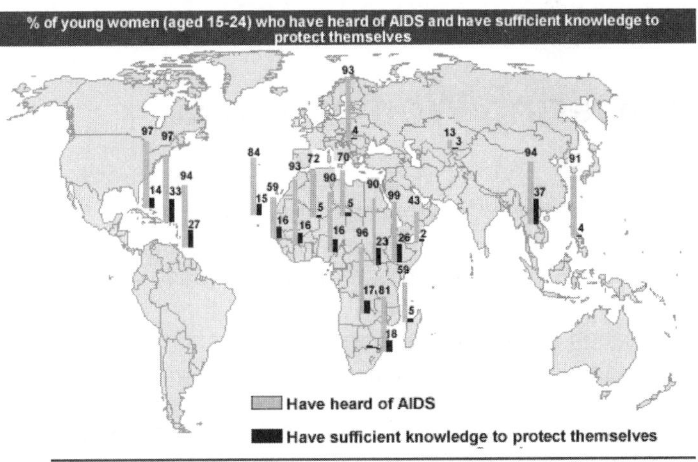

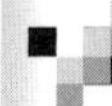

Empowering Women (continued)

- Economic Empowerment
  - Women's economic dependence cripples their ability to take care of themselves and their families.
  - Women need economic independence so that they can escape from high-risk situations, sustain their families, and negotiate their sexual lives.
  - An example of a program that works: In China, a project has successfully raised the incomes of 14,000 women by providing income-generating activities, training in production and business skills, functional literacy, and reproductive health services.

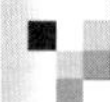

Empowering Women (continued)

- Access to Education, Information, and Skills
  - It is imperative for governments and private organizations to implement policies and programs that increase women's access to education and information.
  - Education and training are catalysts for change.
  - An example of a program that works: A program in Botswana has helped young mothers to continue their education by training them as peer counselors for other girl students. Teenage pregnancies in these schools have dropped significantly.

Glossary

Abacavir: a *reverse transcriptase inhibitor.*

Abstinence: the act or practice of refraining from engaging in sexual intercourse.

Acute HIV syndrome: a flu-like sickness suffered by up to 87% of HIV-infected persons 2 to 4 weeks after exposure to the virus, indicating that their immune systems are fighting the newly introduced HIV. Symptoms last for a few days and include fevers, chills, headaches, night sweats, rashes, and swollen glands.

Adapt: to change a program in order to better address the needs of a new population or setting.

AIDS (acquired immune deficiency syndrome): the symptoms and sicknesses that people infected with human immunodeficiency virus (HIV) eventually develop because of their weakened immune systems. The immune system ordinarily defends the body against illness.

AIDS diagnostic criteria: the Centers for Disease Control and Prevention (CDC) has two different sets of criteria for diagnosing AIDS. If a person has both of the conditions listed in either the first or second set, he or she is said to have AIDS. The first set of conditions includes: HIV infection confirmed by testing, and a CD4+ T-cell count of less than 200 per cubic millimeter of blood. (Healthy adults usually have CD4+ T-cell counts of 1,000 or more.) The second set of conditions includes: HIV infection confirmed by testing, and infection with one or more of the 26 opportunistic diseases associated with AIDS.

AIDS orphan: a child who has lost one or both parents to AIDS, often left in the care of already overburdened relatives or in overcrowded orphanages, or forced to fend for themselves in child-headed households or on the streets.

AIDS risk reduction model (ARRM): a behavioral model developed specifically to organize the many factors that influence whether people change their HIV risk behaviors. ARRM is a stage model, which means that people progress through different levels toward behavior change. According to ARRM, people must first label themselves as vulnerable to HIV infection (stage 1), commit to changing their behaviors (stage 2), and enact the new, less risky behaviors, in part by seeking other people's help (stage 3).

Anonymous testing: testing in which the person being tested is identified in records by a unique code (e.g., a number, or a fictitious name), and the results of the test cannot be associated with the real name, Social Security number, address, or other identifying characteristics of the person being tested, not even by the person administering the test.

Antibodies: immune proteins produced by white blood cells that circulate throughout the body and specifically bind to foreign particles (antigens).

Antiretroviral therapy: treatments for HIV that include three or more drugs. The drugs target different stages of the HIV replication cycle, making the HIV less likely to multiply and mutate.

Asymptomatic period: a period of time in the course of HIV disease when the infected person does not have any symptoms, lasting for a few months to over 10 years; also called *clinical latency*.

AZT (azidothymidine): the first anti-HIV drug approved for use in the United States; belongs to the class of antiretroviral drugs known as nucleoside reverse transcriptase inhibitors; generic name is zidovudine, and brand name is Retrovir®.

Barrier method: a mode of contraception using a device, such as a male or female condom, that prevents sperm from reaching the ovum.

Behavior: an individual's actions or reactions shaped by what is in their mind, including knowledge, attitudes, beliefs, motivation, past experience, and skills. Behavior is also shaped by people's interpersonal experiences—the opinions, advice, support, and behavior of their friends, family, coworkers, and others. In addition, behavior is influenced by the social structures, movements, and policies of communities and their institutions.

Behavior change agent: somebody or something that causes or accelerates behavioral change.

Being faithful: mutual monogamy between partners.

Beneficial disclosure: voluntary and often confidential disclosure of a person's HIV status to others and organizations so that the person gets proper care and HIV becomes less stigmatizing.

Blood products: the parts of blood, including plasma (the liquid in which cells, nutrients, hormones, and enzymes are suspended), platelets (small cells that control bleeding and clotting), and red blood cells (cells that carry oxygen throughout the body).

Blood transfusion: the transfer of blood or any of its parts to a person who has lost blood due to an injury, disease, or operation.

Candidiasis: an opportunistic yeast infection of two main types: localized disease (of the mouth and throat or of the vagina) and systemic disease (of the esophagus, and disseminated disease). The mouth and throat variant (commonly known as thrush or OPC) is not a cause of death, but it can cause oral pain and make swallowing difficult. The main symptom is creamy white lesions in the mouth that can be scraped away. Esophageal (gullet) candidiasis is a more serious condition which can cause pain in the chest that increases with swallowing. Disseminated candidiasis causes fever and symptoms in the organs affected by the disease (e.g., blindness when it affects the eyes), and can be life-threatening.

Capsid: the bullet-shaped core of an HIV particle, where the HIV particle's genetic material is contained.

Case: one instance of a particular disease, health disorder, or condition in a population; sometimes, an individual with the particular disease.

CD4 positive (CD4+) cells: the cells that HIV attacks and hijacks for its own replication. A CD4+ cell, also called a *T-helper cell,* is a kind of T-cell that has a molecule called cluster designation 4 (CD4) on its surface.

Centers for Disease Control and Prevention (CDC): one of the major collectors and distributors of health data in the United States, including data about the HIV/AIDS epidemic. The CDC conducts two kinds of *surveillance*: HIV surveillance and AIDS surveillance. For the HIV surveillance, 29 states and the U.S. Virgin Islands have reported new HIV infections to the CDC since 1998, providing sufficient data to monitor HIV trends over time and to understand better the behaviors that increase HIV infection risk. For the AIDS surveillance, all U.S. states and territories report all AIDS diagnoses to the CDC.

Chronic somatic preoccupation: a psychological symptom of HIV infection characterized by a fixation on physical symptoms.

Clinical latency: see *asymptomatic period.*

Coccidioidomycosis: a fungal *opportunistic infection* that can cause serious lung problems in people with HIV/AIDS and also can spread to other organs, including the bones, joints, lymph nodes, kidneys, or skin. It also can cause disease of the central nervous system, which can be life-threatening if not diagnosed and treated promptly.

Community: a group of people who share something in common such as geographic area, a cultural background, a religious affiliation, or a common set of interests, beliefs, or practices.

Community-level interventions: interventions that influence the knowledge, attitudes, skills, and behaviors of an entire community both directly and indirectly, often through a focus on changing social norms.

Confidential testing: testing in which the person being tested is identified in records by his or her real name, and test results become part of the person's medical record, and therefore can legally be divulged to certain parties (e.g., insurance carriers) under particular circumstances. In contrast, see *anonymous testing.*

Conjunctivitis: an inflammation of the conjunctiva, the clear membrane that covers the white part of the eye and the inner surface of the eyelids, that is caused by infections (such as bacteria and viruses), allergies, or substances that irritate the eyes; commonly known as pinkeye.

Containment-and-control strategy: an approach to HIV/AIDS-related policy and law that focuses on the coercive power of the state to force compliance with laws. It emphasizes the protection of HIV-negative people from exposure to the virus by regulating individual behavior and is enforced by legal and monetary penalties for violation.

Cooperation-and-inclusion: an approach to HIV/AIDS-related policy and law that relies on the participation of all heavily impacted communities. It emphasizes the voluntary participation of HIV+ people in reducing HIV transmission and is enforced through persuasion and material incentives.

Core components: the basic elements of the intervention that are believed to be responsible for its effectiveness.

Cost-effectiveness: analyses that evaluate how well interventions are meeting their goals, in light of how much they cost; also called *cost-benefit*.

Counseling, Testing, and Referral (CTR): an intervention strategy that benefits those who test positive for HIV, as well as those who test negative, by informing people of their HIV status; providing high-quality HIV prevention counseling, to reduce likelihood of transmitting or acquiring HIV; and referring people to appropriate medical, preventive, and psychosocial support services; also known as *Voluntary Counseling and Testing (VCT)*.

Cryptococcosis: an *opportunistic infection* caused by a fungus that primarily infects the brain. It most often appears as meningitis and occasionally as pulmonary or disseminated disease. Untreated cryptococcal meningitis is fatal.

Cryptosporidiosis (crypto): a chronic opportunistic bacterial infection of the intestines caused by protozoan parasites that is easily spread by contaminated food or water, or by direct contact with an infected person or animal. Crypto causes diarrhea, nausea, vomiting and stomach cramps.

Cultural competence: a set of congruent behaviors, attitudes, and policies—including a consideration of linguistic, socioeconomic, and functional concerns that influence behavior—that come together in a system, agency, or among professionals, thus: (1) enabling that system, agency, or those professionals to work effectively with the target population and (2) resulting in services that are accepted by the target population.

Culture: a widely shared set of values, institutions, practices, and beliefs that emerges—and changes—as a group adapts to its environment. Culture is learned through social interactions that provide contexts for behavior and influence behavior; cultural traditions are passed down through generations.

Cytomegalovirus (CMV): an *opportunistic infection* caused by a virus in the herpes family that infects the whole body. It most commonly appears as retinitis, which causes blurred vision and can lead to blindness. CMV also can affect other organs, and is capable of causing fever, diarrhea, nausea, pneumonia-like symptoms, and dementia.

Cytoplasm: the area of the cell outside of the nucleus.

DDL (didanosine): the second drug approved by the FDA for the treatment of AIDS, used in combination with *AZT* by adult patients with advanced HIV infection, accounting for the first successful use of a combination of drugs to treat HIV infection.

Deficiency: the quality or condition of being inadequate, such as a deficiency in one's immune system causing it to no longer work properly.

Delavirdine: a *reverse transcriptase inhibitor*.

Dental dam: a small sheet of latex that acts as a barrier between the vagina or anus and the mouth.

Diffuse: to spread among members of a social group.

Diffusion of innovations theory: a behavioral theory that explains how an *innovation diffuses* among members of a social group. According to this theory, as social groups are unique, the origins, speed, and channels of innovation spread are also unique to each group. The theory also emphasizes that innovations themselves have properties that make them more or less likely to be adopted by different groups.

Disclosure: telling other people of one's own *serostatus*.

Discrimination: unfair treatment of a person or group.

Disparities: in relation to HIV infection, the inequality or difference in the rate of HIV infection and the development of AIDS among different cultural groups resulting from differential access to HIV/AIDS-related prevention and treatment services.

DNA (deoxyribonucleic acid): the chemical that makes up a cell's genes, that controls the cell's operations, and that carries traits from one generation to the next. DNA is usually made up of two strands of molecules twisted together to form a spiral, or helix.

Dry sex: sexual intercourse between a man and a woman for which the woman dries her vagina using special powders, herbs, or douches in order to increase friction. Dry sex is more likely than regular sex to cause small cuts and tears, through which HIV-infected fluids may easily pass.

Economic evaluation: an evaluation that addresses the costs and consequences of HIV prevention programs through techniques such as assessing the resources consumed by the intervention, and balancing the costs of the interventions with the economic and public health effects of the intervention activities.

Efavirenz: a *reverse transcriptase inhibitor*.

Enfuvirtide (T-20): an *entry inhibitor*.

Entry inhibitors: the newest class of anti-HIV drugs, which work by keeping the spikes on the surface of HIV from binding and fusing with host cells.

Enzyme: a protein that begins or speeds up a chemical reaction.

Enzyme-Linked Immunosorbent Assay (ELISA): the first test to determine HIV antibodies' presence in blood or oral fluids, making it possible to screen blood products, to detect HIV infection in people who have not yet developed AIDS, and to identify *seroconversion* in newly infected individuals.

Epidemic: a fast-spreading outbreak of a disease that affects many people.

Epidemiology: scientific study of the incidence, distribution, risk factors, progression, and control of disease in a population.

Ethical partner notification: voluntary and often confidential notification of HIV+ people's sexual and drug-use partners, so that they will get tested and take precautions.

Ethnicity: a grouping of people based on common cultural tendencies or practices, such as language, religion, ancestral origins, customs, or social viewpoint.

Female circumcision: see *female genital mutilation*.

Female condom: a thin, soft, loose-fitting polyurethane plastic pouch that lines the vagina. It has two flexible rings: a smaller inner ring at the closed end, used to insert the device inside the vagina and to hold it in place, and a larger, outer ring that remains outside the vagina and covers the external genitalia.

Female genital mutilation (FGM): a culturally motivated practice that involves partial or complete removal of the external female genitalia, or other injury to the female genitals usually performed in childhood or adolescence; often referred to as *female circumcision*.

Female-controlled prevention method: a way in which women can protect themselves from HIV/AIDS, including *microbicides* and *female condoms*.

Formal theory: theory regarding how a variety of factors interact to influence behavior and behavior change.

Formative evaluation: the collection of data concerning a population's needs and assets, as well as the pilot testing of an initial version of an intervention that addresses those needs and assets.

Fusion inhibitors: a kind of entry inhibitor that prevents HIV replication by keeping the spikes on the surface of HIV from fusing with host cells.

Gay cancer: a phrase used in the early 1980s to describe the unusual immune system failure among gay men in the United States (also used were the terms *gay plague* and *gay-related immune deficiency[GRID]*).

Gay plague: see *gay cancer*.

Gay-related immune deficiency (GRID): see *gay cancer*.

Gender: the socially created, shared, and institutionalized categories of thoughts, feelings, roles, and actions assigned to men and women.

Gender norms: gender-based expectations of "masculine" and "feminine" behaviors and roles that greatly influence social organization, power relations, decision-making authority, and individual responsibility. Gender roles are learned, rather than inherent, and vary from culture to culture.

Gender-based violence: physical, emotional, economic, and sexual abuse rooted in the historically unequal power relations (social, economic, cultural, and political) between males and females, increasing women's vulnerability to HIV/AIDS.

Gene: a segment of DNA that contains the information necessary to make a protein. A gene is the unit of biological inheritance.

Genetic material: molecules (like DNA and RNA) that carry hereditary information.

Glycoprotein 41 (gp41): molecules that make up the stems on the spikes of HIV particles.

Glycoprotein 120 (gp120): molecules that make up the caps on the spikes of HIV particles.

HAART (highly active antiretroviral therapy): the use of three or more anti-HIV drugs in the treatment of HIV/AIDS. Combinations of drugs are more effective than individual drugs because HIV's genetic material mutates very quickly and becomes resistant to individual drugs. Combinations of drugs overwhelm HIV, keeping it from multiplying and mutating as quickly.

Harm-elimination approach: an approach to HIV/AIDS-related policy and law that seeks to strengthen people's ability to abstain from all risk behaviors.

Harm-reduction approach: an approach to HIV/AIDS-related policy and law that tries to make risk behaviors less dangerous.

Harm reduction model: a behavioral model that aims to lessen the negative consequences of risky behaviors, rather than aiming for complete abstinence from these behaviors, both for the people performing them and for the general public, while taking into consideration current attitudes, beliefs, and abilities.

Health belief model: a behavioral model based on the premise that a person must perceive a threat to him- or herself before he or she will take preventive action.

Hemophiliac: a person with hemophilia, an inherited blood disease that causes people to bleed easily and uncontrollably because of a lack of a particular coagulation factor in the blood.

Herpes simplex virus infection: herpes is a general term for two different *opportunistic infections*: one that affects the area around the mouth (oral herpes, also known as cold sores) and another that affects the area around the genitals (genital herpes). Viruses cause both of these diseases. The herpes simplex virus-1 (HSV-1) causes oral herpes; both HSV-1 and herpes simplex virus-2 (HSV-2) cause genital herpes. During an outbreak, or flare-up, the virus becomes active and causes a chain of events leading to a cluster of small bumps to form. The bumps may rupture, heal, and then disappear for an indefinite period of time.

Histoplasmosis: an opportunistic fungal infection that primarily scars the lungs but may also affect other organs. Symptoms can include fever, fatigue, weight loss, and difficulty in breathing.

HIV (human immunodeficiency virus): the virus that causes AIDS. Infecting only humans, HIV attacks and weakens the body's immune system. The immune system normally protects the body against illness.

HIV antibodies: proteins produced by the body in response to HIV. Most tests for HIV are actually tests for HIV antibodies in body fluids or tissues.

HIV antibody testing: tests for the presence of HIV antibodies in a person's body fluids or tissues.

HIV coreceptor blockers: antiretroviral medication that prevents HIV from binding with the host cell membrane.

HIV disease: the time spanning from initial infection with the HIV virus to the diagnosis of AIDS.

HIV encephalopathy: a complication associated with AIDS, also known as *HIV-associated dementia (HAD)*. HIV encephalopathy is one of the only illnesses that can be caused directly by HIV in which HIV passes into the brain and damages nerve cells, affecting the way the brain works.

HIV negative (HIV–): a term used to describe people who are not infected with HIV, also called *seronegative for HIV*.

HIV particles: individual human immunodeficiency viruses.

HIV positive (HIV+): a term used to describe people who are infected with HIV, also called *seropositive for HIV*.

HIV RNA tests: tests used in research and health care settings to diagnose HIV infection very early after exposure, before antibodies are even formed. These tests look for bits of HIV RNA in the blood.

HIV wasting syndrome: a complication associated with AIDS causing a loss of body mass or size, most notably muscle mass.

HIV-1: human immunodeficiency virus type 1.

HIV-2: human immunodeficiency virus type 2.

HIV-associated dementia (HAD): a progressive neurological disorder that can affect HIV+ people, and that is characterized by cognitive, motor, and behavioral impairments.

Home HIV antibody testing kits: a type of HIV test that allows consumers to interpret their own HIV test results at home in a few minutes. The Federal Trade Commission, however, has warned that these home-use HIV test kits, many of which are available on the Internet, supply inaccurate results. Only one home test kit, Home Access Express HIV-1 Test System, has been approved by the U.S. Food and Drug Administration. Blood samples collected in the home are mailed to an outside lab for testing. Results can be obtained by calling a toll-free number and using a personal identification number.

IDUs: injection drug users; injection drug use.

Immune system: a collection of organs, cells, and proteins that works to protect the body from foreign substances and cancerous cells.

Impact evaluation: outcome evaluation that is conducted over an extended period, to assess the very long-term impacts of an intervention.

Impulsivity: the tendency to do things suddenly, without thinking about the consequences of the action.

Incidence: the number of new instances of a disease in a population for a specified period of time, usually expressed as the proportion of new cases relative to the total population.

Individual-level interventions: interventions that are delivered to individuals in one-on-one settings by professionals, peers, and/or media and are commonly based on psychological theories of behavior. These interventions and seek to directly influence the knowledge, attitudes, skills, and behaviors of persons who participate in intervention activities.

Inflammatory infections: sexually transmitted infections that do not cause sores, such as gonorrhea and chlamydia.

Information-motivation-behavioral skills (IMB) model: a model of behavioral risk reduction that attributes HIV risk-related behavioral change to three factors. First, information regarding HIV/AIDS transmission and prevention must be relevant to HIV/AIDS and easy to apply in the person's environment. Second, motivation to change HIV/AIDS-risk behavior must come from both from the person's own attitudes toward the change and from other people's support. Third, the person must have behavioral skills for performing specific HIV/AIDS-preventive acts and believe in his or her ability to perform the act.

Innovation: a new idea, object, or behavior practice.

Integrase: an enzyme that HIV uses to splice its newly formed strands of DNA with host cell DNA.

Integrase inhibitors: antiretroviral medication that prevents HIV's newly formed DNA from being spliced into the host cell's DNA.

Integration: the process in which the newly reverse-transcripted HIV DNA makes its way into the host cell's nucleus, and is spliced into strands of the host cell DNA once inside with the aid of an enzyme called integrase.

Interpersonal: relating to the interactions between individuals.

Intrapersonal: occurring within the individual mind or self.

Isosporiasis: a chronic *opportunistic infection* of the intestines caused by protozoan parasites that is easily spread by contaminated food or water, or by direct contact with an infected person or animal. Isosporiasis causes diarrhea, nausea, vomiting, and stomach cramps.

Kaposi's sarcoma (KS): Kaposi's sarcoma is a kind of opportunistic cancer that causes dark blue lesions, which can occur in a variety of locations including the skin, mucous membranes, gastrointestinal tract, lungs, or lymph nodes. The lesions usually appear early in the course of HIV infection.

Langerhans cells: cells contained on the inner surface of the penis's foreskin that are particularly receptive to the HIV virus. These cells are likely to be the primary point of viral entry into the penis of an uncircumcised man.

Leadership-focused model: a behavioral model that emphasizes the role of leaders in changing the behaviors of their groups.

Lentivirus: a retrovirus that has a long delay between the time it initially infects a person and the time the person starts to show serious symptoms.

Lipid: fat.

Lipid membrane: see *viral envelope*.

Long-term goals: the changes in behaviors and health status (e.g., sexual risk-taking behavior, injection drug use behavior, HIV status, *viral load*) that the program will seek to achieve over a long period of time (perhaps 6 months to a year after completion of the intervention).

Lymphatic system: the system that produces, stores, and carries white blood cells to fight infection and disease. These organs and tissues include the spleen, thymus, lymph nodes, tonsils, and adenoids.

Lymphocyte: cells that the body's immune system makes to fight off invaders; also called white blood cells.

Lymphoid interstitial pneumonia/pulmonary lymphoid hyperplasia (LIP/PLH): diseases of the lungs associated with AIDS that may lead to the formation of cysts in the lungs and to lymphoma.

Male condom: a flexible sheath, usually made of thin rubber or latex, designed to cover the penis during sexual intercourse for contraceptive purposes or as a means of preventing sexually transmitted infections/diseases.

Messenger RNA (mRNA): the form of RNA that carries information from DNA in the nucleus to the ribosome sites of protein synthesis in the cell; the template for protein synthesis.

Microbicides: creams, gels, or foams that can be inserted into the vagina or rectum that kill or disable HIV, helping prevent sexual transmission of HIV and other STIs/STDs.

Minor cognitive-motor disorder (MCMD): a psychological disorder associated with HIV, which includes mild impairments in memory, movement, and concentration; mood disorders, like depression; anxiety disorders; and brain tumors.

Molecule: the smallest unit of a substance that retains all the physical and chemical properties of that substance, consisting of a single atom or a group of atoms bonded together.

Morbidity: a diseased state; also, the proportion of diseased people in a population, expressed as either incidence or prevalence.

Mortality: the death rate, usually expressed as the proportion of deaths relative to the total population.

Mother-to-child transmission: see *vertical transmission.*

MSM: men who have sex with men.

Mucous membrane: the linings of certain cavities (such as the nose, mouth, vagina, and anus) that produce a protective layer of mucus.

Mucus: a slippery substance produced by mucous membranes for lubrication and protection.

Mutate: to change. HIV's genetic material mutates through mistakes in replication, giving rise to new strains of HIV that are resistant to antiretroviral therapy.

Mycobacterium avium complex/intracellulare (MAC/MAI): a opportunistic disease that generally affects multiple organs; symptoms include fever, night sweats, weight loss, fatigue, diarrhea, and abdominal pain. The germs of the mycobacterium avium complex/intracellulare (MAC/MAI) are related to the germ that causes tuberculosis.

Narcissism: preoccupation with the self.

National Institutes of Health (NIH): a part of the U.S. Department of Health and Human Services; the primary federal agency for conducting and supporting medical research.

Needs and assets assessment: the process of collecting and assessing data that describe the nature and magnitude of a community's needs, as well as its resources or assets (e.g., financial, organizational, intellectual, institutional, and human).

Nevirapine: a *reverse transcriptase inhibitor.*

Non-Hodgkin's lymphoma (NHL): a cancer of the *lymphatic system* associated with AIDS.

Non-nucleoside reverse transcriptase inhibitors (NNRTIs): anti-HIV drugs that slow down HIV replication by chemically binding to reverse transcriptase, making it unable to convert the HIV RNA into DNA.

Nonoccupational exposure: exposure of people to HIV through activities not associated with one's occupation, including consensual sex, nonconsensual sex, exposure to mother's body fluids, and injection drug use.

Nonoxynol-9 (N-9): a common spermicide formerly believed to be a potentially effective barrier against HIV that was later shown to significantly increase the risk of HIV transmission.

Norm: a rule or standard for behavior that each member of a social group is expected to follow. Also known as social norm.

Nucleoside reverse transcriptase inhibitors (NRTIs or "nukes"): anti-HIV drugs that are faulty versions of reverse transcriptase. When the HIV attempts to turn its RNA into DNA, NRTIs replace real reverse transcriptase, resulting in the creation of incomplete DNA and, in turn, inactive HIV particles.

Nucleus: the part of the cell that contains DNA and RNA and that is responsible for cell growth and reproduction.

Occupational exposure: the exposure of health care workers to HIV through needlestick injuries or other accidental contact with body fluids.

Opinion leader: people who are capable of influencing others and of disseminating an intervention throughout their social networks.

Opportunistic infections (OIs): infections that do not ordinarily affect people with healthy immune systems, or that become much more severe than they do in people with healthy immune systems. A hallmark of AIDS is the presence of one or more opportunistic infections.

Outcome evaluation: an evaluation that assesses whether or not an intervention achieved its intended objectives and goals—that is, whether it achieved the desired changes in the target population.

Outreach intervention: a relatively low-cost intervention that targets a large number of people in their natural environment, where they may not otherwise be exposed to HIV-prevention messages. Outreach intervention activities include providing both prevention information and prevention materials (e.g., condoms, clean needles, bleach for sterilizing drug injection equipment) where they are needed, and also often serve as a means of alerting the community to the existence of other prevention (or treatment) programs and services and recruiting new program participants.

Pandemic: a widespread outbreak of a disease that affects many people over a large area.

Parent-to-child transmission: see *vertical transmission*.

Partner notification programs: programs that locate, counsel, and test the partners of HIV-infected people.

Pathogen: things that cause disease, including viruses, bacteria, fungi, and protozoa.

Perceived behavioral control: how much control a person thinks he or she has over performing a certain behavior, such as using a condom or cleaning injection drug paraphernalia.

Perinatal transmission: see *vertical transmission*.

Plasma: the watery, liquid part of the blood in which the red blood cells, white blood cells, and platelets are suspended.

Plasma viral load: HIV levels in an HIV+ person's body; also called plasma viremia tier.

PLWAs: people living with AIDS.

Pneumocystis Carinii Pneumonia (PCP): an *opportunistic infection* caused by a parasite that infects the lungs, which was formerly called pneumocystis carinii but has now been renamed pneumocystis jiroveci. PCP is a frequent HIV-associated opportunistic infection in industrialized countries but appears to be less common in Africa. The symptoms are mainly pneumonia along with fever and respiratory symptoms such as dry cough, chest pain, and dyspnea.

Policy: a plan or course of action created by governments or by nongovernmental bodies; policies are clarified through the legal system.

Population: the total number of inhabitants at a given time in a given area (usually a city, county, state/province, or country).

Positive prevention: HIV prevention efforts targeted at HIV+ people to prevent them from giving HIV to others.

Postexposure prophylaxis (PEP): the giving of antiretroviral therapy to people after they have been exposed to HIV, in an attempt to prevent HIV infection.

Prevalence: the total number of people in a population with a particular disease at a particular time; usually expressed as the proportion of infected people relative to the total population.

Prevention intervention: a program designed to reduce rates of disease transmission, such as HIV transmission.

Primary infection: the first stage of HIV disease, when the virus first establishes itself in the body.

Primary prevention: HIV prevention efforts focusing on *HIV– people*; encouraging safer sex and safer drug use among people who are not infected with HIV.

Primary stage: the first stage of HIV disease, when HIV establishes itself in the body. At the beginning of the primary stage, most people have a short, flu-like illness. People are very contagious during the primary stage because there is a large amount of HIV in bodily fluids. However, HIV-infected people may not test positive for HIV during the primary stage because the body may not yet be producing antibodies to the virus.

Process evaluation: an evaluation that addresses who was served by an intervention, with what activities or services, as compared to what was planned. It also can assess satisfaction among program staff and clients with the intervention as delivered.

Prognosis: the probable outcome or course of a disease.

Progressive multifocal leukoencephalopathy (PML): a life-threatening *oppotunistic infection* of the brain, caused by a virus. The infection continues to get worse and often leads to serious brain damage.

Protease: an enzyme that cleaves proteins. Near the end of HIV's replication cycle, protease finalizes the creation of mature HIV particles by cutting up the long strands of proteins that replication has so far produced.

Protease inhibitors: anti-HIV drugs that chemically bind to protease so that it cannot cleave the HIV proteins into mature viral particles.

Protein: a large, complex molecule made up of chains of amino acids. The sequence of the amino acids—and thus the function of the protein—is determined by the DNA of the gene that encodes it. Proteins are required for the structure, function, and regulation of cells, tissues, and organs.

Provirus: the name for HIV's form when it has combined its DNA with the host cell's DNA.

Public service announcement (PSA): a noncommercial advertisement in a variety of mass media (newspaper and bus advertisements, billboards, informational brochures, and radio and television spots) broadcast for the public good. In regards to HIV prevention messages, PSAs can help raise awareness of HIV/AIDS and how it is transmitted, reduce stigma against people who are infected with HIV, promote HIV testing, and keep HIV/AIDS in the public eye.

PWAs: people with AIDS.

Race: a classification of people, often based on physical traits.

Rapid serum HIV antibody test: a type of HIV test that produces fast results, allowing clinicians and patients to make decisions about medical management more quickly.

Replicate: to reimplement interventions that have already been rigorously evaluated and shown positive findings with similar groups and in similar settings; to make copies of oneself.

Replication: the process of making copies. The HIV provirus must replicate itself in order to survive.

Resistance, drug-resistance: the state of HIV when drugs no longer stop or slow its replication. HIV reproduces and mutates quickly, and in so doing evolves new forms that are not affected by drugs.

Retroviruses: viruses that carry RNA instead of DNA as their genetic material. Retroviruses do not "proofread" their genetic material during replication, and therefore mutate more quickly than do DNA-based viruses.

Reverse transcriptase: an enzyme that allows HIV RNA to change into DNA, so that it can pass into a host cell's nucleus, commandeer the host cell, and begin reproducing itself.

Reverse transcriptase inhibitors: anti-HIV drugs that interfere with reverse transcriptase's ability to change HIV RNA into DNA, either by replacing the HIV's reverse transcriptase with a faulty decoy (nucleoside reverse transcriptase inhibitors) or by chemically binding with the HIV's reverse transcriptase (non-nucleoside reverse transcriptase inhibitors). Most anti-HIV drugs are reverse transcriptase inhibitors, and include *AZT*, ddC, ddI, d4T, 3TC, *nevirapine, delavirdine*, *abacavir*, and *efavirenz*.

Reverse transcription: the process in which RNA is converted into DNA.

RNA (ribonucleic acid): the genetic material in retroviruses. RNA is a chemical that is similar to DNA, but different in structure. Whereas DNA has two strands of molecules, RNA has only one. Because RNA does not "proofread" itself as it replicates, it mutates more quickly than does DNA.

RNA polymerase: an enzyme that separates the two halves of DNA like a zipper in order to create a new strand of *messenger RNA*.

Safer sex: sex that reduces the likelihood of transmitting HIV and other STIs/STDs by preventing or reducing contact with bodily fluids, including blood, semen, preejaculate, vaginal fluids, anal fluids, and the discharge from sores caused by STIs/STDs. Using condoms, dental dams, and adequate lubrication all contribute to safer sex.

Saliva- and urine-based antibody test: alternative HIV tests that do not require that an individual's blood be drawn.

Salmonella septicemia: a bacterial *opportunistic infection* causing patients to be very ill with chills and high fever, with a danger of septic shock if there is a delay in treatment.

Saquinavir: the first approved *protease inhibitor*.

Secondary prevention: prevention for HIV+ people aimed at reducing barriers to HIV testing, providing access to quality medical care, and providing ongoing prevention services to people living with HIV/AIDS.

Self-efficacy: belief in one's own ability to perform a task.

Seroconversion: the time when the body begins producing antibodies to the virus. Most people undergo seroconversion within 3 months of infection with the HIV virus, often accompanied by flu-like symptoms.

Serodiscordant: describes couples in which one person has tested positive for HIV and the other has not.

Seronegative for HIV: see *HIV negative.*

Seropositive for HIV: see *HIV positive.*

Seroprevalence: the proportion of people in a given population at a given time who are infected with a given virus, such as HIV.

Serostatus: positive or negative results of a test for certain antibodies in the blood, such as the antibodies that form in response to HIV infection; whether one is HIV+.

Sex: either of the two biological categories (male or female) into which most organisms are divided, based on their reproductive roles; a biological distinction between men and women, defined by physical features including a person's chromosomes (genes), internal and external anatomy, and hormones.

Short-term objectives: the immediate changes in knowledge, attitudes, beliefs, skills, intentions, behaviors, and other factors that the intervention will seek to achieve.

Small group-level interventions: interventions delivered to couples, small groups, or families by professionals, peers, and/or media that seek to influence the knowledge, attitudes, skills, intentions, and behaviors that are most closely linked to HIV transmission.

Social cognitive theory: a behavioral theory that views people's lives as made up of interactions between their internal state and events, which are their thoughts, feelings, and personality (P); their behaviors (B); and their external social and physical environments (E). Because these three components interact with one another, changes to each component are essential to achieving behavior change.

Social influence interventions: community-level interventions that seek out people who are capable of influencing others and of disseminating an intervention throughout their social networks. Social influence interventions are commonly based on theories about behavior and behavior change that focus on the importance of social norms, such as the theory of reasoned action, social cognitive theory, and the diffusion of innovations theory.

Social marketing: the use of commercial marketing methods to promote HIV antibody testing and safer sex.

Social movement theory: a behavioral theory proposing that behavior change takes place when large groups of people unite to address the behavioral problem, often in opposition to local leaders or common practices.

Social norm: see *norm.*

Socioeconomic status (SES): a person's relative rank in society, based on his or her education, income, or occupation.

Spikes: the complex proteins that protrude through HIV's surface. Spikes attach the virus to a host cell and fuse the two together.

Stages of change model: see *transtheoretical model.*

STI/STD: sexually transmitted infection and sexually transmitted disease.

Stigma: the qualities or conditions, such as being a racial/ethnic minority or having HIV, that decrease a person's worth in society's eyes.

Stigmatization: the association of a quality or condition with lower social worth.

Stress: a state of mental or physical strain or suspense.

Stressor: an activity, experience, condition, or situation that causes stress.

Structural barrier: a barrier to reducing risk behaviors and increasing protective behaviors for HIV, which can be reduced through advocacy efforts that mobilize community members, lawmakers, policy makers, and other stakeholders to effect changes to relevant laws, policies, structures, and institutional practices.

Structural intervention: interventions that indirectly influence risk behavior by effecting changes to policies, laws, organizational practices, or other structures that are related either to risk behaviors or to access to behavioral prevention information, tools, or services.

Superinfection: infection with two or more different strains of HIV at the same time.

Surveillance: the ongoing, systematic collection, analysis, interpretation, and sharing of health data.

T-cell: a kind of lymphocyte, or white blood cell, that the body's immune system makes to fight off infections.

T-helper cell: see *CD4 positive (CD4+) cell.*

Technology transfer: the process of transferring the best science-based prevention interventions to prevention providers, which involves identifying them, putting them in a format that can be readily used by service providers, disseminating these materials widely, and supporting their use.

Theory of gender and power: a theory that attributes three major structures to the gendered relationships between men and women: the sexual division of labor, which concerns economic inequities favoring males; the sexual division of power, which concerns inequities and abuses of authority and control in relationships and institutions favoring males; and cathexis, which concerns social norms and affective attachments. The three structures are overlapping but distinct, and serve to explain the gender roles assumed by men and women. Together, they constrain women's daily practices by producing gender-based inequalities in earning potential, control of resources, and expectations of roles. These factors, in turn, lead to socioeconomic circumstances, interpersonal conditions, and behaviors that increase the likelihood of HIV infection.

Theory of planned behavior: similar to the *theory of reasoned action*. This theory, however, additionally takes into account the fact that some behaviors are easier to control than others, and includes a new component—perceived behavioral control.

Theory of reasoned action: a behavioral theory asserting that behavior change is the last link in a causal chain that also involves beliefs, attitudes, norms, and intentions. The chain begins with two kinds of beliefs: people's beliefs about the consequences of a given risky behavior, and their beliefs about other people's opinions of the risky behavior. Beliefs about the consequences of the act combine with evaluations of those consequences to form an attitude toward the behavior. Similarly, beliefs about other people's opinions combine with motivations to comply with other's expectations to form subjective social norms. If a person's attitudes and subjective norms regarding the risky behavior are sufficiently negative, he or she may develop the intention to change the risky behavior. The intention to change behavior, in turn, is necessary for behavior change.

Toxoplasmosis (toxo): an opportunistic parasitic infection caused by a protozoan found in uncooked meat and cat feces. This microbe infects the brain and can cause headache, confusion, motor weakness, and fever. In the absence of treatment, disease progression results in seizures, stupor, and coma.

Transcription: the conversion of DNA to RNA during the *replication* process.

Transfusion: the transfer of blood or any of its parts to a person who has lost blood due to an injury, disease, or operation.

Transgender: individuals that have a persistent and distressing discomfort with their birth sex, and so may assume the roles of the other sex through such behaviors as dress, occupation, or even sex-reassignment surgery. These persons constitute an often ignored gender group that is at risk for HIV infection.

Translation: the conversion of RNA into proteins during the replication process.

Transmission of HIV infection: the process by which the HIV virus invades a person's body.

Transplant: transferring a healthy tissue or organ to replace a damaged tissue or organ.

Transtheoretical model: a behavioral model asserting that people move through a series of stages toward behavior change. A person's advancement to a higher stage marks an increase in her or his motivation for, confidence about, and commitment to a change in behavior. People do not always advance straight through the stages, however. Because changing complex, intimate behaviors can be difficult, people often relapse to previous stages; also known as the *stages of change model*.

Tuberculosis (TB): an opportunistic bacterial infection that primarily infects the lungs. Tuberculosis is the leading HIV-associated opportunistic disease in developing countries.

Ulcerative infections: sexually transmitted infections that cause sores on the genitalia, such as syphilis and herpes.

Unprotected sex: any act of sexual intercourse in which the participants use no form of protection against sexually transmitted infections/diseases.

Vaccine: a medicine made of dead or weakened *pathogens* (viruses, bacteria) that, when injected or eaten, strengthen the body's immune system against a particular disease.

Vertical transmission: Transmission of a disease-causing agent (such as HIV) from mother to infant during pregnancy, childbirth, or breast-feeding; also known as *parent-to-child transmission*, *perinatal transmission*, and *mother-to-child transmission*.

Viral envelope: the outer coat of a virus composed of two layers of fat molecules, also called the *lipid membrane*.

Viral load: the amount of HIV RNA per unit of blood plasma. Viral load indicates how much HIV there is in the blood, how quickly it is replicating, and how quickly a patient is progressing toward AIDS and subsequent death.

Virus: a tiny, relatively simple, nonliving substance, usually made up of little more than a few strands of genetic material and a protein shell, that enters cells and causes disease.

Voluntary Counseling and Testing (VCT): see *Counseling, Testing, and Referral (CTR)*.

Western Blot: a highly specific supplemental test that detects the presence of HIV antibodies in the blood. The Western Blot test is less sensitive than the *ELISA* test but it hardly ever gives a false positive result; therefore, it is used for confirming the *ELISA* test.

White blood cell: see *lymphocyte*.

Wife inheritance: a traditional practice in many parts of Africa whereby a young widow is inherited by a brother in-law or any other suitor chosen by the village elders.

Zero tolerance: the policy or practice of not tolerating and punishing undesirable behavior, such as all forms of gender-based violence against women and girls, in an effort to effectively reduce such behavior.

Index

NOTES

NOTES

NOTES

NOTES